Medical Instrumentation For Health Care

Medical Instrumentation For Health Care

LESLIE CROMWELL
California State University
Los Angeles

MORT ARDITTI
Cedars-Sinai Medical Center
Los Angeles

FRED J. WEIBELL and ERICH A. PFEIFFER
Veterans Administration Biomedical
Engineering and Computing Center
Sepulveda, California

BONNIE STEELE
California State University
Los Angeles

JOSEPH LABOK
Los Angeles Valley College

Prentice-Hall, Inc. *Englewood Cliffs, New Jersey*

Library of Congress Cataloging in Publication Data
Main entry under title:

Medical instrumentation for health care.

Bibliography: p.
Includes index.
1. Medical instruments and apparatus. I. Cromwell, Leslie.
[DNLM: 1. Biomedical engineering—Instrumentation. QT34 M489]
R856.M377 610'.28 75-35505
ISBN 0-13-572602-6

10 9 8 7 6 5 4 3 2 1

Printed in the United States of America

PRENTICE-HALL INTERNATIONAL, INC., *London*
PRENTICE-HALL OF AUSTRALIA PTY. LTD., *Sydney*
PRENTICE-HALL OF CANADA, LTD., *Toronto*
PRENTICE-HALL OF INDIA PRIVATE LIMITED, *New Delhi*
PRENTICE-HALL OF JAPAN, INC., *Tokyo*
PRENTICE-HALL OF SOUTHEAST ASIA (PTE.) LTD., *Singapore*

Contents

Preface

As the world's population grows, the need for health care increases. In recent years progress in medical care has been rapid, especially in such fields as neurology and cardiology. A major reason for this progress has been the marriage of two important disciplines: medicine and engineering.

The opening paragraph of this preface is not new. It has appeared in print before, in a book also published by Prentice-Hall, Inc. and entitled *Biomedical Instrumentation and Measurements.* This book was first put on the market in early 1973 and became widely adopted in a short time. Interest came from many sources. Engineers and biomedical engineering technicians were the primary market, but many physicians and other health care personnel bought the book and found some appeal. However, one group expressed particular interest: the critical care nurses. There was a problem, however. The earlier book assumed a background of electricity and electronics, and this knowledge was lacking in the education of the typical nurse.

Consequently, the publisher and the authors were approached about writing a supplement to the other book, and so out of a series of meetings the present text emerged in skeleton form. At first it was thought that much of the original work could be used; then it was realized that a different approach would be necessary. Also, many new disciplines were developing, disciplines that can be loosely categorized under the heading of "paramedical." Much of their background and needs paralleled that of the nurses. With these points in mind, the ultimate form of this book was shaped.

The authors decided that their own scope was limited. This field is a very complex one, and so others were invited to participate. A team was formed. To the original team were added: one nurse with particular experience in critical care nursing, one teacher of instrumentation for nurses at beginning college level, and one biomedical engineer in a hospital, who was working on a day-to-day basis with all the people for whom this book was to be written.

When six persons of diverse backgrounds get together to write a book, there are problems. Hopefully, all these problems have led to good results. Everyone was concerned for the quality of the work, and, as a result, everyone edited everyone else. There were long debates and much rewriting, but all agreed on the basic theme. It had to be a fundamental book but sophisticated enough to be meaningful in an everchanging field. It had to have breadth to cover a wide range of the field of medicine, but it had to have depth where it mattered. The authors all agreed that it had to be down to earth. Also, the approach was to be such that this book could be a building block on which to build further knowledge as the field expanded.

Essentially, it evolved into a three-part work. First, the fundamentals, then the most important clinical applications, and, finally, the applications to many of the specialities involved were considered.

What is medical instrumentation? The first two chapters attempt to answer that question. The reader is given some of the broader aspects of the entire subject matter. Many definitions and ideas are presented, but in order to understand how these instruments work and how they are used, a knowledge of electricity is necessary. Chapters 3 and 4 are concerned with that subject. Every topic is approached fundamentally. Finally, to complete the first part of the book, the physiological variables that must be measured are explained.

The second part deals with the major clinical applications, and comprises six chapters. They deal, in turn, with the topics of electrodes, electrocardiography, indirect measurement of blood pressure, direct measurement of blood pressure, defibrillators and pacemakers, mobile intensive care, and instrumentation in special care units and neonatal care. All these chapters deal with their subjects in some depth.

The final part covers a wider scope but with less depth. The chapters include blood flow and volume, cardiac output, biotelemetry, respiration instruments, X rays and cardiac catheterization, the surgical suite, electroencephalography, electromyography, ultrasonics, and fetal monitoring. The last three chapters are universal and cover safety in the hospital, computers in medicine, and the care and use of electronic equipment.

The information for this book has been collected from a variety of sources. It has been presented in part in courses given at California State University, Los Angeles, in both nursing and engineering; at Los Angeles Valley College in both nursing and technician courses; at the various centers and hospitals of the United States Veterans Administration, at Cedars of Lebanon Hospital, and the Cedars-Sinai Research Center in Los Angeles.

In a work of this nature, it is essential to illustrate commercial systems in common use. There are many manufacturers who produce similar equipment, and it was difficult to decide which to use as illustrative material. All companies and hospitals have been most cooperative, and we apologize for the fact that it is not possible to illustrate alternate examples. The authors wish to thank all companies that were willing to supply this material. All are acknowledged in the text in the appropriate places.

The authors also wish to thank Mrs. Irina Cromwell, who typed the bulk of the manuscript; Mrs. Elissa J. Schrader and Mrs. Erna Wellenstein for their help on some of the chapters and necessary correspondence; Mr. Leonard Suidor of UCLA for advisory assistance and Mr. William Gibson and Prentice-Hall, Inc. for their encouragement.

Los Angeles, California

Leslie Cromwell
Mort Arditti
Fred J. Weibell
Erich A. Pfeiffer
Bonnie Steele
Joseph Labok

1

Understanding Medical Instrumentation

The ultimate objective of those concerned with health care is to use directly or to facilitate the use of all available resources to assist the patient in obtaining optimal health. The practitioner accomplishes this goal by continually assessing and reassessing the patient as physiological and other pertinent data become available. In large part, these data are obtained through instrumentation. Much of this comprises the diagnostic task that nurses have practiced since the days of Florence Nightingale. For example, in critical care practice a depth of knowledge and specialized skill are demanded by an increasingly expanded role. Similar statements could be made for paramedical personnel in a variety of settings.

The commitment of caring personnel to patients has never been stronger. The one-to-one relationship of the critical care practitioner to his or her charge and the tremendous responsibility of emergency medical crews are good examples. This same commitment may be reflected in all acute care settings where caring personnel focus on patient problems by a willingness to make decisions and act on them and a readiness to be held accountable for their actions. With increased assessment skills in the realm of physical diagnosis, the health care practitioner becomes an integrator as well as a prime collector of patient data and assumes a focal position in the health care system because of this knowledge and what is done with it.

Medical instrumentation is directly related to the attainment of optimal health and, as such, is an important step in achieving health care goals. As a result of intensive coronary care and technological advances in all spheres of acute care, the practitioner is continually challenged to deal directly with new monitoring equipment and automated treatment methods. Lack of a knowledge base may predispose the health care practitioner to undue preoccupation with the equipment and less personalized patient care. Because health care personnel are generally avid learners, the "black box" from which important physiological parameters are documented becomes a source of inquiry, raising such questions as: What is the nature of "damping"? How does a biochemical phenomenon become a bright spot on an oscilloscope? What is the nature of electrical current flow?

Increased understanding in this area must ultimately bring about positive patient outcomes; the setting and the level of the individual's practice are of less importance than the total expertise mobilized for the patient's benefit.

1.1 Early Involvements

The field of medical instrumentation is by no means new. Many instruments were developed as early as the nineteenth century—for example, the electrocardiograph first used by Einthoven at the end of that century. Progress was rather slow until after World War II when a surplus of electronic equipment became available. At that time many technicians and engineers, both within industry and on their own, started to modify existing equipment for medical use. This process occurred primarily during the 1950s, and although the results were disappointing, the efforts of this decade provided the groundwork for the subsequent movement of the 1960s: the designing of equipment specifically for medical use.

Much help was provided by the U.S. government, in particular, by NASA (National Aeronautics and Space Administration). Some of the concepts and features of patient-monitoring systems presently used in hospitals throughout the world evolved from astronaut monitoring. The use of adjunct fields, such as biotelemetry, also finds some basis in NASA programs.

An important landmark in medical instrumentation was the establishment of the first coronary care units in the early 1960s. Previously, cardiac surgery included some nursing in this area, although to a limited extent because of the relatively early state of the field at that time. Two units were established in 1962 by Dr. Hughes Day at Bethany Hospital, Kansas City,

Kansas, and by Dr. Lawrence Meltzer and Dr. J. R. Kitchell at the Presbyterian-University Hospital of Pennsylvania Medical Center. Dr. Day began his unit on noting only a 4% survival rate from resuscitative methods on patients who arrested on general wards; his interest was primarily in cardiopulmonary resuscitation, and his figures probably reflected the national average at that time. Drs. Meltzer and Kitchell established their unit as a result of a research project they conducted on more than 700 male patients with acute myocardial infarctions. The salient findings included the following: 47% of the 171 deaths were due to arrhythmias, and 70% of all deaths occurred during the first five days after admission.

With this information, Meltzer and Kitchell initiated the prototype for intensive coronary care programs. They combined a method of continuous electrocardiographic monitoring with a prepared method for terminating ventricular fibrillation and ventricular standstill for patients with acute, or suspected, myocardial infarction during the first critical days following the event. With the advent of coronary care units across the nation and the inclusion of defined pharmacological intervention by nursing staff to prevent life-threatening arrhythmias, based on electrocardiographic data, the in-hospital mortality rate of acute myocardial infarction diminished from 30 to 15%.

In a very real sense, this situation brought the field "home" to nursing personnel. No longer was bioelectrical patient assessment limited to the researcher or the technical expert performing along functional lines in fields of radiology, electrocardiography, electroencephalography, laboratory technology, and the like. Now personnel conventionally assigned to patient care had diagnostic and interventive responsibilities based on the assessment of physiological parameters via bioelectrical monitoring systems.

1.2 The Challenge of Today

Although many areas of medical care are involved, perhaps the best example of the relationship between health care and instrumentation is the way intensive coronary care and technology bridged the gap between engineering and medicine that formed the field of medicine and nursing known as *critical care*. Patient-monitoring systems and extended roles for nursing and paramedical personnel became an integral part of care wherever the person in physiological crisis could be found: surgery and recovery rooms, intensive postsurgical areas, emergency departments, respiratory care units, neonatal intensive care, medical intensive care, and even in the home via mobile care ambulances. It was no longer academically desirable, but highly feasible, to monitor sophisticated physiological assessment parameters at the bedside of the acutely ill patient. In addition to the use of electrocardiographic (EKG or ECG) monitoring, defibrillators, and pacemakers, the routine use of floatation catheter monitoring of right heart and pulmonary artery pressure, cardiac output by Fick and dye dilution methods, circulation time, left atrial and arterial pressure monitoring, blood pH, skin temperature, and renal clearance studies are documented by bioelectrical instrumentation accurately and repetitively on a clinical basis. Computers, too, have been used for improved patient care. Figure 1-1 illustrates a central computerized monitor.

At least 75% of all hospitals with 100 or more beds have both intensive and coronary care units where nurses bear primary responsibility for patient monitoring. At the same time, hospitals are focusing their inpatient resources to meet the many diagnostic, treatment, and ongoing monitoring and patient-care needs of the more acutely ill. The most obvious reasons for this trend include: (a) the skyrocketing costs of medical care and hospitalization, mandating improved utilization of existing facilities and personnel, (b) the increased emphasis on primary care and outpatient facilities to maintain health through diagnostic screening and treatment of minor problems before they become major concerns, (c) the enhanced effectiveness and availability of medical and surgical therapeutics for various common ailments—for example, myocardial revascularization techniques for intract-

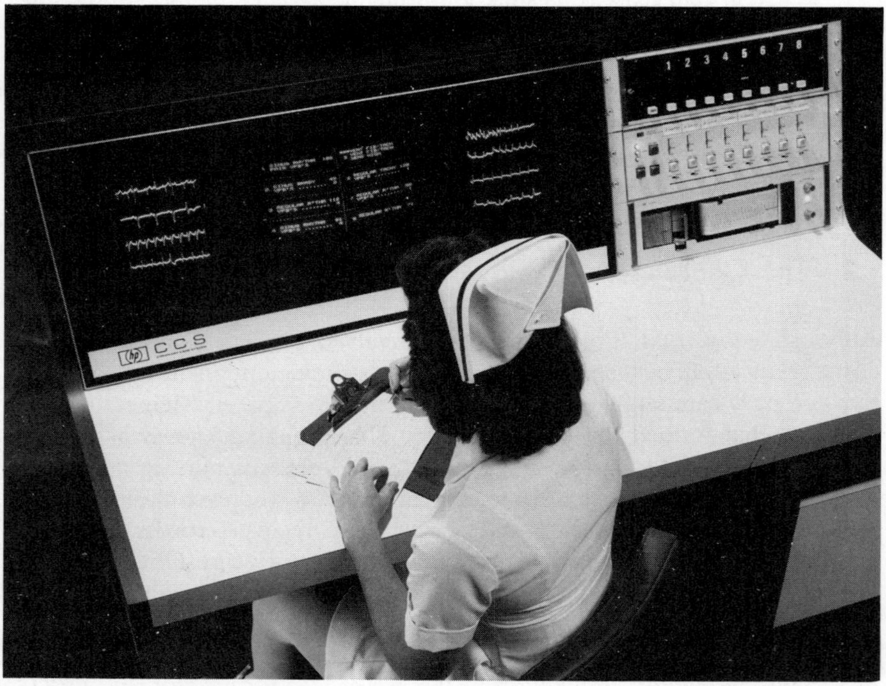

Fig. 1–1 The nurse in an environment of medical instrumentation. (*Courtesy of Hewlett–Packard Company.*)

able angina, renal transplantation and hemodialysis for chronic renal failure, and (d) the expanding role of the hospital as a center for a community-wide comprehensive system for emergency medical services. To underscore this last phenomenon, consider the following: approximately one million people experience acute myocardial infarctions each year, and more than 650,000 die annually of heart disease. Of the latter figure, about 350,000 deaths occur outside the hospital within two hours after the onset of symptoms. Similarly, many drowning, electrocution, drug intoxication, and automobile accident victims could be saved during the prehospital period through the prompt and proper application of emergency cardiac care that uses countershock, monitoring, and communication systems with the base facility.

Actually, almost every patient in an acute care setting is a potential or actual recipient of critical care services, including some form of biomedical instrumentation.

1.3 The Knowledge Base for Critical Care

The knowledge and skills necessary for the nurse involved in critical care have been defined by the American Association of Critical Care Nurses. This body has made great progress in establishing beginning or entrance-level standards of practice as well as methods to qualify practitioners according to established criteria. Additional standards will probably evolve from other disciplines preparing paramedical personnel.

Most educational programs are postgraduate in nature, based on basic "generalist" preparation conventionally defined within the framework of undergraduate nursing programs. With the increased demand for technological expertise and related physiological, biochemical and physical science knowledge, the question arises as to how adequate conventional preparation is as a base on which to build. With special reference to biomedical instrumentation knowledge, the student anticipating further study in the area of critical care might well include basic electronics. This book incorporates the belief that monitoring/interventive skills must be built on the basic understanding of such principles. In addition, physical diagnosis with support courses in physics, biochemistry, and advanced physiology could be taken prior to or concurrent with the actual critical care and other health care courses.

1.4 New Directions in Medical Instrumentation

Medical instrumentation falls largely, but not exclusively, within the context of critical care. In fact, certain trends may greatly expand involvement in areas other than the acute care setting.

One striking area of application includes primary care in terms of automated multiphasic screening operations. Preventive medical programs already widely utilize nurse practitioners in pediatric, maternity, and adult health care. Hospital corpsmen are also being used in such physician-assistance programs as Medex. Moreover, it is possible that significant inroads will be made in the fight against chronic, debilitating conditions by prevention and/or early detection methodologies. Computer science and automated laboratory assessment are integral parts of such a system. Similarly, nurses and other health workers will be increasingly involved with the important follow-up care of persons who have implanted pacemakers and artificial organs via telemetry networks and other monitoring systems so as to detect and offset significant problems.

In the critical care areas, advances in biomedical engineering and surgical techniques will undoubtedly increase the use of artificial organs and organ systems in humans. These and other wonders need no longer be viewed with fear and suspicion; our society may want to accept the possibilities offered by science and technology for the prolongation of human life.

1.5 The Objectives of This Book

The purpose of this book is to relate instrumentation principles and practices to a broad spectrum of health care fields. The early chapters are devoted to fundamentals, including the basic concepts of electricity and electronics and a discussion of those physiological variables that are measured.

The major clinical applications are then discussed in some depth, followed by other special applications. The concepts of computers in medicine and safety in the hospital are given the attention they deserve. The final chapter is concerned with the care and use of electronic equipment in general.

The subject matter is presented in such a way that it could be extended to classes of instruments that will be used in the future. Thus the material can be used as building blocks for the health-care instrumentation system of tomorrow.

2

Introduction to Medical Instrumentation

The term *instrument* has a number of meanings. Basically, an instrument is a tool or implement. The surgeon's scalpel and the dividers used by the draftsmen are both examples of instruments in common use. A device used in the measurement of length, weight, pressure, or some other physical quantity is also an instrument. The term *instrumentation* denotes a group of instruments employed for a particular purpose or function.

A wide variety of instruments are used in the diagnosis and treatment of disease in health care settings. Some of these devices are quite simple; others are complicated. Many utilize the principles of electricity and electronics. Together they constitute the realm of *medical instrumentation.*

In a broad sense, medical instrumentation includes all types of instruments used in connection with the various aspects of clinical medicine and medical research. This book, however, deals primarily with electrically powered instruments used in clinical diagnosis and the treatment of hospital patients. Laboratory instruments and instruments for medical research are largely excluded.

Of necessity, this overview chapter contains some technical terms with which the reader may be unfamiliar. Such terms are explained in Chapters 3, 4, and 5.

2.1 Physiological Measurements

A major function of medical instrumentation is the measurement of physiological variables. *A variable* is any quantity whose value changes with time. A variable associated with the physiological processes of the body is called a *physiological variable.* Examples of physiological variables are body temperature, the electrical activity of the heart (ECG), arterial blood pressure, and respiratory airflow. The measurement of physiological variables is required both in the diagnosis of disease and in monitoring the progress of treatment. In either case, measured values are compared with so-called normal values obtained through measurement of the same variables in large numbers of healthy persons. The physiological variables most often measured in relation to patient care are described in Chapter 5.

In order to be useful in diagnosing a given disease, a physiological variable must undergo a significant change from its normal values whenever that disease occurs. Equally important, it must be easily measurable and the method of measurement must cause a minimum of discomfort to the patient. Some physiological variables, such as body temperature and pulse rate, meet both requirements and have long been used for diagnostic purposes. Other variables that provide meaningful information are not as readily accessible and require complex electronic equipment for their measurement.

Several physiological variables, such as body weight and temperature, change their values relatively slowly and therefore require less frequent measurement. Others, however, vary continuously at a rather rapid rate and require instruments that can respond quickly enough to measure or record them. In certain physiological variables, such as the ECG voltages, the momentary value has little meaning. To be useful, the variable must be recorded over some interval of time in order to produce a pattern from which meaningful information can be obtained. In the case of the ECG, for example, the voltage must be recorded for at least one complete cardiac cycle. In some cases, clinically important information occurs infrequently, and a physiological variable must be recorded over a long period of time in order to detect significant events.

Sometimes important diagnostic information can be obtained through measurement of physiological variables only when a certain *stimulus* is applied. A stimulus is a condition or treatment purposely imposed on the patient, such as the glucose given for a glucose tolerance test or a specified program of exercise for an exercise electrocardiogram measurement. The changes that occur in the physiological variables of a patient as a result of a stimulus are his *response* to the stimulus.

2.2 Components of a Medical Instrument

Regardless of its simplicity or complexity, every medical instrument for measurement of physiological variables can be divided into three basic components: a transducer, signal-conditioning equipment, and some form of display. In addition, several instruments also include a means of generating a stimulus. In some instruments these components are easily discernible, whereas in others the functions are not clearly defined. In the following paragraphs each of these basic components is described and explained.

2.2.1 *The Transducer*

The transducer is the part of an instrument that is able to sense the physiological variable to be measured. In the transducer, the variable is converted into an *electrical signal,* a voltage that changes its value in exactly the same way as the variable being measured. For example, if arterial blood pressure is being measured, the voltage produced by the transducer increases as the pressure increases and decreases as the pressure decreases, closely following the pressure pattern. (The concept of voltage is explained in Chapter 3.) Even those physiological variables that occur essentially in electrical form, such as the electrocardiogram and the electroencephalogram, require transducers, called *electrodes,* to convert ionic voltages into electrical voltages.

Because the transducer must, in most cases, be attached to the patient or introduced into some part of his body, it is often separate from the main unit of the instrument. Application of the transducer to the body is often critical to proper operation of the instrument. In fact, unless a suitable signal is obtained by the transducer, the instrument cannot produce useful results regardless of how well the other components are designed.

The fact that the measured information produced by a transducer is represented in the form of an electrical signal means that some knowledge of basic electricity is needed for the understanding of medical instrumentation. The basic concepts of electricity are covered in Chapter 3.

2.2.2 *Signal-Conditioning Equipment*

In most instruments the electrical signal produced by the transducer must be modified in some way before it is suitable for its eventual use. This modification is called *signal conditioning,* and all parts of an instrument required for this purpose constitute the *signal-conditioning equipment.*

The electrical signal produced by most transducers is small and must be made larger by a process called *amplification*. This process is accomplished through the use of electronic devices, devices in which the movement of electrons is controlled. Chapter 4 is intended to give the reader a basic understanding of the concepts involved in electronics and amplification.

The signal-conditioning equipment in an instrument may consist of nothing more than a simple amplifier, or it may include a large number of devices that modify the signal in a number of ways. Usually the signal-conditioning equipment is hidden within the case or cabinet of the instrument. In many cases, controls that affect this equipment are found on the front panel to allow the operator to adjust certain characteristics of the instrument. Sometimes controls are hidden as a protection against "dial twisters."

2.2.3 *Display*

If the results of a measurement are to be meaningful, they must be presented in such a way that they can be perceived by one or more of man's senses. The part of an instrument capable of converting the modified electrical signal produced by the signal-conditioning equipment into a perceivable form is called the *display* or *readout*. The display might be some form of indicator light, a meter reading, a warning buzzer, a paper chart recording, an oscilloscope screen (a cathode-ray tube of the type used as a television screen), or any other appropriate method by which the measured information can be presented. Sometimes more than one form of display is used in the same instrument. For example, a patient monitor might display the ECG pattern on an oscilloscope, the heart rate on a meter, and an indication of danger to a patient by means of a warning buzzer.

2.2.4 *Stimulus*

Certain instruments also include a means of producing or controlling stimuli to be applied to the patient. For instance, in the measurement of nerve conduction times, an electrical stimulus (a slight electric shock) is required. This stimulus is applied to the nerve of interest. The response to that stimulus (either a muscle response or activity in another part of the nervous system) is measured by an appropriate transducer and the results are displayed on an oscilloscope screen.

2.3 Block Diagram of a Medical Instrument

The functions of an instrument are often described by a *block diagram*. In such a diagram each box, or *block*, represents a component or major function of the instrument. Arrows indicate the direction in which a signal or information travels between blocks. Figure 2-1 is a block diagram showing the basic components of a medical instrument as described in Section 2.2. Here a stimulus is being applied to the body. The transducer (sometimes there is more than one) senses the physiological variable being measured and produces an electrical signal that is modified by the signal-conditioning equipment. The modified electrical signal is converted into perceivable information by the display. When more than one instrument is used to obtain a required set of measurements, an *instrumentation system* is formed. An instrumentation system may include several transducers, an assortment of signal-conditioning equipment, and various forms of display. Often the information from several transducers is recorded side by side on a single chart recording or is displayed on a single oscilloscope screen. The measurement from each transducer is called one *channel* of information. An instrumentation system may also include equipment (such as a tape recorder) to record several channels of information for future playback.

2.4 Important Characteristics of a Medical Instrument

It is imperative that people who select and use medical instruments understand the important characteristics of such instruments. In doing so, they are better able to interpret manufacturers' literature and make knowledgeable comparisons between similar devices. They will also be better equipped to select the specific instruments best suited to their needs and understand instructions for their operation. The following paragraphs briefly define and discuss several of the more important characteristics of instruments. Certain characteristics that are more technical in nature have been purposely omitted.

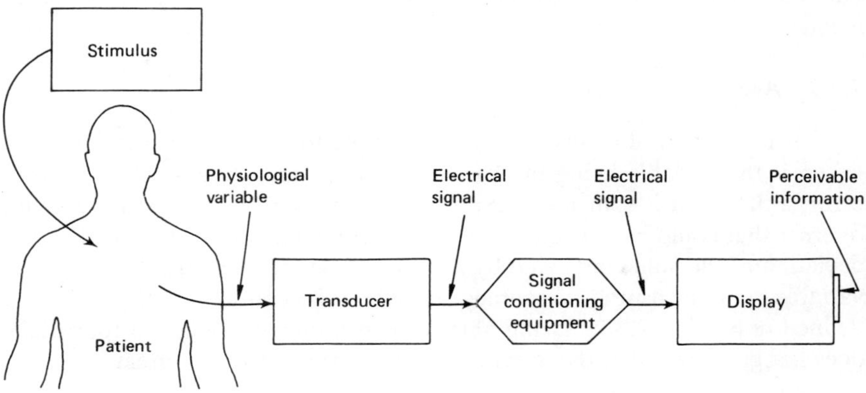

Fig. 2–1 Block diagram of a typical medical instrument.

2.4.1 Range

The range of an instrument is the complete set of values over which the instrument is designed to operate properly. In an instrument that measures a physiological variable, the range extends from the lowest value of the variable that the instrument is capable of accurately measuring to the highest. For example, a heart rate monitor may have a range of from 0 to 250 beats per minute. Such an instrument, then, would be expected to operate properly in measuring and indicating any heart rate between these two limits.

2.4.2 Sensitivity

There are two ways in which the term *sensitivity* is used in connection with medical instrumentation. It is, first of all, an indication of the ability of an instrument to detect small changes in the variable being measured. Thus a more sensitive instrument is capable of detecting and displaying smaller variations than a less sensitive one. The sensitivity of an instrument is partly dependent on the *resolution* of the display. Resolution is an indication of the smallest change that can be read from the display. For example, if the display is a meter, an instrument having a large meter face with well-marked graduations between numbers can be read much more closely than one with a small meter and has higher resolution.

The second definition of *sensitivity* relates the value of the measured physiological variable to the size of the paper graph recording or the height of the pattern on a monitor display screen. A monitor display, for example, may have a sensitivity of 1 millivolt (mV) of ECG voltage for each centimeter of the pattern's height. By knowing this sensitivity, it is easy to determine that a pattern on the screen measuring 3 cm in the height of the R wave represents an ECG in which the R wave has a 3-mV peak value. Often a "sensitivity" control is provided to adjust the sensitivity of the instrument.

2.4.3 Accuracy

The accuracy of an instrument is its ability to indicate correctly the true value of the variable being measured. Accuracy also means freedom from error, although it is sometimes expressed in terms of the maximum amount of error that could be expected from the instrument. *Error* is defined as the deviation of the value indicated by an instrument from the true value of the variable being measured. Accuracy should not be confused with resolution, defined in Section 2.4.2. Being able to read a digital display to four digits does not guarantee that the accuracy of an instrument is that great.

2.4.4 Ease of Calibration

Calibration is a procedure by which an instrument is adjusted to make its indicated values correspond as closely as possible to the actual values being measured. Sometimes calibration is accomplished by measuring a set of known values and adjusting the instrument accordingly. In other types of instruments calibration is performed by comparing the readings of that instrument with those of another instrument that serves as a *reference* or *standard*. Some instruments are relatively easy to calibrate, whereas others may require a difficult and time-consuming process. Proper calibration of an instrument when required greatly improves the accuracy of the instrument. Figure 2-2 shows an electrocardiogram with a 1-mV standardization signal shown as the rectangular pulse. The voltages of all parts of the ECG can be determined accurately when the sensitivity of the instrument is adjusted so that the 1 mV pulse is the correct height on the graph.

2.4.5 Stability

Once calibrated, an instrument will maintain its accuracy only as long as it does not deviate from its calibrated condition. A gradual degradation of the accuracy after calibration is called the *drift* of the instrument. The *stability* of an instrument is its ability to maintain its accuracy over a given interval of time after calibration. A stable instrument seldom requires recalibration, but one with poor stability must be recalibrated frequently.

2.4.6 Frequency Response

Some physiological variables change their values slowly, whereas others change rapidly. Many variables, such as the electrocardiogram, have patterns that include both rapid and slow changes. In order to represent such a pattern accurately, a medical instrument must be able to follow all the changes, both fast and slow. As explained in Chapter 3, a complex

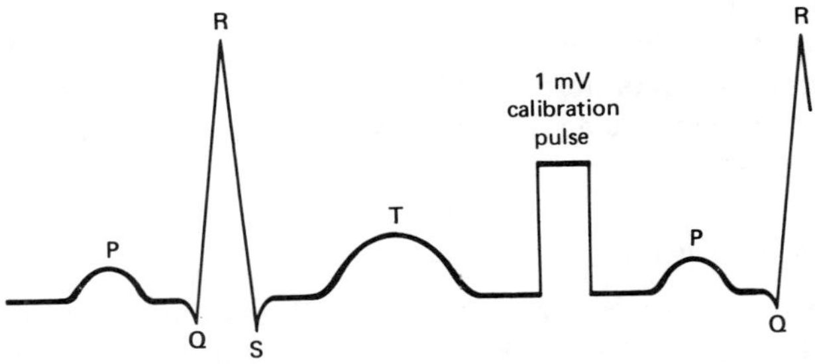

Fig. 2–2 Electrocardiogram showing standardization pulse.

pattern of variations can be represented by a range or *band* of *frequencies.* The concept of frequency is also explained in Chapter 3. At this point it should be sufficient to state that frequency is expressed in cycles per second or *hertz* (Hz) and that the range of frequencies over which an instrument is able to follow changes in the measured variable constitutes its *frequency response.* Thus the frequency response of an instrument must correspond to the band of frequencies included in the variations being measured in order to represent the variable adequately.

2.4.7 Freedom from Noise and Artifact

In Section 2.2 the signal produced by a transducer was defined as variations in voltage corresponding to the information being measured. Often, however, other variations in voltage appear along with the signal. These unwanted variations, usually called *noise, interference,* or *artifact,* also contribute to the results presented in the display. An artifact is any artificial change in the measured variable, such as that produced in the electrocardiogram when the patient moves. If the display is a pattern on a monitor screen, the interference may appear as high-frequency variations in the tracing that give the pattern a fuzzy appearance. In a meter or certain other types of display, the interference may cause an erroneous indication.

Noise or interference can originate from a number of sources. In the measurement of EEG, ECG, or other bioelectric potentials, the patient's body can act as an antenna to pick up 60-Hz energy from electric lights, wiring, and other electrical equipment. This 60-Hz energy can also be picked up by long input cables to instruments. Aspects of powerline noise are discussed in Chapter 3. Sometimes noise is generated internally in the instrument. In many cases, undesired voltage fluctuations occur when the patient moves during the course of the measurement. Also, unwanted variables can be picked up by a transducer along with the desired information. For example, if an ECG electrode is placed over a muscle, activation of that muscle will cause an unwanted EMG signal to be combined with the electrocardiogram.

Some instruments contain special features to eliminate or reduce the effect of certain types of noise or interference. In many cases, proper knowledge of the instrument enables the operator to use procedures that can reduce interference.

2.4.8 Ease of Use

Another instrument characteristic of particular interest to hospital personnel is its ease of use. This factor applies in a number of areas. Perhaps the most important is the ease with which the transducer can be applied to the patient. Simplicity of controls is also important. So is the ease with which the display can be read and interpreted. Other related characteristics pertain to any physical care and cleaning that may be required. Such features include the ruggedness (the ability of the instrument to withstand continued use, and possibly abuse, without breaking or failing in other ways), cleanability (how often the instrument needs cleaning), and the expected life of its most delicate parts. The care and use of electronic instruments are discussed in Chapter 20.

2.4.9 Patient Safety and Comfort

In measuring a physiological variable, it is often necessary to apply or connect a transducer to a location within the body from which the variable can be obtained. Many variables can be measured by placing transducers outside the body or on the surface of the skin. A measurement of this type is said to be *noninvasive.* Some measurements, however, require *invasive* techniques, in which a transducer or catheter is placed within the body. For example, a catheter leading to a transducer must be entered into an artery in order to measure arterial blood pressure. Invasion of the body usually means a certain amount of risk for the patient and often considerable discomfort. Consequently, measurements that can be obtained by noninvasive techniques are used whenever possible. If a suitable noninvasive method is not available, however, invasive procedures must be used.

Instrumentation intended for invasive use within the body must meet certain special requirements. It must be able to withstand sterilization. Also, it should be designed to minimize trauma and discomfort to the patient as much as possible. If invasion of the cardiovascular system is involved, that portion of the instrument that enters the bloodstream must also be nonthrombogenic (does not produce clots) and nonpyrogenic (does not generate heat).

Fortunately, developments in the late 1960s and 1970s have made it possible to replace some of the older invasive clinical techniques with new noninvasive methods of obtaining similar information. For example, echocardiography, in which ultrasonic energy is used to obtain functional information about the heart, is often used in place of certain clinical diagnostic procedures that require catheterization. Much of the emphasis in new instrumentation design and development is on noninvasive methods of measurement that will, hopefully, further reduce the number of invasive procedures still in clinical use.

Even the use of noninvasive instrumentation can present considerable discomfort to the patient. For example, long-term application of ECG electrodes can cause skin irritation. Patient discomfort is an important consideration both in the design and the use of instruments. The degree of discomfort often largely depends on the length of time required for a given procedure. Caring personnel should be trained to perform uncomfortable procedures as quickly as possible and should learn to apply instrumentation in a way that will minimize patient discomfort.

Another type of danger in using medical instrumentation with patients should be mentioned at this point. Whenever equipment that receives power from the electric power line is used with patients, a possible electrical safety hazard exists. This danger is considerably greater when the patient is connected to the instrument (as in the case of an electrocardiograph or ECG monitor) or when an electrically conductive path leads from outside the patient's body to the inside (especially to the heart). Electrical safety hazards are discussed in detail in Chapter 18.

3

The Fundamentals of Electricity Applied to Medicine

People in the industrialized world use electricity almost as readily as they do water. Although the behavior of water is generally well understood, most people know little about electricity. They realize that electricity operates home appliances, illuminates the world, and does much more. It is conveniently at hand, ready to serve at a simple flip of a switch. They also realize, because of an accidental electric shock experience at home or at work, that electricity is both an abstract phenomenon (since it is never seen) and an entity commanding a good deal of respect, since it can cause undesired damage or, at least, an unpleasant sensation. It could be said that users of electricity need not understand what it is or how it behaves in order to use it satisfactorily. It could also be argued that a driver need not understand how an engine behaves in order to operate an automobile. Many stranded motorists, however, have benefited from a basic understanding of an engine's behavior. Similarly, the user of electricity, especially in the critical care area of a hospital, can benefit from understanding what it is, how it behaves, and how it is used effectively and safely.

3.1 Electricity—What It Is

Strictly defined, electricity is a basic property or characteristic of all matter, for matter is composed of atoms that contain, among other particles, *electrons*. The electron, illustrated in Figure 3-1, is a tiny *electrically charged* particle that normally orbits around an atom's electrically charged nucleus much as a satellite orbits the earth. The atom represented in Figure 3-1 is hydrogen, the simplest of over 100 known chemical elements.

The electron (shown with a minus sign) is held in orbit partly by a force of attraction that exists between it and its electrically charged nucleus, a proton (shown with a plus sign). Understanding the nature and behavior of the electron (and of electric charges) is a vital first step in understanding electricity.

3.1.1 Electric Charge Behavior

As shown in Figure 3-2(a), the electron is a negative electric charge identified by a minus sign. A positive charge is shown by a plus sign. The signs connote that the charges behave differently in nature. The term *charge* means that a particle (or object) possesses electrical *energy*. Any object or substance having the capacity to do work possesses energy. For example, when someone uses his energy to move a hospital bed a certain distance, work is done. The amount of energy expended or utilized equals the amount of work done. Therefore energy and work done are, for practical purposes, the same. There are two kinds of energy: *potential energy* and *kinetic energy*. Potential energy is possessed, for example, by a 100-pound (lb) object raised one foot above the floor. When released, it will do work upon

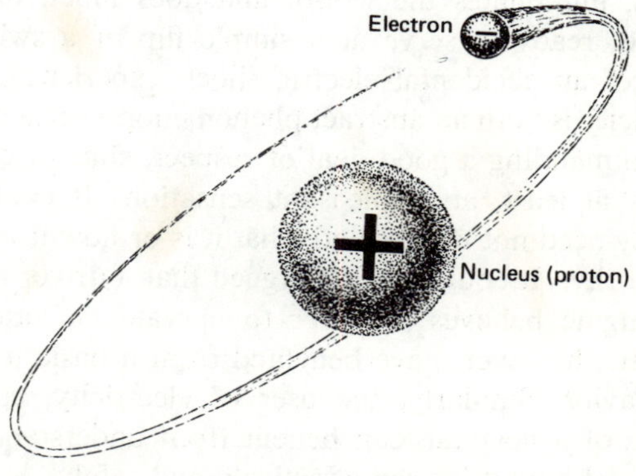

Fig. 3–1 Representative structure of the hydrogen atom.

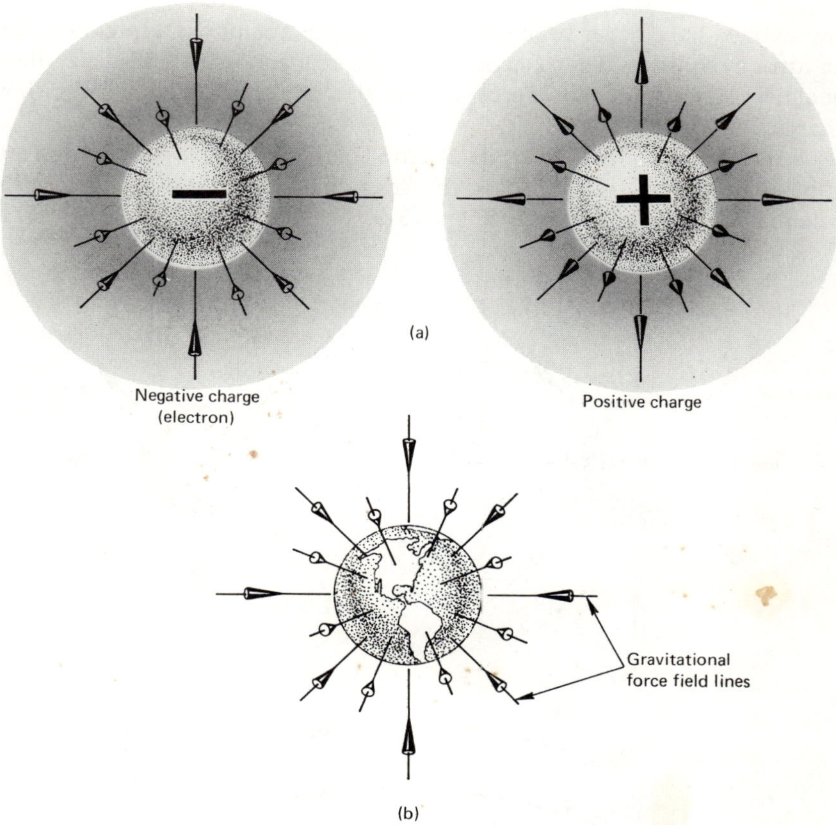

Fig. 3–2 Force (energy) fields found in nature: (a) electric fields surrounding charges; (b) gravity field surrounding earth.

impact with the floor (damage, perhaps). While suspended, the object stores potential energy; that is, it has the potential to do work. Kinetic energy is energy in motion. When the 100-lb object is released, its potential energy reverts to kinetic energy. Potential energy is stored in many substances. Fossil fuels (coal, oil, gasoline) contain potential energy. When released, their energies are used to generate heat and electricity. An electric charge possesses potential energy in the form of a *force field* that surrounds it. Thus it is able to do work. The electrified force field is shown as an aura in Figure 3-2(a). The geometry of the electric force field is similar to the gravitational force field surrounding the earth in Figure 3-2(b). Directional arrowheads placed on these force lines (representing the attractive force of gravity) signify that if an object were dropped above the earth's surface, it would travel along the lines of force toward the earth. It should be noted that the aura shown surrounding the electric charges and the lines representing the gravity field have never been seen. They are the author's interpretation and an artist's rendition. The sketches allow the reader to better visualize these qualities; hence lines show force, arrows show direction, and spheres show charges.

Because of its force field, an electric charge is capable of moving (and of being moved by) other electric charges. Thus, as noted, a charge has the potential to do work. Consider Figure 3-3.

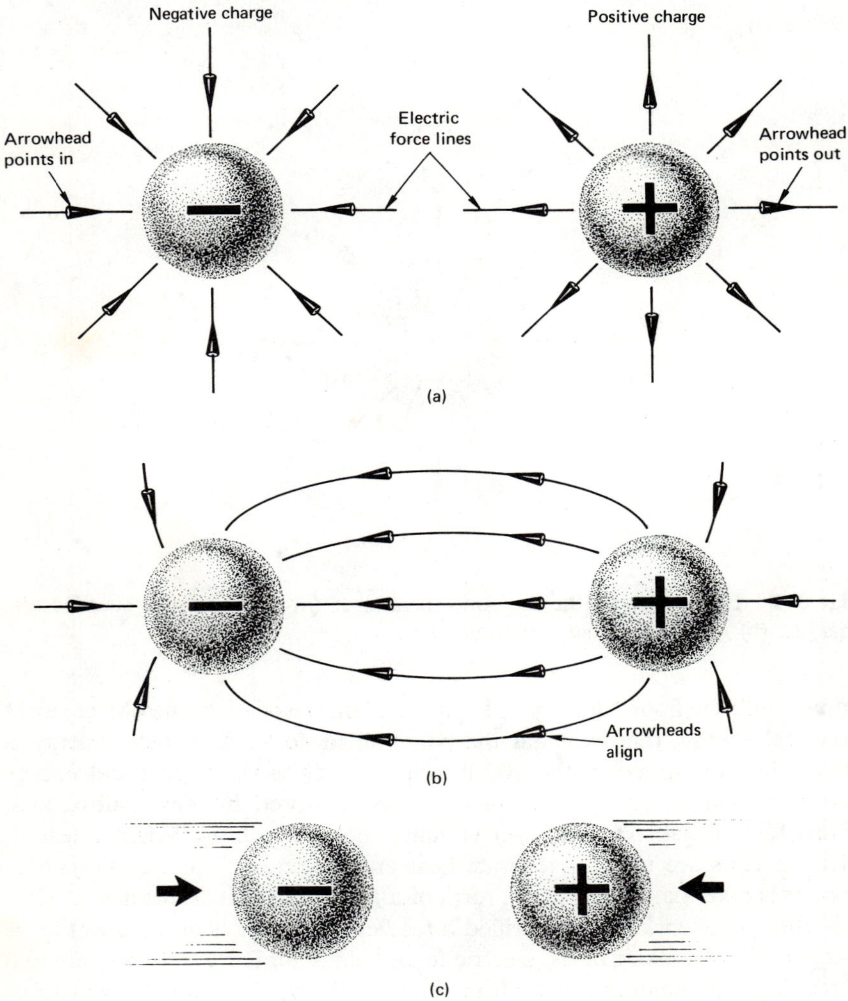

Fig. 3–3 Unlike electric charges: (a) separated; (b) attracted to each other; (c) resulting charge motion (towards each other).

The charges from Figure 3-2(a) are redrawn without their auras but with their force lines.

Arrowheads on the force lines in Figure 3-3(a) point in opposite directions, toward the negative charge and away from the positive charge. For the negative charge, the arrowheads denote that if a positive charge is placed near it (and the positive charge could move), the positive charge will be attracted to the negative charge. The positive charge will move toward the negative charge along the lines of force because unlike (negative and positive) charges attract each other. Their electric fields interact, resulting in charge motion and hence in work. The way their fields interact is shown in Figure 3-3(b). The force lines tend to align, forcing the two mutually attracted charges to come together just as two properly positioned magnets come together. Their relative movement is shown in Figure 3-3(c) without their fields.

Similar (like) charges behave differently from opposite (unlike) charges. The fields of two negative charges in Figure 3-4(a) are identical. Since, as noted, a negative charge will attract a positive charge, it will *repel* a like negative charge, as shown in Figure 3-4(b). The force lines tend to oppose each other rather than become aligned. Thus, as shown in Figure 3-4(c), like charges repel each other.

Two positive charges behave the same as two negative charges [Figure 3-4(d)]. Electric charge behavior in these three basic combinations is easily summarized:

Unlike charges attract each other.

Like charges repel each other.

The generation or movement of electric charges is called *electricity*. Charge behavior is very predictable. In order to understand why charges behave as they do, it is necessary to examine the structure of the atom. Only those atomic properties pertinent to electricity will be examined.

3.1.2 The Structure of the Atom

Atoms form molecules, molecules form compounds and mixtures, and so on. Normally atoms are electrically inert (neutral). They each possess equal amounts of negative and positive charges. Therefore matter is, by nature, electrically neutral.

When energy in various forms (heat, light, electric) is applied to an atom, its normal energy state changes. A proper amount of applied energy will cause electrons to escape from their usual orbits, leaving an atom with fewer electrons than usual. Then the atom, stripped of one or more electrons, is electrically unbalanced and becomes electrically *charged*. A

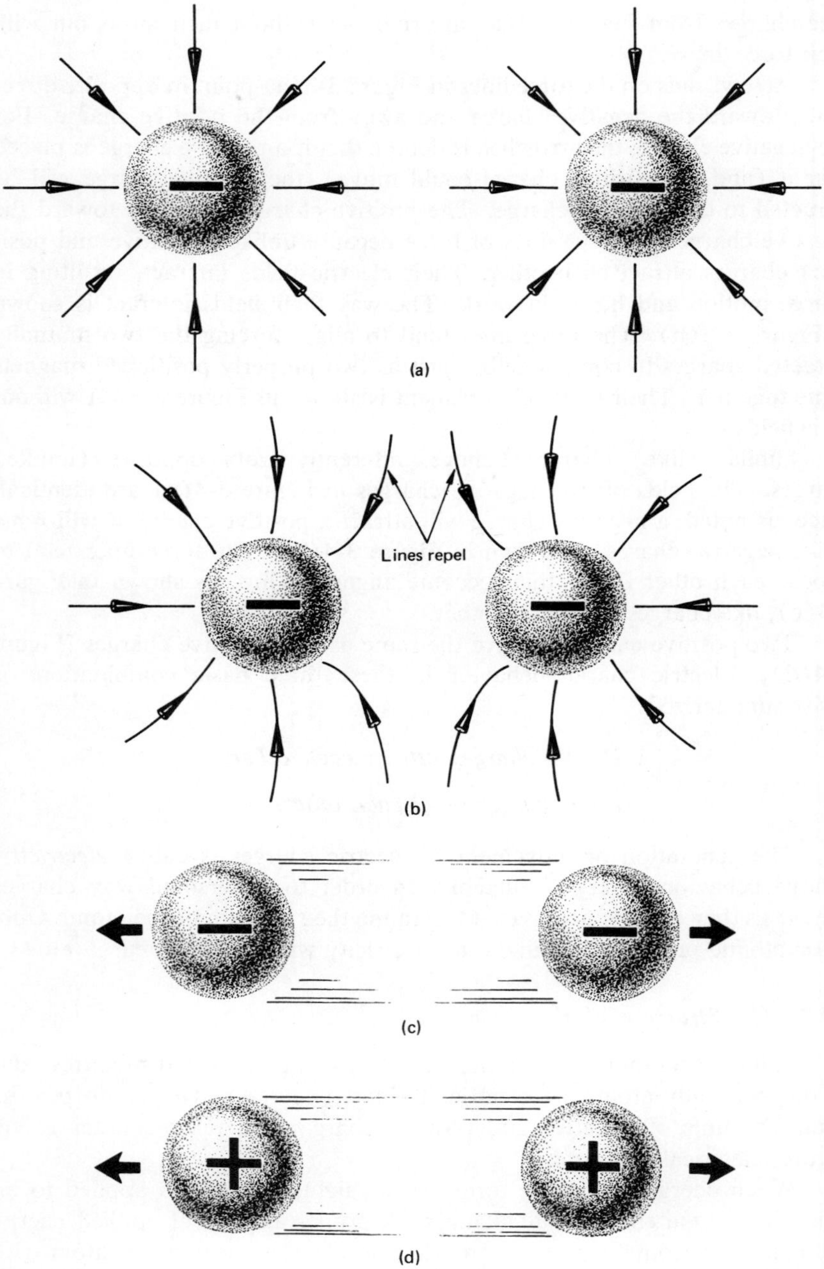

Fig. 3–4 Like charge behavior: (a) negative charges separated; (b) each repels the other; (c) resulting charge motion; (d) like (positive) charges repel each other.

charged atom behaves like a fundamental charge already described. Conversely, an atom may be forced to gain one or more electrons, again becoming electrically unbalanced. Atoms that lose or gain electrons are called *ions,* or electrically charged atoms. There are two types of ions—negative and positive. A *negative ion* or *anion* is formed whenever an atom *gains* electrons. When an atom loses electrons, it becomes a *positive ion* or *cation.* The formation of a positive ion is illustrated in Figure 3-5.

The sodium atom is shown in Figure 3-5(a) with its full complement of electrons and protons. The outermost electron, the *valence* electron, differs from the others in two respects. First, because it is farther away (in the outermost orbit) from the nucleus, it has more potential energy than the others. This is similar to the difference in potential energy between an object 100 feet (ft) from the ground and an identical one only 10 ft from the

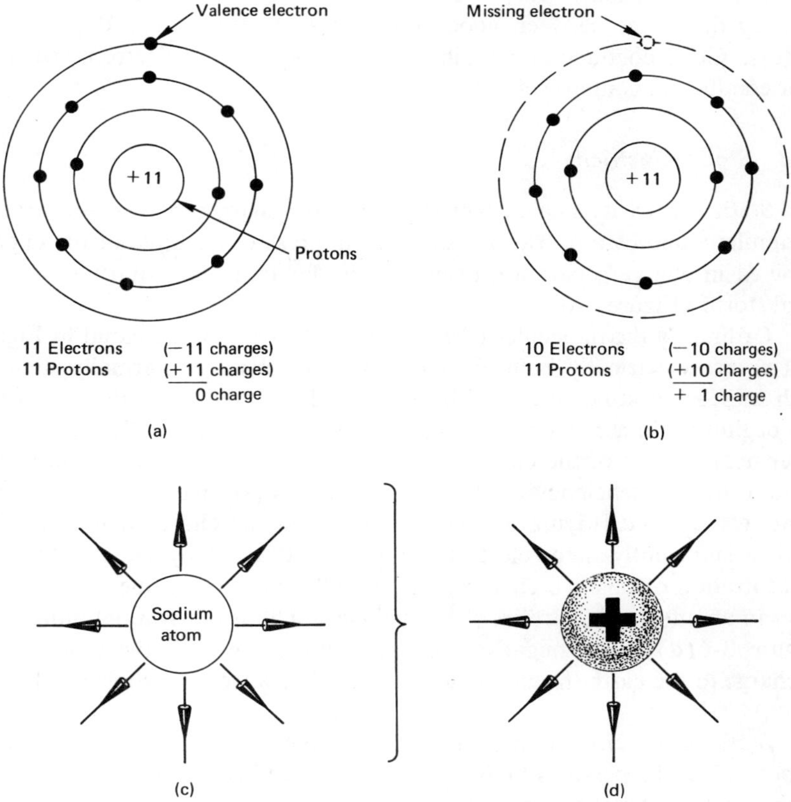

Fig. 3–5 Forming an ion: (a) balanced sodium atom; (b) missing valence electron; (c) resulting positively charged ion; (d) resulting positive charge.

ground. The higher object possesses more energy than the other. Secondly, because the valence electron is more remote from the nucleus than the others, the electric attractive force between it and the nucleus is relatively weak. So the electron is loosely bound to its nucleus and is relatively free to move. For these reasons, little externally applied energy or force is required to cause the valence electron to leave the atom.

The easily displaced valence electron is shown missing in Figure 3-5(b). Now electrically unbalanced, the entire atom is a positively charged atom (ion), shown in Figure 3-5(c), and will behave in every way like the positive charge shown in Figure 3-5(d). Thus when electrically neutral atoms (or complex molecules, such as proteins) gain or lose electrons, they become electrically charged (possess electric energy) and behave accordingly.

It is noteworthy that an atom's protons are immobile; they are solidly locked into its nucleus. Only electrons are mobile. This important property is a key difference between good conductors of electricity and poor conductors. Good conductors contain an abundance of free electrons, whereas poor conductors contain very few.

3.1.3 Static Electricity

Static electricity occurs whenever electric charges become separated, accumulate, and cannot travel easily. An impressive example of the energy involved in charge separation results in the lightning flash during an electrical storm (Figure 3-6).

Ordinarily the molecules of water droplets forming the cloud in Figure 3-6(a) are electrically neutral. Therefore the cloud is normally neutral. With increasing atmospheric turbulence, and as larger rain droplets form and begin to fall, a concentration of electrons (forming negative ions) may occur near the top of the cloud [Figure 3-6(b)], causing the bottom of the cloud to have a deficiency of electrons, shown as positive ions. Winds may separate the cloud [Figure 3-6(c)]. Then when the charge concentrations become sufficiently high, electrons, strongly attracted by an equally high concentration of positive charges, will literally jump from one cloud to the other in an effort to neutralize the imbalance. The result is a lightning flash [Figure 3-6(d)]. The negatively charged cloud may, on the other hand, discharge to the earth through a high object (like a tree) as shown in Figure 3-6(e).

Static electricity often forms when someone walks across a nylon carpet. Then the person's body becomes energized with excess charges that discharge to a touched metal object (like a doorknob). The discharged energy can be felt, heard, and sometimes seen as a spark.

Similarly, static charges accumulate on the apparel of operating room

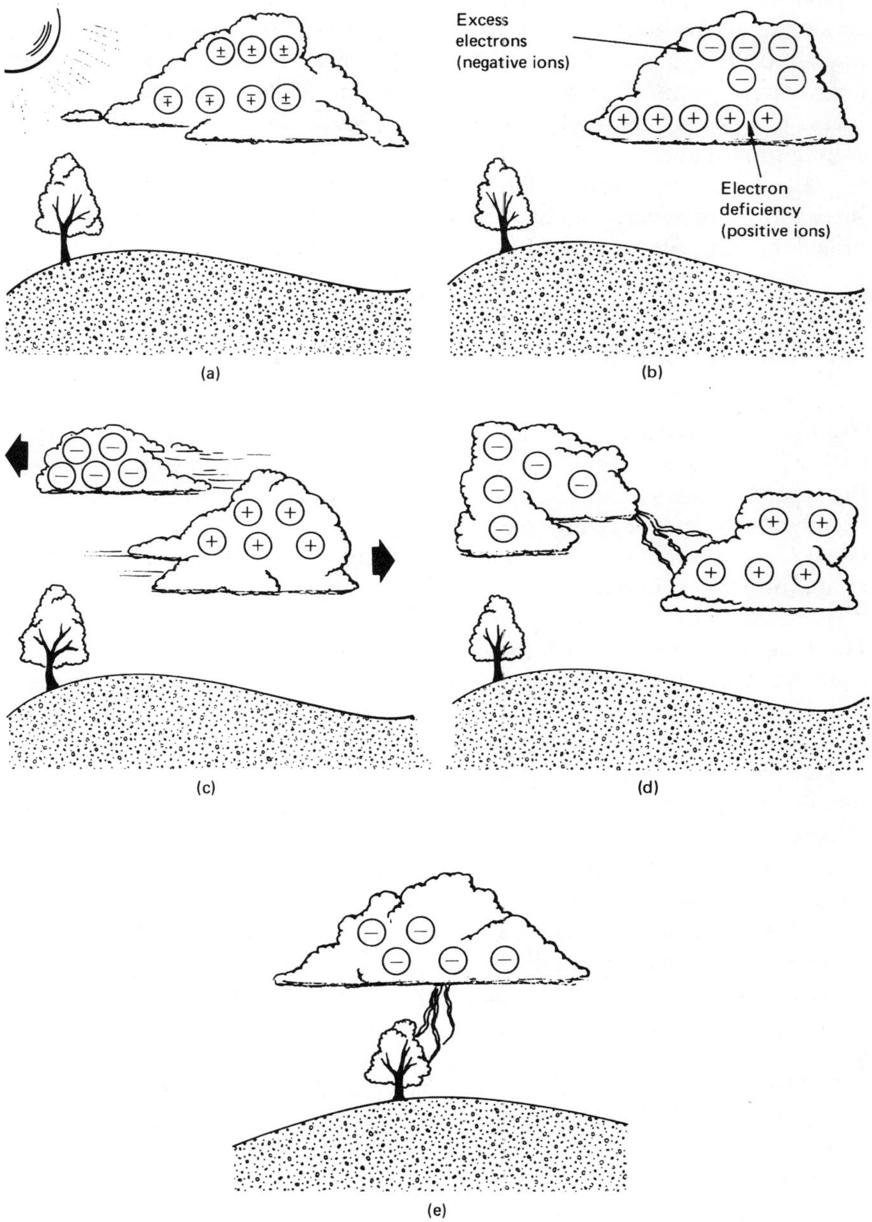

Fig. 3–6 Static electricity in nature: (a) electrically neutral cloud (b) charge separation; (c) cloud separation; (d) lightning between clouds (e) lightning to earth.

personnel. Ensuing spark discharges may be hazardous in the presence of anesthetic agents, such as cyclopropane and ether, that become flammable when mixed with air. To prevent charges from accumulating, personnel wear cotton gowns or gowns with a 1% stainless steel fiber content. Any excess charges are allowed to disperse to ground (earth) through the operating room floor.

Electricity used to provide light and operate appliances involves the generation and separation of electric charges with their continuous controlled motion. Electric charges in motion constitute electric current.

3.2 Electric Current

Electric current is illustrated in Figure 3-7. Two electrically neutral spheres, each with an equal amount of unlike charges, are shown in Figure 3-7(a). Because they are not charged, each lacks the potential to do work electrically; thus they are at zero electric potential. Their electric potentials are equal (*equipotential* or *isopotential*). In Figure 3-7(b) the atoms of sphere *A* are forced to gain more electrons than they normally have (negative ions are formed). The atoms of sphere *B* have lost an equal number of electrons (forming positive ions). The spheres are now electrically (and oppositely) charged. Thus the potential of *A* is negative and the potential of *B* is positive. There now exist *different electric potentials* at *A* and *B*. If a conducting pathway (charge conductor) were suddenly to bridge the spheres [Figure 3-7(c)], excess electrons, attracted to positive charges, would rapidly transfer to *B*. The transfer of charge is electric current. Soon both spheres are again electrically neutral, and no difference in potential exists between them. Once more they are equipotential as shown in Figure 3-7(d). Once an equipotential condition is achieved, current cannot travel.

This principle can also be explained by use of a hydraulic (fluid) analogy (see Figure 3-8). Fluid analogies are helpful in understanding electrical phenomena because physical factors involved in electricity are often similar (analogous) to factors involved in hydraulics. This chapter uses several fluid analogies to explain electrical principles.

The containers in Figure 3-8(a) have equal levels of water. In Figure 3-8(b) some water is added to *A*, while an equal amount is drained from *B*. There now exists a difference in water levels between *A* and *B*. If, as shown in Figure 3-8(c), a conducting pathway (pipe) were suddenly connected, the water pressure at *A* (greater than the pressure at *B*) would force water to flow from *A* to *B* until the water levels equalize. Water would then stop flowing because no difference in water pressure would exist between *A* and *B* [Figure 3-8(d)]. Thus equal water pressure is analogous to equal electric

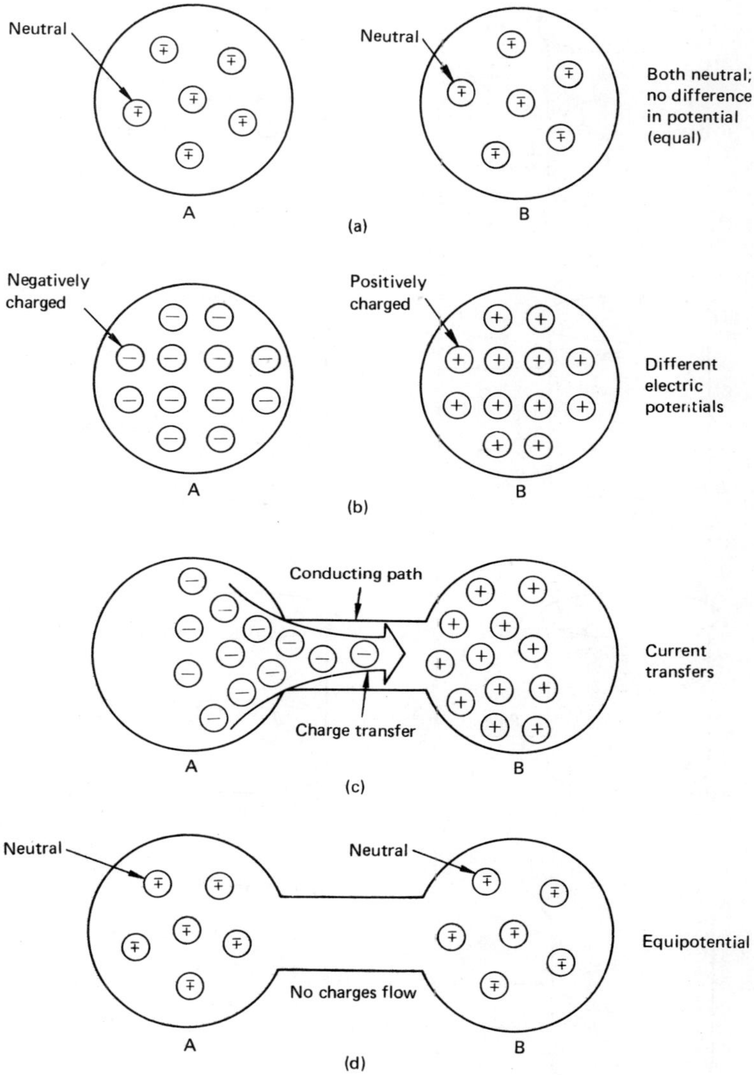

Fig. 3–7 Electric charge flow is electric current: (a) electric potentials equal; (b) electric potentials different; (c) current flows (d) no current flow.

potentials, and water flow can be compared to the flow of electric charges (electric current) in Figure 3-7(c).

Water flows because of the difference in water pressure between containers *A* and *B*. Similarly, electrons flow because of the difference in electric

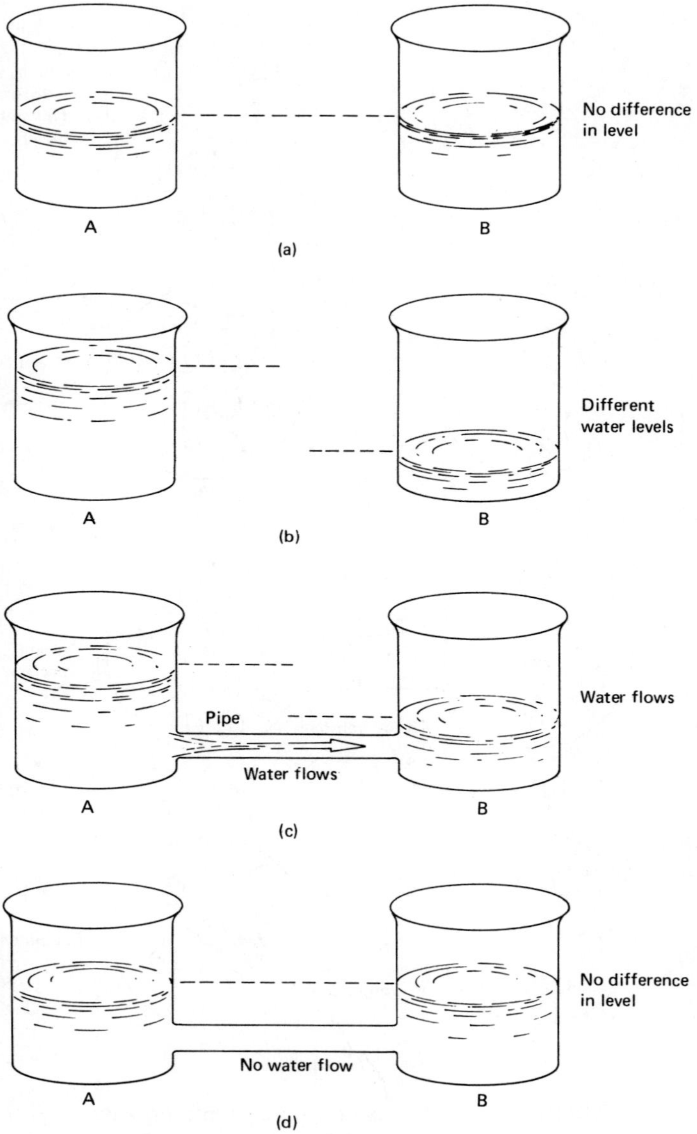

Fig. 3–8 Water flow: (a) water levels equal; (b) water levels different; (c) water flows; (d) no water flow.

potentials between spheres *A* and *B*. A difference of electric potential is called *voltage* (see Section 3.4).

Whenever electric charges are put in motion, the result is electric current. Current is analogous to fluid flow and, like fluid flow, can be measured in appropriate terms or units. Blood flow is measured in liters of blood passing, for example, through the ascending aorta as shown in Figure 3-9(a) during a one-minute interval. Thus blood flow is measured in *liters per minute* (l/min).

Electric current is measured in the number of charges that flow past a point (in a conductor) in a one-second time interval as shown in Figure 3-9(b). When 6,250,000,000,000,000,000 (about six billion billion) electric charges flow past a point in one second, the value of the current is 1

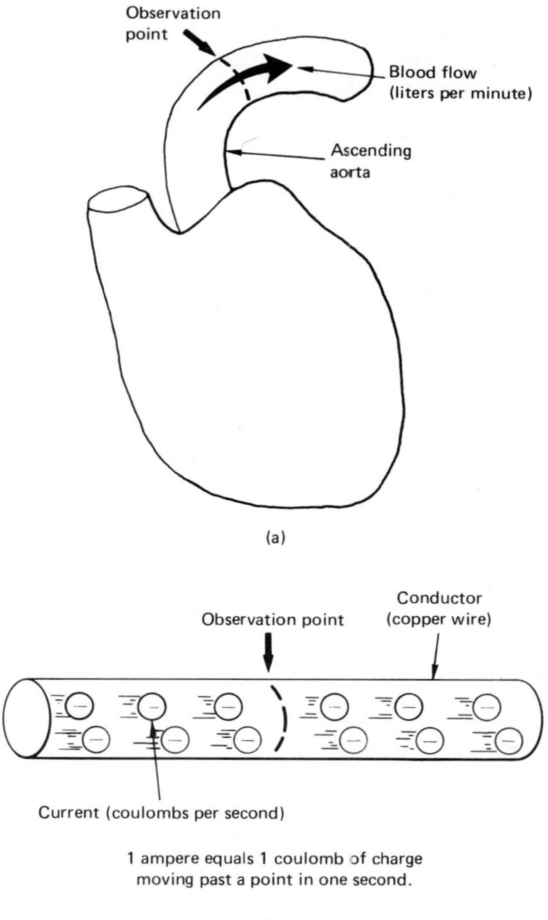

Fig. 3–9 Fluid and electric analogies: (a) blood flow; (b) current.

ampere (abbreviated A). The ampere is a practical unit that denotes the *rate* at which electric charges flow, just as the unit liters per minute denotes the rate of blood flow.

The large number of charges quoted above is called a *coulomb* (abbreviated C). Thus 1 ampere equals the flow of 1 coulomb per second. A 100-watt (W) light bulb requires about 1 A, a toaster about 10 A.

Because the ampere is a comparatively large amount of current and personnel involved with medical equipment are often concerned with much smaller values, current values are given in *milliamperes* and *microamperes* when appropriate. A milliampere is 1 one-thousandth (1/1000) of an ampere, while a microampere is equal to 1 one-millionth (1/1,000,000) of an ampere. The prefixes *milli* and *micro* are often denoted as m and μ (the Greek letter mu), respectively. Thus a milliampere is abbreviated 1 mA and a microampere as 1 μA. The minute magnitude of the microampere is often difficult to appreciate. It may easily be put into focus if remembered as an allegory.

> One microampere is to one ampere as one dollar is to one million dollars.

It will be shown in Chapter 18 that critical care personnel should be aware of electric current values that range from a few microamperes to many amperes. It will also be shown that a relatively small value of electric current flowing into the human body can, under certain circumstances, be hazardous.

Summarizing briefly, electric current is the movement or flow of electric charges forced by an electric potential difference or voltage. It is analogous to the flow of fluid (blood) forced by hydraulic pressure (blood pressure). The charges that are able to move in most conductors of electricity are electrons, although current may also consist of ions in motion. Actually, electrons move rather slowly from atom to atom. However, their electric fields propagate at nearly the speed of light. This is why many of the effects of electricity seem to occur almost instantaneously.

3.3 Electric Conductors, Insulators, and Resistance

The idea of *conductors* of electricity was presented early in this chapter. The converse of a conductor is an *insulator*. Common to both is the property of electric *resistance;* furthermore, both are materials that form elements in the electrical environment—wires, equipment, and the human body.

3.3.1 Electric Conductors

Many materials are able to conduct electric current, some more easily than others. Among the better conductors are metals (such as copper, silver, gold, aluminum, and carbon) and electrolytes (salt or acid solutions and blood).

Metals are good conductors of electricity because the atoms of which they are composed give up electrons easily. Their valence electrons are loosely bound to the atoms' nuclei and are able to move with very little applied force. Thus electrons can easily be made to flow. Copper is a material widely used in wires to carry current to and from appliances and devices. Figure 3-9(b) illustrates loosely bound valence electrons drifting through a section of copper wire. Copper and other good conductors of electricity offer little *resistance* to current.

Electrolytes are solutions that are able to conduct electricity. Common examples are salt and acid solutions.

The human body is essentially composed of a salt solution (about 60% water with a salt content). It may be considered as a volume of electrolytic solution in a leatherlike container (the skin). The human body, then, is a *volume conductor* of electricity.

The earth (ground) is also a good conductor of electricity. It accepts all electric charges, like those that form a lightning bolt. Just as a large body of water will accept a waterfall without changing its water level, the earth will accept electric charges without changing its electrical level. Since charges entering the earth are unable to accumulate and concentrate (they quickly disperse), the earth is electrically neutral. The earth is considered an equipotential or zero potential reference.

3.3.2 Electric Insulators

Materials that are poor conductors of electricity are called *insulators*. They are composed of atoms that contain very few loosely bound valence electrons. In insulators, electrons cannot flow easily; therefore insulators resist current. Among the good insulators are such nonmetals as glass, air, wood, and plastics. Teflon and plastic materials are commonly used to insulate copper conductors so as to isolate them electrically from other conductors. It should be realized, however, that no insulator is perfect.

3.3.3 Electric Resistance

Whether conductors or insulators, all materials offer a certain amount of resistance to the flow of electricity. All resist current to some degree. The unit of electric resistance is the ohm (Ω), a term used to honor the nineteenth-century physicist Georg S. Ohm. The letter designation for resistance is *R*.

The resistance of materials ranges from very low values (very good conductors) to an almost infinite amount (very good insulators), as illustrated in Figure 3-10.

A fairly long piece of copper wire, a good conductor (shown at the extreme left of the scale), may offer less than 1 Ω of resistance. Insulating materials may have resistance values of several million ohms. The human body may offer resistance to current ranging from as little as 50 to as many as one million ohms, depending on various factors.

Wire resistance depends on several physical factors, one of which is the type of material from which the wire is made. For example, metals form better conductors than nonmetals; and, among the metals, copper is a better conductor than aluminum. Silver is a better conductor than copper.

The resistance of a wire is directly proportional to its length. That is, the resistance increases as the length of the wire increases because electricity must flow through more of the material. A long wire has more resistance than a short wire, just as a long vessel offers more resistance to blood flow than does a short vessel.

The cross-sectional area or diameter of a wire also influences its resistance value. A narrow (small-diameter) wire offers more resistance than does a wire whose diameter is large, just as a small-diameter vessel offers more resistance to blood flow than does a large-diameter vessel. The resistance of wire is inversely proportional to its cross-sectional area.

The resistance properties of wire are used in a typical blood pressure transducer. A transducer is a device that converts one form of energy to

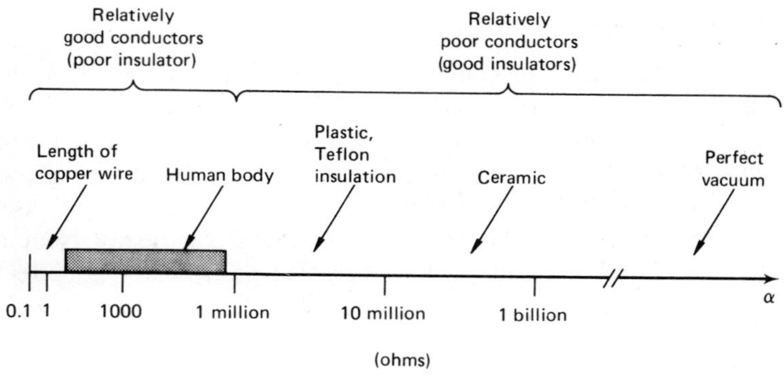

Fig. 3–10 Range of resistance values of materials.

another. In the resistance type of transducer, changes in blood pressure bend a metal diaphragm on which is mounted a thin wire. As the wire is strained (stretched), its length increases while its diameter decreases. The resistance value of the wire changes (increases) as a function of blood pressure. This resistance value is further processed to provide a blood pressure display. Details of blood pressure transducers are given in Chapter 9. Manufactured components (parts) called *resistors* are widely used within electrical devices. Details of resistors are given in Section 3.6.1.

3.4 Voltage—Electric Force

Electricity will flow when only two conditions are met. One is the presence of a conductor. The other is the presence of a difference of electric potential called *voltage* or *electromotive force* (*EMF*). The unit of voltage is the *volt*. The letters *E* and *V* are used interchangeably to indicate EMF or voltage. It must be remembered that voltage can only exist as the difference in electric potential between two points. Voltage cannot flow. Only current flows when a difference of potential exists and a conductor is present. It follows that a conductor must make at least two points of contact with a source of voltage in order for current to travel. If the electric potentials at two points (or across a conductor) are the same, there is no potential difference (zero voltage) and current cannot flow. These concepts are illustrated in Figure 3-11.

A source of constant voltage with terminals *A* and *B* is shown enclosed within the dashed lines in Figure 3-11(a). Because terminal *A* has an accumulation or an excess of negative charges while terminal *B* has a deficiency of negative charges (positive charges), there is a difference of electric potential between the terminals. The voltage is given as 6 V. When a conductor is connected between the terminals, electrons flow from the more negative terminal (*A*) to the less negative terminal (*B*). If, as shown in Figure 3-11(b), both terminals were equally negative, there would be no difference in electric potential because both terminals have equal potentials (equipotential). Therefore electricity cannot flow even though a conductor is present, for there is no difference of potential. This condition corresponds to zero volts. Note that the only entity in motion in Figure 3-11(a) is current. Voltage, the difference of potential, can only exist between two points, as stated.

Very small values of voltage, like very small values of current, are of concern to personnel in critical care areas. These voltage values are on the order of millivolts (mV) and microvolts (μV).

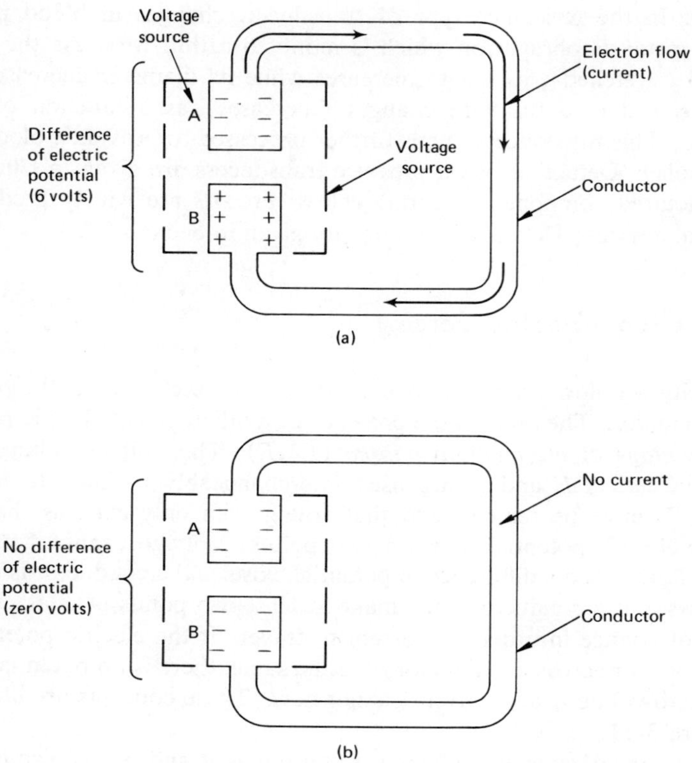

Fig. 3–11 Difference of electric potential: (a) potential difference forces current to flow; (b) no potential difference, no current flows.

3.5 Relationships of Current, Resistance, and Voltage

A brief review of the three key characteristic parameters of electricity discussed so far is given in Table 3-1. Electric current (designated by the letter *I*) is the flow of electric charges and is measured in amperes. It is analogous to the flow of blood. Resistance, *R*, is the property of materials that resists or impedes current. It is measured in ohms. Electrical resistance is analogous to the resistance to blood flow offered by a partially occluded vessel. Voltage, *E* or *V*, is the electric force that causes current to flow. It is a difference in electrical potential, analogous to a difference in blood pressure between two points in the circulatory system—for example, between the arterioles and venules on either side of a capillary bed.

Table 3-1 Key Electrical Parameters

Parameter	*Unit*	*Designation*	*What It Is*	*Comparable To (Blood Flow Analogy)*
Current	ampere	I	Movement or flow of electric charges	Flow of blood
Resistance	ohm	R	Opposition to current	Opposition to blood flow
Voltage	volt	E or V	Electric force or difference of potential	Blood pressure differential

In order for current to flow, a difference of electrical potential must exist between two points with a complete conductive path in between, just as a difference in blood pressure and a complete circulatory path are needed for continuing blood flow. The amount of current that flows depends on the voltage between the two points and the resistance of the path between them. In the same way, the amount of blood that flows in a circulatory path depends on the difference in blood pressure between two points and the resistance of the vessels between them. The relationships between voltage, current, and electrical resistance are covered in the following section.

3.5.1 Ohm's Law

As stated, the current in a conductor depends on voltage and resistance. The value of current is directly proportional to the value of voltage. This statement means that

1. When voltage increases, current increases.
2. When voltage decreases, current decreases.
3. When voltage is zero (difference of potential is zero), current is zero.

The value of current is inversely proportional to the value of resistance. That is,

1. When resistance increases, current decreases.
2. When resistance decreases, current increases.

These important relationships are expressed in a basic electrical law called *Ohm's law,* which states that the value of current equals the value of the voltage divided by the value of the resistance. Expressed symbolically,

$$I = \frac{E}{R},$$

where I is current in amperes, E is voltage in volts, and R is resistance in ohms. When a difference of potential of 1 V is applied to a resistance of 1 Ω, the current equals 1 A. These relationships are illustrated in Figure 3-12. Here three batteries, each with a different voltage, are applied to 1-Ω

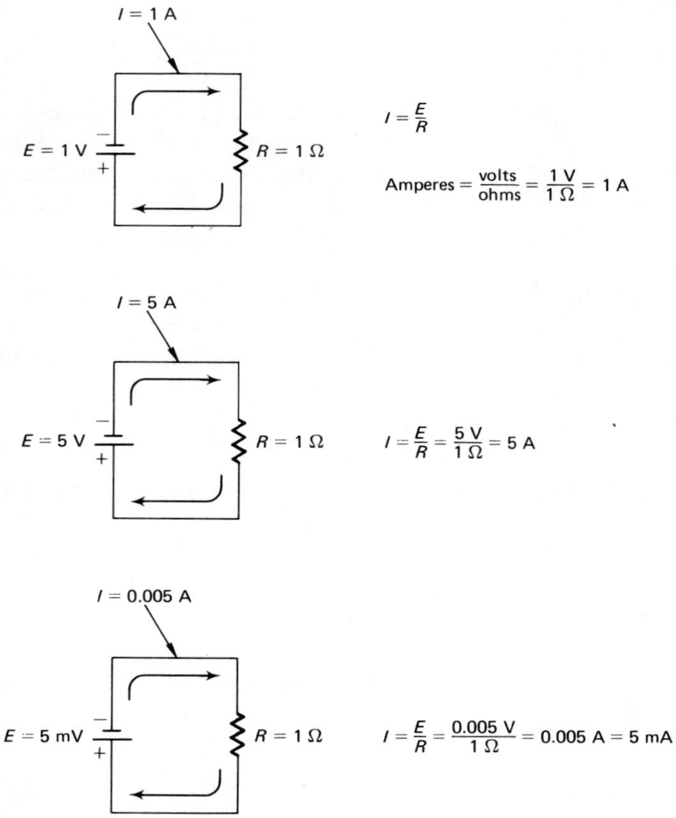

Fig. 3–12 Ohm's Law applied. Resistance is held constant; voltage is changed.

resistors. The resulting currents, according to Ohm's law, are directly proportional to the voltage values.

On the other hand, when voltage is held constant and resistance is changed, current is inversely proportional to resistance, again obeying Ohm's law. Figure 3-13 illustrates Ohm's law with different values of resistance.

Ohm's law can also be used to calculate the amount of voltage across a resistance when the value of the resistance and the amount of current through it are known. In this version, Ohm's law states

$$E = IR.$$

When the resistance of a device is unknown but the voltage and current can be measured, a third version of Ohm's law can be used to calculate the value of resistance:

$$R = \frac{E}{I}.$$

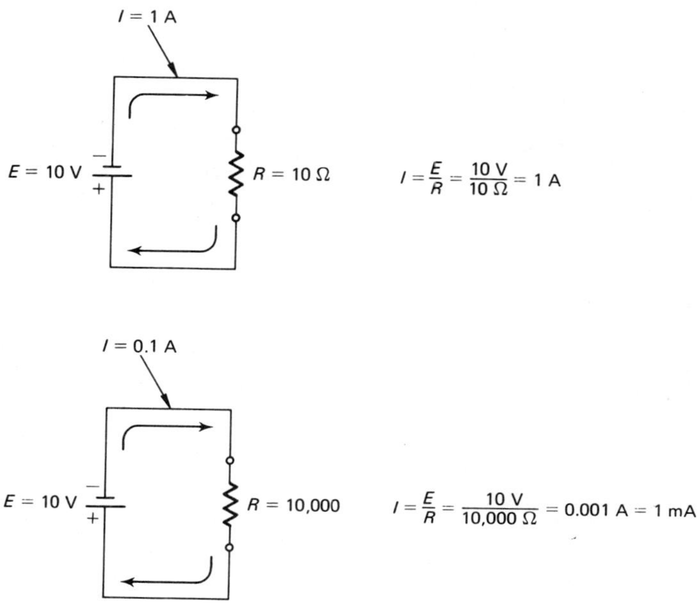

Fig. 3–13 Ohm's Law applied. Voltage is held constant. Resistance is changed.

3.6 Direct and Alternating Current

Voltage sources can either be man-made devices or appear as part of natural processes. Common voltage sources are ordinary batteries and electric generators. Batteries are used to energize a variety of useful items, among which are flashlights, artificial heart pacers, defibrillators, and patient monitors. In addition, they are used to start automobiles and to supply electricity for other portable devices.

3.6.1 Direct Current

The electrical symbol for the battery is shown in Figure 3-14. The shorter of the two parallel lines is the battery's negative terminal or pole;

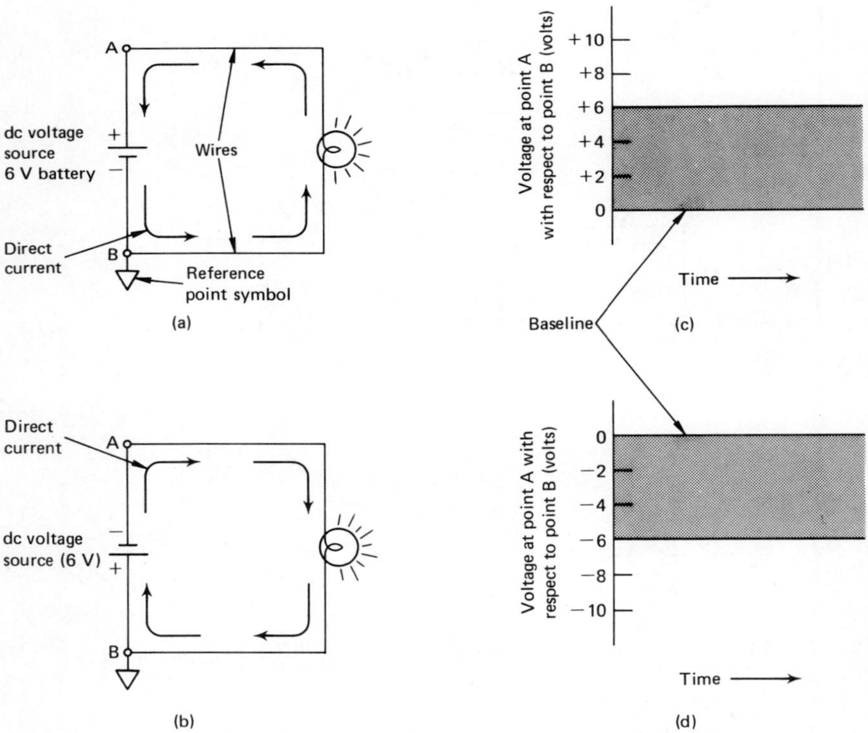

Fig. 3–14 DC voltage source with graphs: (a) direct current, counterclockwise; (b) dc, clockwise; (c) polarity and value at point A; (d) reversed polarity at point A.

the other is its positive pole. Thus a battery is polarized. Batteries provide a unidirectional form of current, called *direct current* (dc), that travels in one direction only. It is analogous to unidirectional blood flow in a vein. The notation *dc* is also applied to a voltage that remains at a given polarity. Such a voltage is called a *dc voltage*.

In Figure 3-14(a) a 6-V battery is shown wired to a lamp. Since a dc voltage and a complete conducting path are present, current flows counterclockwise (in one direction) from the negative terminal of the source, through the lamp, and finally returns to the positive terminal. When the battery is reversed [Figure 3-14(b)], current will flow clockwise. In either case, the result is the same. Energy is transferred from the source to the lamp because of electric charge motion; the lamp glows.

The battery terminals are identified as points *A* and *B*. If point *B* in Figure 3-14(a) is used as a point of (voltage) reference, then point *A* is positive with respect to point *B*; and point *A* is negative with respect to point *B* in Figure 3-14(b). In each case, polarity of point *A* is indicated with respect to point *B*. The arrowhead drawn at point *B* symbolizes the point of reference. It is frequently called *ground*. For a clearer visualization of the concept of polarity, see Figure 3-14(c) and (d).

Figure 3-14(c) shows a graph of the dc voltage with the reference (point *B*) at the negative side of the battery [see Figure 3-14(a)]. The graph shows the value as well as the polarity of voltage at point *A* plotted as a function of time. Positive values are, by convention, shown upward from the baseline, whereas negative values are shown downward. Figure 3-14(d) shows the same voltage level (6 V) for point *A* in Figure 3-14(b) but with an opposite polarity because point *A* is negative with respect to point *B*.

Direct current can be produced in three different forms: *pure, pulsating,* and *transient*.

3.6.2 Alternating Current

Almost all electric energy distribution systems carry *alternating current* (ac) from alternating voltage generators. For instance, the voltage available at household and hospital electric wall outlets is 120 V ac. Special outlets provide 240 V ac for portable X-ray units.

Unlike direct current, ac alternates in direction. That is, it constantly changes or reverses its direction, as illustrated in Figure 3-15. The term *ac* is used to denote either a voltage or a current that alternates.

Figure 3-15 shows an ac voltage source (with terminals labeled *A* and *B*) connected to a lamp. The voltage at the generator's terminals continuously changes, alternating periodically from one polarity to the other. Changes in polarity are noted as events 1, 2, 3, and 4. At event 1 [Figure 3-15(a)] terminal *A* is positive with respect to terminal *B* (the point of

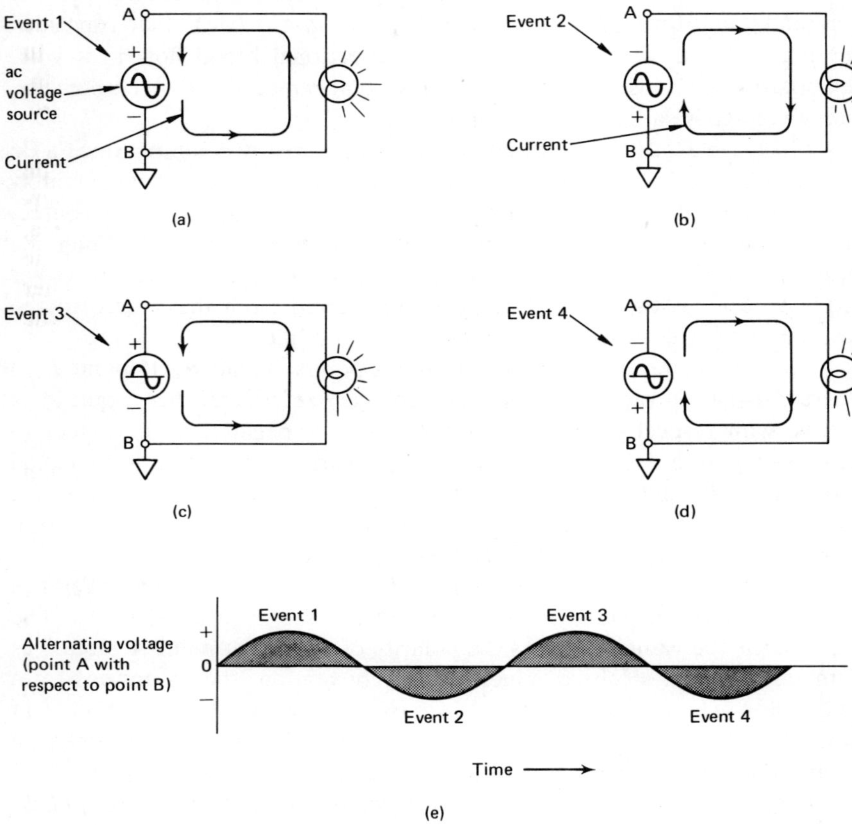

Fig. 3–15 Alternating voltage: (a) counterclockwise current; (b) clockwise current; (c) repeat of a; (d) repeat of b; (e) resulting waveform.

reference). Therefore current travels counterclockwise through the lamp. For event 2 [Figure 3-15(b)], the generator terminals take on opposite polarities; current now travels clockwise. At event 3 [Figure 3-15(c)] the generator terminal polarities are again as they were during event 1; thus current again travels counterclockwise. Event 4 [Figure 3-15(d)] is the same as event 2, and current travels clockwise. So as the polarity of the ac sources alternates, current reverses direction. The waveform of the ac voltage used in household and hospital power systems is shown in Figure 3-15(e). This waveform is called a *sine wave.* It is biphasic with periodic excursions above and below baseline. The first upward (positive) excursion indicates that, for event 1, terminal *A* of the voltage source is positive with respect to terminal *B*. The event 2 excursion shows that at event 2 terminal *A* is negative.

Note that in the sine wave shown in Figure 3-15(e) the voltage changes continually in a recurring pattern. The value of the voltage (its height above and below baseline) is called its *amplitude*. One complete sequence of amplitude variations [consisting of events 1 and 2 in Figure 3-15(e), for example] is called a *cycle*. The number of cycles that occur each second is called the *frequency* of the ac voltage. Frequency is expressed in *cycles per second* (*cps*) or *hertz* (Hz). The voltage available at wall outlets in the United States occurs at 60 Hz. Thus 60 complete cycles occur each second. The time required for each cycle is 1/60 of a second. This time is called the *period* of the waveform. The period is just the inverse or reciprocal of the frequency. Hence the higher the frequency, the shorter the period.

Although the standard power line frequency is 60 Hz, sine waves can be produced or generated at any frequency. For example, Figure 3-16 shows a sine wave with a frequency of 1 Hz. Its period is therefore 1 second.

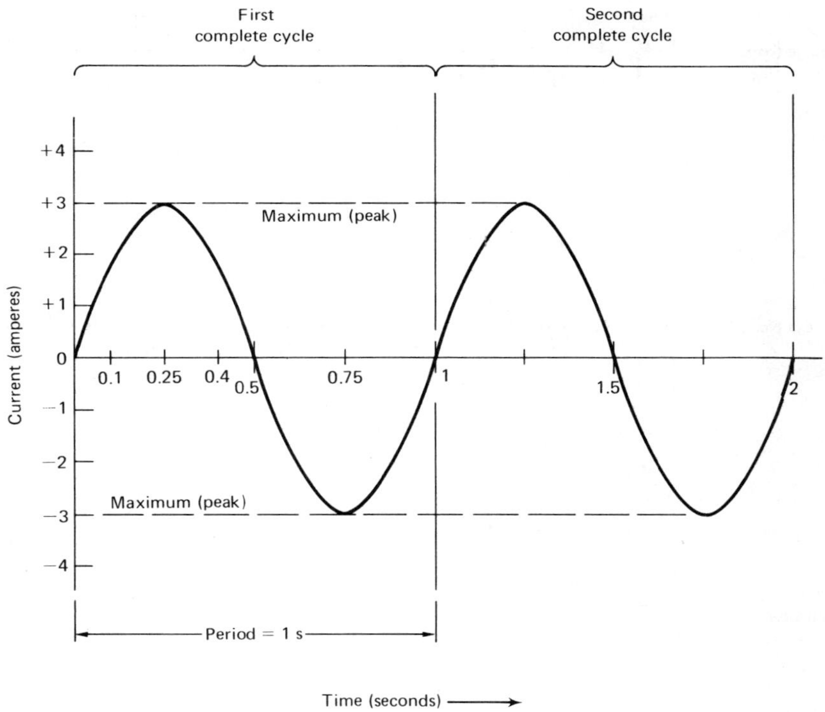

Fig. 3–16 Typical 1-Hz sinewave.

If the time at which the voltage begins to rise in its positive polarity from zero is designated as a reference, it should be noted that the voltage reaches its positive *peak* (its maximum positive value) ¼ second later. This shows that any sine wave reaches its positive peak ¼ cycle after the reference time. At ½ cycle (½ second after the reference time) the waveform returns to zero and begins to increase in the negative direction. At ¾ cycle the negative peak is reached and the voltage returns to zero at the completion of the cycle in order to begin the next one.

The sine wave is a basic type of waveform. However, many other waveforms are encountered in medical instrumentation, some of which appear in Figure 3-17. Figure 3-17(a) shows a square wave in which the voltage changes suddenly from one polarity to the other. The waveform in Figure 3-17(b) forms a triangular pattern and is called a triangular waveform. Figure 3-17(c) shows the waveform of the electrocardiogram, which is described in Chapter 5.

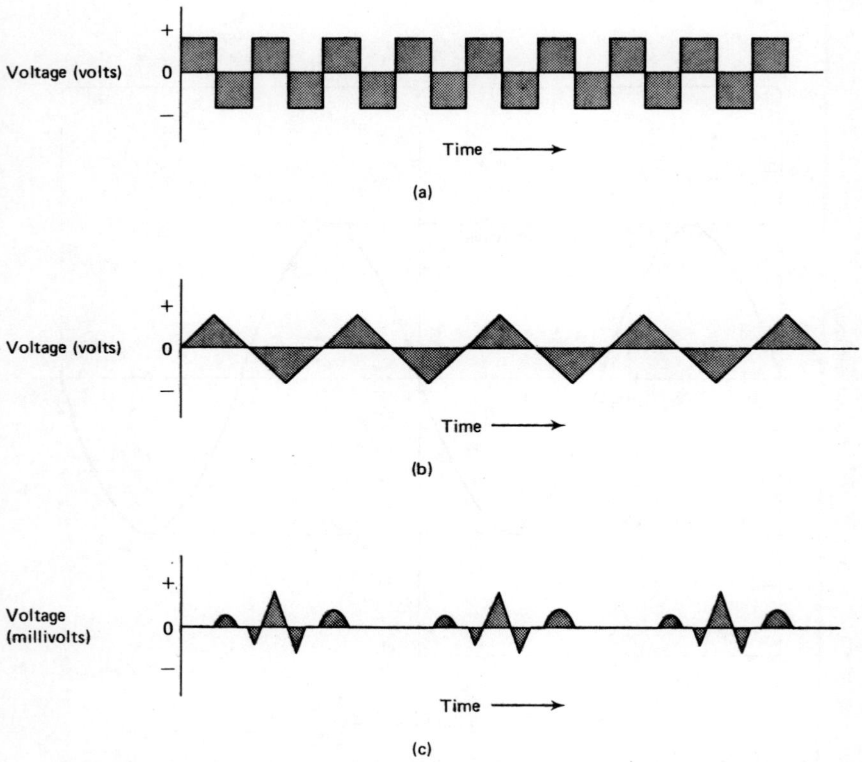

Fig. 3–17 Non-sine waves: (a) square wave; (b) triangular; (c) ECG wave.

Voltages and currents whose amplitudes vary but do not change polarity are designated by the term *fluctuating* or *pulsating dc.* Fluctuating dc has characteristics of both ac and dc and can actually be considered a combination of both. Two examples of fluctuating dc are shown in Figure 3-18. The voltage waveform representing arterial blood pressure is shown in Figure 3-18(a). This is a typical output of a direct blood pressure measurement as described in Chapter 9. Since the pressure is always positive, the voltage waveform does not change its direction. Figure 3-18(b) shows a waveform that consists of a series of dc *pulses* that are similar to those produced by an artificial pacemaker.

3.7 Electric Components

This section describes electric components or parts that are common to virtually all electrical instruments. They are the *resistor, capacitor, inductor,* and *transformer.*

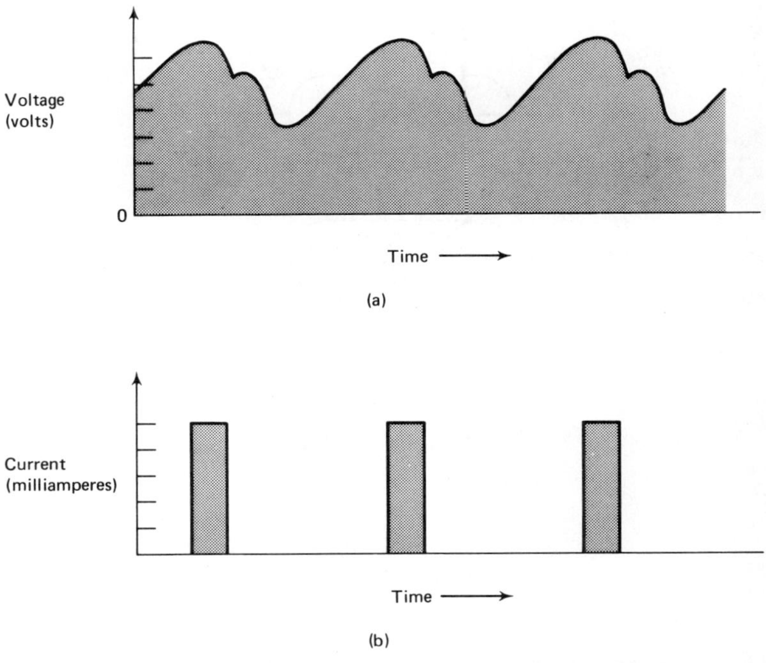

Fig. 3–18 Examples of fluctuating or pulsating dc: (a) voltage representing arterial blood pressure; (b) series of dc pulses.

3.7.1 The Resistor

The resistor is used to provide a certain amount of resistance in an electric circuit. A typical *fixed resistor* is shown in Figure 3-19(a) and its diagrammatic (schematic) symbol in Figure 3-19(c).

Contained inside a tubular insulating body is a composition of conductive material (usually carbon) and a nonconducting binder. The proportions of conductor and nonconductor allow resistors to be manufactured with widely ranging resistances. Very low resistance wire is used as connecting leads.

The symbol is used to represent an actual resistor or the resistance inherent in any physical quantity. For example, the resistance of a human body may be represented by the resistor symbol.

The numerous resistor types fall into two general categories—*fixed* and *variable.* The type in Figure 3-19(a) through (c) is fixed, since its manufactured value cannot be adjusted. Resistors whose values are easily varied are called *potentiometers.* The schematic symbol of a variable resistor is shown in Figure 3-19(d). Actually, a potentiometer is a special type of variable resistor. It is frequently used as a control element. The volume

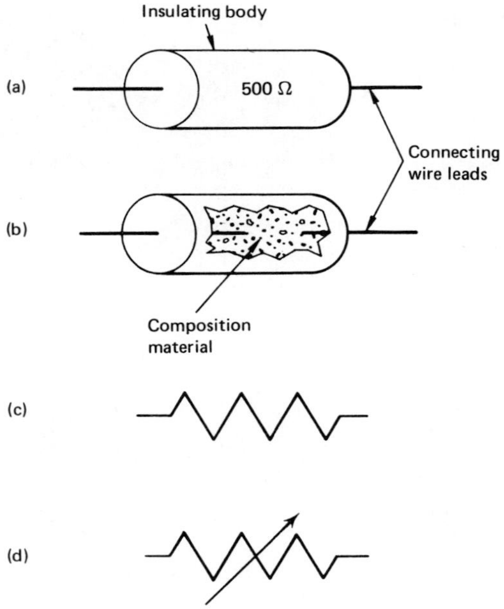

Fig. 3–19 Composition resistor: (a) external construction; (b) internal construction; (c) schematic symbol; (d) variable resistor symbol.

control of a radio, for example, is usually a potentiometer, as is the gain or sensitivity control of a patient monitor.

The physical size of a resistor is determined not by the amount of resistance but rather by the amount of heat it can dissipate into the air without burning out. This heat is the result of the power dissipated in the resistor. The concept of power is discussed in Section 3.10.

3.7.2 The Capacitor

A capacitor consists of two parallel metal plates separated by an insulating medium (called a *dielectric*), as shown in Figure 3-20(a). It has the ability to store electric charges; and since electric charges are forms of energy, the capacitor is able to store *energy*.

An electron forced into plate 1 will travel no farther than shown in Figure 3-20(b) because the dielectric material is a nonconductor. However, in approaching its final destination, its electric field propagates through the dielectric separator and repels an electron away from plate 2. In its wake there exists a positive ion—a positive charge. Because unlike charges attract, the deposited electron and its associated positive charge mutually attract and hold each other in place.

In practice, many electrons are deposited or stored on one capacitor plate. Only a few are shown in Figure 3-20(c). They are held in place by positive charges on the other plate. Their electric fields exist in the dielectric medium. Energy is stored in the capacitor's dielectric in the form of a stable electric field. Note that the electric field sketched between opposite charges is similar to the field between charges shown earlier in Figure 3-3(b). The capacitor is charged (plate 1 negative with respect to plate 2); a difference of potential exists. Therefore a voltage exists across the terminals of a charged capacitor.

Electrons, or electricity, stored in a capacitor are analogous to air stored under pressure in a balloon or water stored in a tank. Both stored quantities can be discharged. Similarly, a charged capacitor is discharged when electrons are provided a path to travel, from the plate where they are in excess to the other plate where they are deficient.

The charge-discharge ability of a capacitor is widely used in electricity and in medical equipment. This principle is demonstrated in the dc defibrillator shown in Figure 3-21.

Electric energy is stored in the capacitor in Figure 3-21(a) because electrons are in excess on one plate and deficient on the other. The switch is open. Properly applied to a patient's torso are paddles or *electrodes* (metal contact plates with insulated handles), which, together with the patient's torso and wires, provide a complete conducting pathway. When the switch closes, current rushes through the patient. Electric energy is

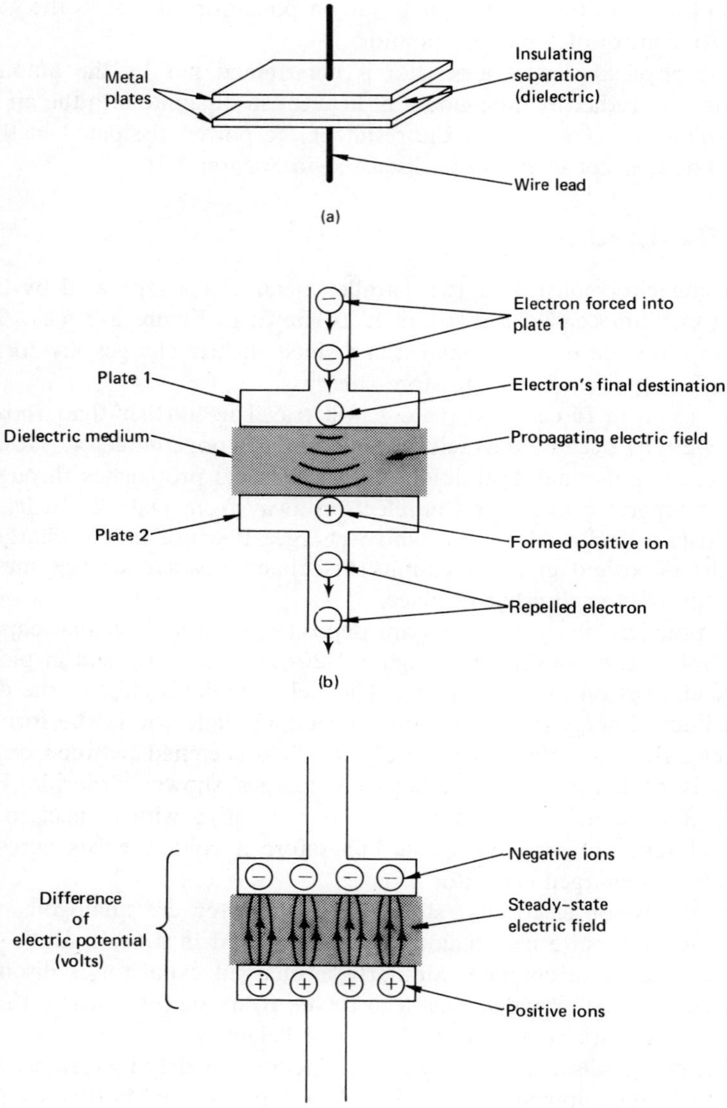

Fig. 3–20 The capacitor: (a) representative construction; (b) capacitor charging, electric field action; (c) charged capacitor.

quickly transferred from the defibrillator to the patient to affect a therapeutic procedure.

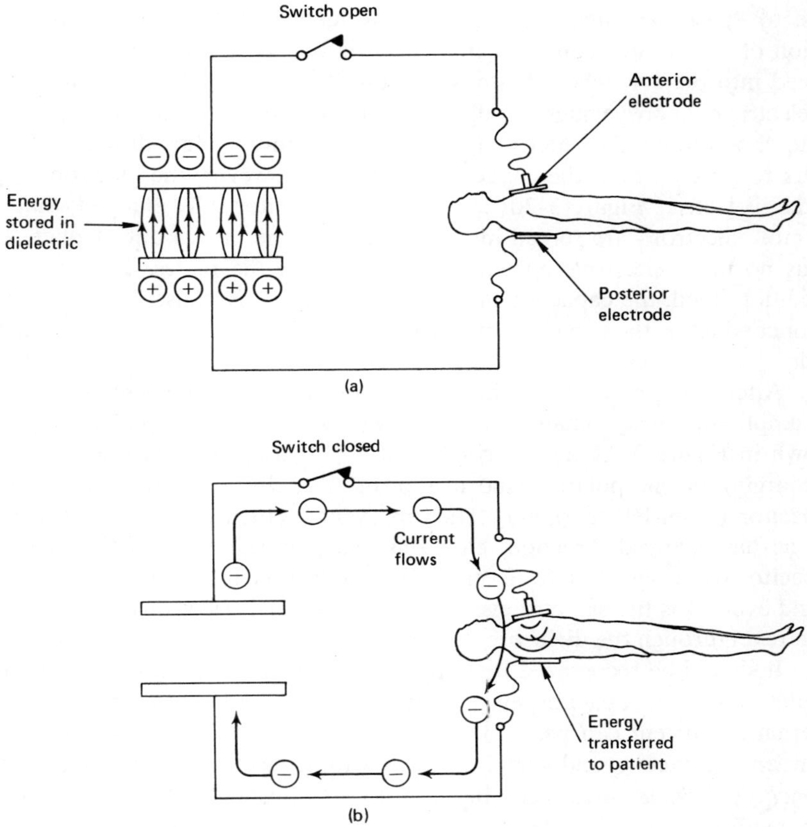

Fig. 3–21 Capacitor charge-discharge example: (a) charged defibrillator capacitor; (b) discharges through patient.

The ability of a capacitor to store electric charges is called *capacitance,* noted as *C*. The unit of capacitance is the *farad* (F), used to honor Michael Faraday, a nineteenth-century British scientist. A farad is a large amount of capacitance. Consequently, practical capacitor values rarely approach one farad. Instead capacitors with values on the order of 1/1,000,000 farads (*microfarads*) and 1/1,000,000,000,000 farads (*picofarads*) are used. For example, a 0.01 microfarad (0.01 μF) capacitor has a value of one-hundredth of one-millionth of a farad, or 0.00000001 farad.

As noted, the basic function of a capacitor is to store electricity. It does so by accepting electrons on one plate while simultaneously ejecting electrons from the other plate. Because of this characteristic, a capacitor stops or "blocks" any direct current (from passing through it) although it is able to "pass" an alternating current. Referring to Figure 3-20(b), the action of a capacitor can be seen while it is being charged. An electron is forced into plate 1, where it stops because it can go no farther. However, its electric field propagates through the dielectric and repels an electron from plate 2. Although the entering electron travels only a short distance, it appears to pass through the capacitor. Actually, however, the electron stops at the dielectric. Figure 3-20(c) shows the capacitor fully charged; that is, no more electrons are forced into plate 1 (so none moves out of plate 2). Thus no more electrons appear to pass between the plates. In a charged condition, then, the capacitor blocks direct current. Because its dielectric is a nonconductor, the capacitor appears as an open circuit or incomplete path to dc.

Alternating current, on the other hand, has two important properties. Its amplitude always changes and it reverses its direction periodically, as shown in Figure 3-22(a). During event 1 [Figure 3-22(b)] the capacitor is charging in one polarity, and it appears that electrons flow through the capacitor (from left to right). Then in event 2 [Figure 3-22(c)], because the ac has changed direction, electrons again appear to pass through the capacitor from right to left. Event 3 [Figure 3-22(d)] is the same as event 1 and event 4 is the same as event 2. Thus although electrons do not actually travel through the dielectric, the capacitor passes the alternating current.

It should be recognized that any two conductive surfaces separated by insulation form a capacitor, even if they are not intended to do so. Because alternating current can pass through a capacitor, current is able to "leak" between conductors and metal surfaces within electrical equipment. This *capacitive leakage current* can be hazardous to hospital patients under certain conditions (see Chapter 18). Because air can serve as the dielectric in an unintentional capacitor, coupling of ac between electrically operated devices and wiring is also responsible for 60-Hz interference in medical instrumentation.

3.7.3 The Inductor

A capacitor stores energy in the form of an electric field. The *inductor* also stores energy but in the form of a *magnetic* field, not unlike the magnetic field around an ordinary bar magnet.

When moving through a conductor (wire), electrons develop a magnetic field around the wire as shown in Figure 3-23(a). Since a magnetic field stores energy, a current-carrying wire has energy stored around it. The field shown around a straight wire is relatively weak.

However, when the wire is wound into a *coil* [Figure 3-23(b)], the weak force lines are able to link together, concentrating in the coil's center

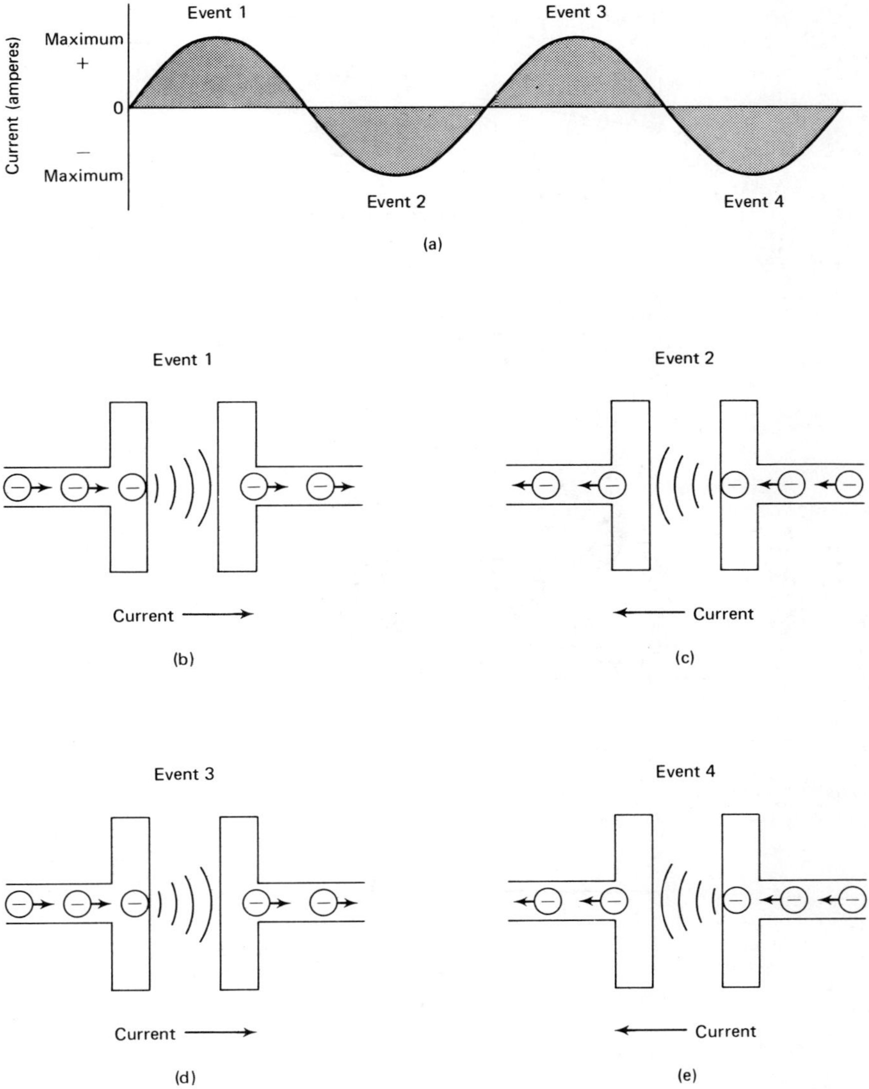

Fig. 3–22 Capacitor passing ac: (a) applied ac; (b) current *appears* to flow; (c) current again appears to flow; (d) same as event 1; (e) same as event 2.

as shown in Figure 3-23(c). Thus the stored energy field is concentrated in the center of the coil.

If the current through the coil were suddenly stopped, the magnetic

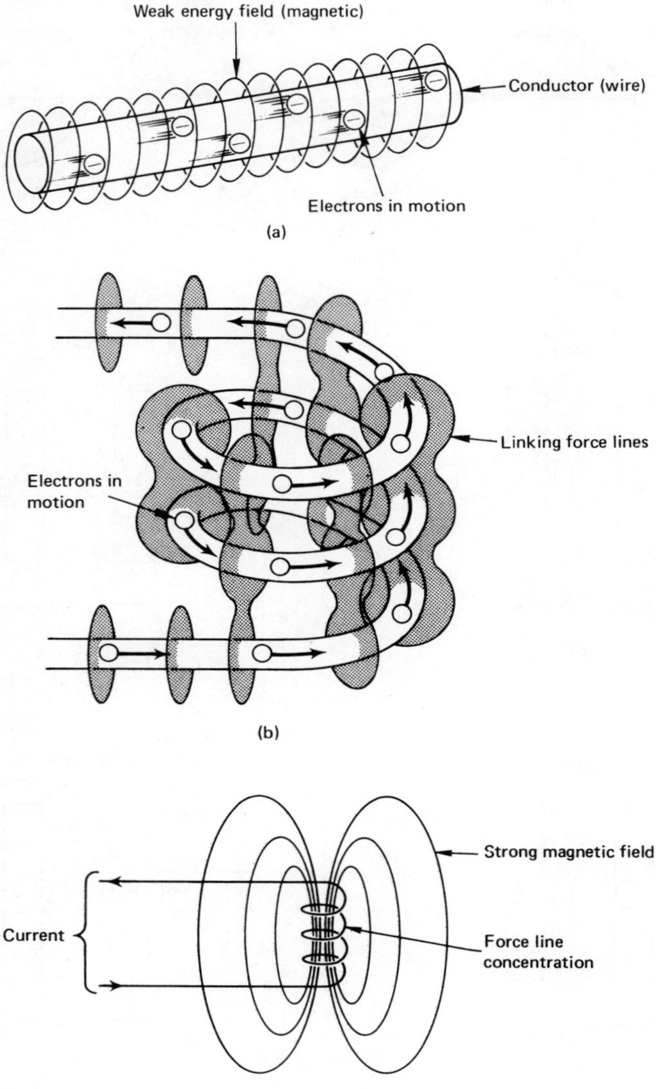

Fig. 3–23 Magnetic energy field: (a) around a straight wire; (b) force lines link up when wire is coiled; (c) magnetic field around a coil.

field would quickly disappear, collapsing within the coil where it originated. When current again flows into the coil, the magnetic field develops once again and expands to envelop the coil. In this way, a current changing from zero to some fixed value creates a changing magnetic field. The energy stored in the magnetic field produces within the coil an opposition to any *change* in current flow. This characteristic of a coil is called its *inductance,* and is used in many ways in electrical and electronic equipment. A coil especially built to provide a given amount of inductance is called an *inductor.* The unit of inductance is the henry (H), used to honor the nineteenth-century American scientist Joseph Henry. Its letter designation, *L,* connotes the linking of magnetic force lines.

3.7.4 The Transformer

The changing magnetic field caused by changes in the current through a coil of wire can induce a voltage in another coil, if the two are close together. The two coils constitute a *transformer.* The principle of the transformer is shown in Figure 3-24.

In Figure 3-24(a) two coils are shown in proximity. Note that they do not touch each other. In Figure 3-24(b) coil *A* is connected to a source of alternating current; coil *B* is connected to a lamp. As changing current travels through coil *A,* a changing magnetic field propagates to and links up with the turns of coil *B,* thereby inducing a changing current in coil *B*. Thus energy is transferred from the ac source and coil *A* to coil *B* and the lamp

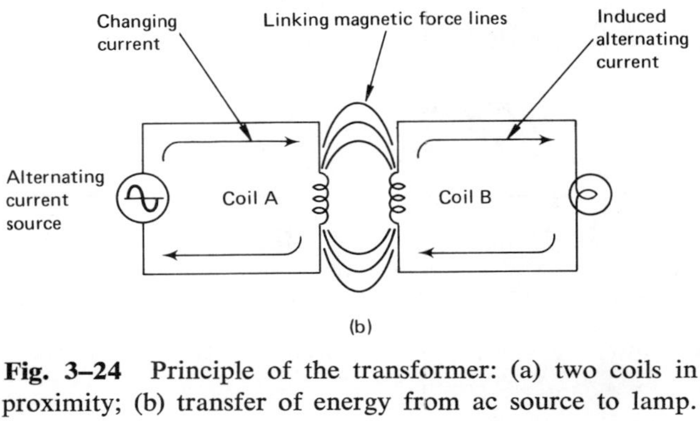

Fig. 3–24 Principle of the transformer: (a) two coils in proximity; (b) transfer of energy from ac source to lamp.

via the changing magnetic field. The lamp glows. This important principle of energy transfer forms the basis of the transformer.

The efficient use of electric energy often requires the conversion of supplied forms of energy to a form needed to accomplish a task. For example, it may be necessary to transform the energy available at wall outlets (120 V ac) to energy at a higher voltage (say 300 V ac) for use in electronic equipment. Or the 120 V may need to be transformed to a lower voltage (such as 50 V). A *transformer,* utilizing the principle of induction already described, is used to accomplish these tasks.

Figure 3-25(a) shows two separated inductors wound around a steel core. Inductor *A* constitutes the *primary* winding and inductor *B* the *secondary*. The coil wires are insulated so that they cannot contact the steel core or each other. Since this type of transformer is used in the 60-Hz power distribution system, a steel core is used to enhance the effect of induction. Its schematic symbol appears in Figure 3-25(b). A practical application of the transformer is shown in Figure 3-26.

In Figure 3-26(a) a 120-V ac source is connected to the primary of the transformer. The secondary is connected to a device needing 300 V ac. The changing primary current produces a changing magnetic field, which is efficiently linked by the steel core to the secondary coil. Here the changing magnetic field induces a changing current in the secondary coil at a potential difference of 300 V. The secondary voltage is "stepped up" from the available 120-V ac source because there are more wire turns in the secondary coil than in the primary. This is called a *step-up* transformer, represented as a functional block in Figure 3-26(b).

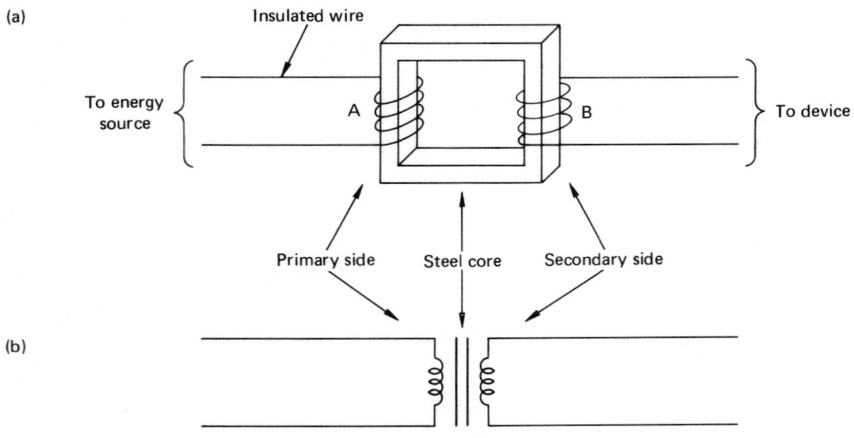

Fig. 3–25 Power transformer: (a) pictorial; (b) schematic symbol.

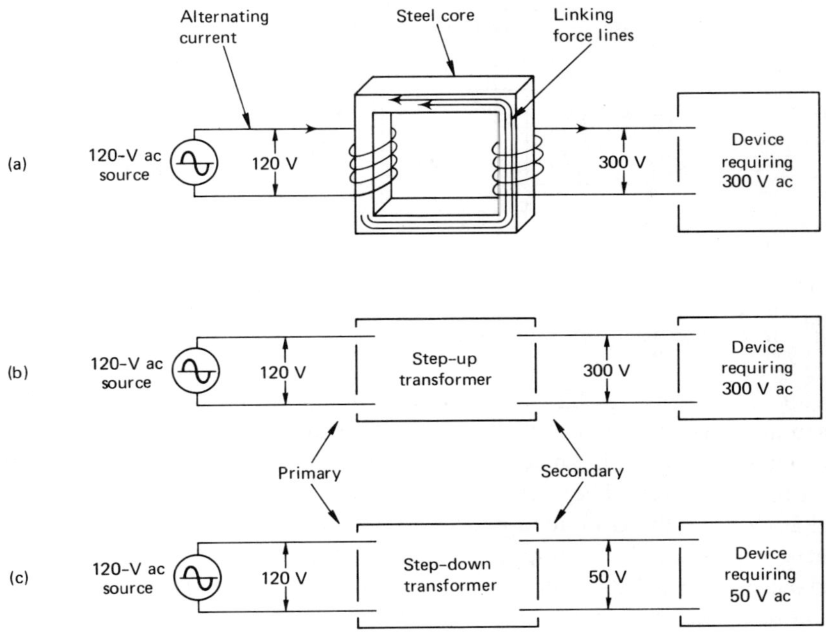

Fig. 3–26 Power transformer operation: (a) voltage step-up; (b) voltage step-up simplified; (c) voltage step-down.

A transformer whose secondary coil contains fewer turns than its primary coil is called a *step-down* transformer, and it provides a secondary voltage that is less than that applied to the primary, as in Figure 3-26(c).

When, however, the number of turns in both primary and secondary are the same, the transformer is neither step-up nor step-down. The secondary voltage is the same as the applied voltage. It can be used, however, as an *isolation* transformer whose purpose is to isolate *electrically* anything connected to the secondary from the primary (and from the energy source). An isolation transformer is shown in Figure 3-27.

Note that there are no direct wire connections between primary and secondary coils. Nevertheless, because of transformer action, electric energy still appears as needed at the secondary. Thus energy is transferred to the secondary; yet the secondary is isolated (no direct contact) from the primary source.

Isolation transformers are used at times to provide 120 V ac for equipment in critical care areas and are used to provide electrical energy in operating rooms.

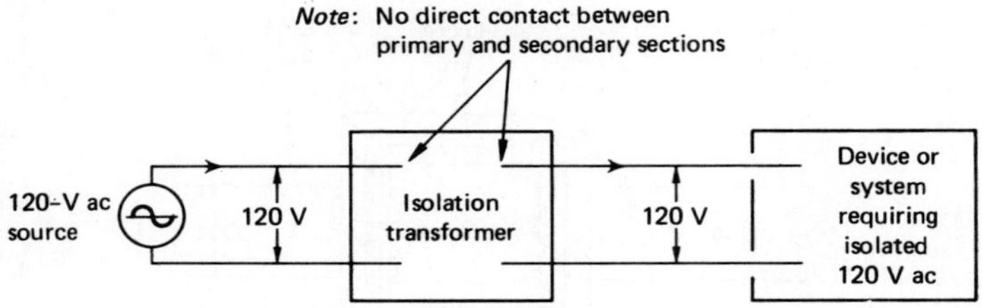

Fig. 3–27 Isolation transformer operation.

3.8 Impedance

As noted in Sections 3.7.2 and 3.7.3, capacitors and inductors act differently when an ac voltage is applied than when connected to a source of constant dc. Thus the current in an ac circuit with a given voltage is affected by more than the resistance. The opposition to ac current flow is called *impedance,* which includes the combined effects of capacitance, inductance, and resistance. The symbol for impedance is the letter Z. Like resistance, impedance is measured in ohms. Impedance in an ac circuit can be thought of in the same way as resistance in a dc circuit. By substituting impedance for resistance, the relationship expressed by Ohm's law still applies. For example, in an ac circuit

$$I = \frac{E}{Z}, \quad E = IZ, \quad \text{and} \quad Z = \frac{E}{I}.$$

With a given voltage, increasing the impedance decreases the current, whereas decreasing the impedance increases the current.

3.9 Series and Parallel Circuits

An arrangement of batteries and resistors with their connecting wires forms a complete (closed) conducting path through which current is able to circulate continually. This arrangement [shown in Figure 3-28(b)] is called a *circuit.*

A physiological analogy of an electric circuit appears in Figure 3-28. The cardiovascular circuit in Figure 3-28(a) is the hydraulic analogy of the electric circuit in Figure 3-28(b). In the vascular circuit, the heart(pump) produces a difference in blood pressure between its terminals. At the aorta there exists about 100 mm Hg of pressure (the average of systolic and diastolic pressures). At the right atrium, the pressure is almost zero. The

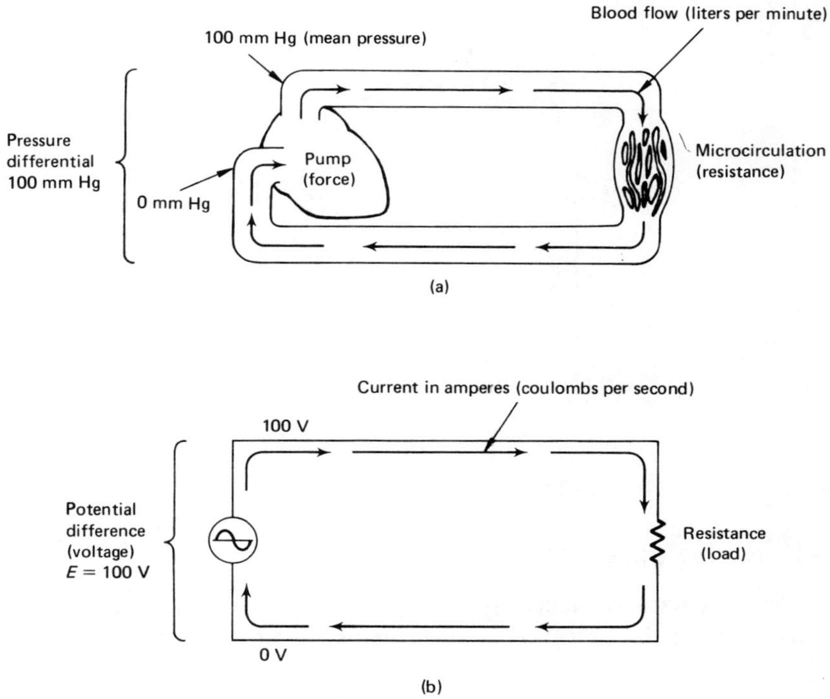

Fig. 3–28 Series circuit analogies: (a) the cardiovascular circuit; (b) the electric circuit.

difference in pressure (about 100 mm Hg) is the systemic pressure gradient forcing blood through the microcirculation, which provides resistance to blood flow. Similarly, in Figure 3-28(b) the difference in electric potential (100 V) forces current to flow from the source through a resistor and then back to the source. In Figure 3-28(a) the microcirculation is the resistance "load" for the heart. Similarly, the resistor is the load for the source voltage in the electric circuit.

3.9.1 Series Circuits

There are two basic types of electric circuits: *series* and *parallel.* Figure 3-29 shows a series dc circuit. In a *series* circuit, current travels from the battery, through wires, and then through each resistor in turn in order to return to the battery. Since current elements are connected in series, the same current travels through the battery and each resistor. In a series circuit, the total resistance is the sum of the values of the resistors in the circuit.

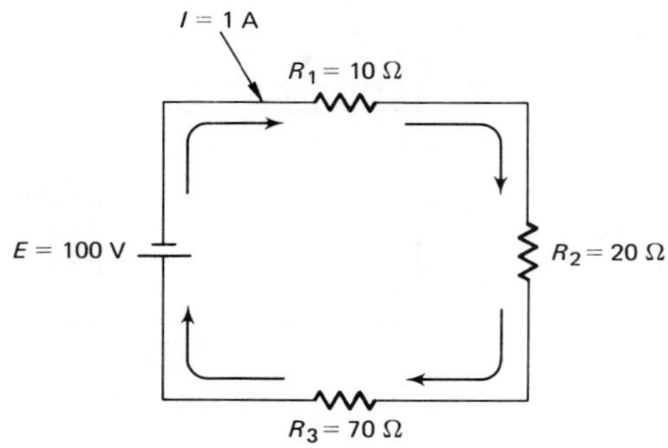

$$R\text{ (total)} = 10\ \Omega + 20\ \Omega + 70\ \Omega = 100\ \Omega$$

$$I = \frac{E}{R} = \frac{100\text{ V}}{100\ \Omega} = 1\text{ A}$$

Fig. 3–29 Series dc circuit.

3.9.2 *Parallel Circuits*

When circuit elements are arranged so that each receives the same source voltage, they form a *parallel* circuit. Figure 3-30(a) shows three

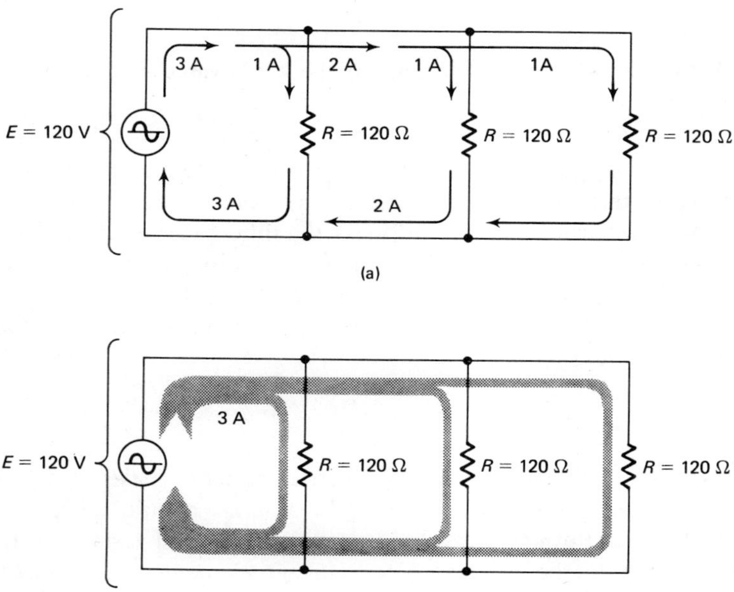

Fig. 3–30 Parallel circuit: (a) three parallel-connected resistors; (b) current from source divides.

120-Ω resistors connected in parallel so that the same source voltage (120 V) is applied to each. By Ohm's law, the current through each resistor is 120 V/120 Ω = 1 A. Since each load requires (draws) one ampere, the source must supply 3 A, as shown in Figure 3-30(b).

Elements connected in parallel provide multiple paths through which current will travel; the largest amount of current will always take the path of least resistance (see Figure 3-31).

Figure 3-31(a) shows two parallel resistors connected to a 100-V source. By Ohm's law, the current through the 500-Ω resistor is 200 mA, ten times the current (20 mA) through the 5000-Ω resistor. Figure 3-31(b) shows a water analogy. More water will flow through the large-diameter pipe because it offers less resistance than the smaller pipe. Water from the pump takes the path of least resistance. Similarly, current from a source takes the path of least resistance.

An interesting parallel circuit application appears in Figure 3-32. In Figure 3-32(a) resistors R1 and R2 are connected in series while R3 is in series with variable resistor R4. The four resistors form two branches of a parallel circuit. A voltage indicating meter (*voltmeter*) "bridges" points *A* and *B*. This type of circuit is called a *bridge circuit* and points *A* and *B* are the bridge output terminals. The circuit is energized (excited) with 10 V dc.

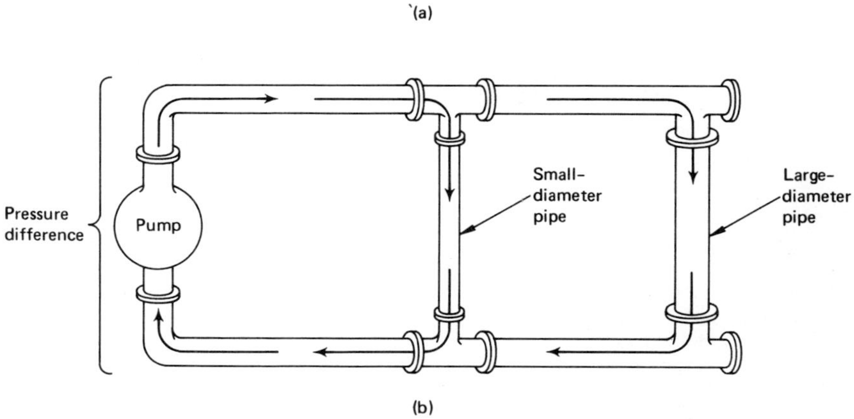

Fig. 3–31 Parallel circuit: (a) current takes the path of least resistance; (b) water analogy.

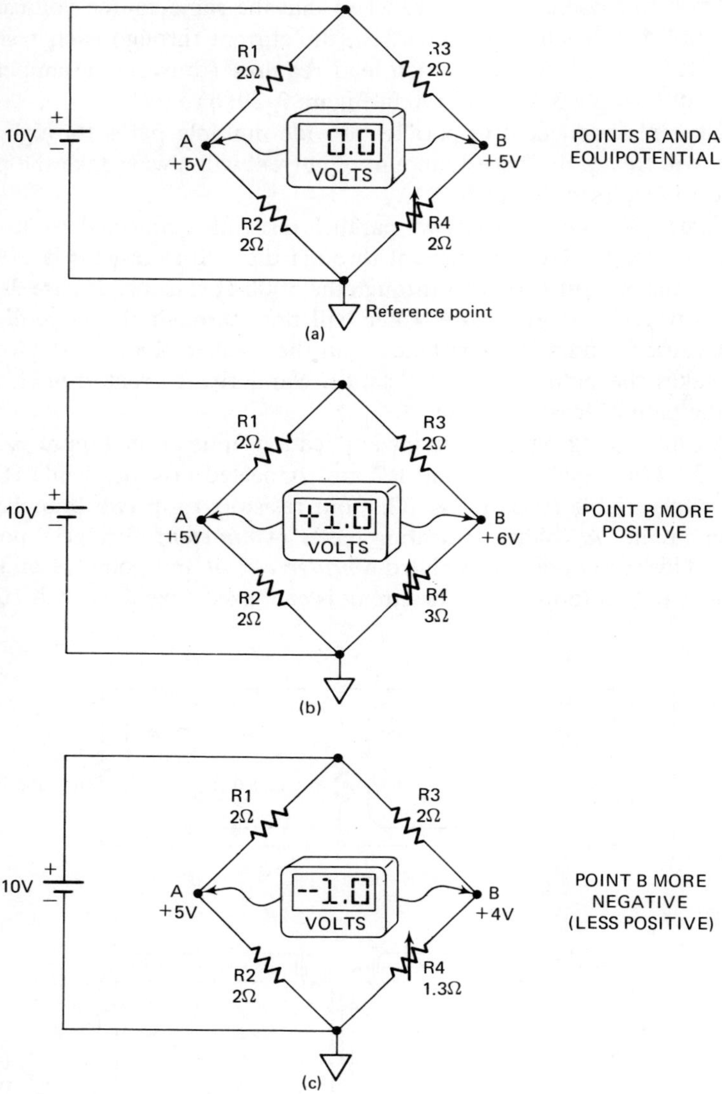

Fig. 3–32 Electric bridge circuit: (a) balanced bridge condition; (b) unbalanced condition, positive readout; (c) unbalanced condition, negative readout.

When the branch resistors are equal in value (2Ω), points *A* and *B* are at equal electric potentials (5V) with respect to the reference point in accordance with Ohm's law. Therefore the difference between the potentials at the voltmeter terminals is zero (5V — 5V = OV), and the voltmeter shows zero volts. This is a *balanced bridge* condition.

However, if the value of R4 increases [Figure 3-32(b)], point B becomes more positive (6 V) than it was whereas the voltage at point A remains the same. The resulting difference of potential at the bridge terminals causes the voltmeter to show +1V (6V −5V = +1V), indicating that point B is more positive than point A. Thus the bridge is *unbalanced.* Conversely, when the value of R4 decreases [Figure 3-32(c)], point B will become less positive (4V) than point A. The difference of potential at the bridge terminals will cause the voltmeter to show −1V indicating that point B is less positive (or more negative) than point A. The bridge is again unbalanced. In this way, a bridge circuit is able to provide voltage variations at its output terminals proportional to changes in the resistance of one (or more) of its branch resistors. This principle is widely used in blood pressure transducers.

Electrical equipment plugged into the power distribution system is connected in parallel as shown in Figure 3-33. In Figure 3-33(a) a vacuum cleaner and toaster are shown plugged into the power line and

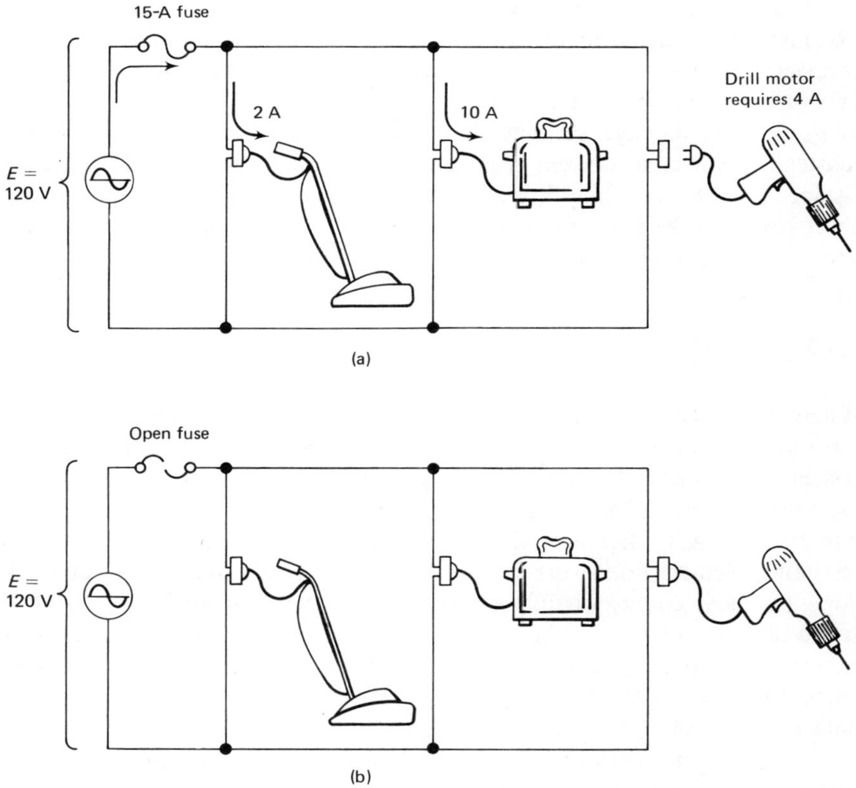

Fig. 3–33 Parallel-connected appliances and overcurrent; (a) fuse is intact; (b) fuse is open.

turned on. A drill motor is about to be connected. Together the vacuum cleaner and toaster draw 12 A from the source. The circuit has a 15-A *fuse,* an overcurrent device which melts and opens the circuit if the current exceeds its rated value. When the drill motor (requiring 4 A) is connected and operated, as shown in Figure 3-33(b), the total current drawn by all appliances will reach 16 A. The fuse element, designed to melt when current exceeds 15 A, opens one of the power lines and disconnects the voltage from all the appliances. Then current from the source becomes zero. Without overcurrent protection, excess heat in the wires may melt their insulation, thus creating a fire hazard. Overcurrent protection is provided by circuit breakers as well as with fuses. Whereas a fuse is consumed when it acts, a *circuit breaker* will "trip," thereby opening the circuit and disrupting current. Then when the overload is removed (or the problem corrected), the circuit breaker can be reset. Both devices act to produce an *open circuit* to remove power from the circuit.

A *short circuit* occurs whenever the normal resistance value of equipment, devices or of wire insulation, for example, becomes nearly zero. Then, according to Ohm's law, current becomes extremely high in value. For instance, imagine in Figure 3-33(a) that only the vacuum cleaner is connected to the power line and operating. Next, suppose that the toaster (about to be connected) has a short in its line cord (the insulation has worn away through damage so that the conductors are touching). When the toaster is connected, current from the source, taking the path of least resistance (nearly zero ohms), greatly exceeds 15 A and the fuse opens. The short circuit in the toaster's power cord results in an open circuit, thus preventing overheating and damage.

3.10 Electric Power and Energy

When current flows through a resistance material, work is done as heat (a form of energy) is generated in the material. For example, a resistor becomes heated when electrons are forced to flow through material that resists their flow. A sort of "electric friction" causes the resistor to dissipate heat into the air. A toaster uses this principle as the heat dissipated from its resistance element does work in toasting bread. When the amount of work done (or heat energy dissipated) is measured each second, the result is called electric *power, P.* The unit of power is the *watt* (W). One watt of power is dissipated when a potential difference of one volt causes one ampere to flow. A toaster may dissipate 1000 W, whereas a common light bulb may dissipate 100 W.

Power is the rate at which electric energy is expended, just as current is the rate at which charges flow. Energy, as stated, is the amount of work done. The unit of electric energy is the *watt-second* (W-s) or the *joule* (J).

For example, the energy stored in a capacitor may be expressed in watt-seconds or joules.

To illustrate the difference between electric power and energy, consider a mechanical allegory. Imagine that two identical but separate brick walls are to be constructed by two masons. They begin together, but one worker completes construction in a day, the other in 5 days. Both workers expended the same amount of energy, for the same amount of work was done by both in building identical walls. However, the mason finishing first exerted more "power" than the other because he finished in one-fifth the time. In this example, the rate at which energy is used is of interest. Energy is a quantity, whereas power is the rate at which the quantity is used.

3.11 The Power Distribution System

Electric energy used in homes and hospitals is generated and distributed as shown in Figure 3-34. In Figure 3-34(a) the energy source (actually a transformer secondary) has two terminals across which is produced 120 V ac. One terminal, A, is connected to a conductor embedded below the earth's surface (ground). Therefore terminal *A* is *grounded* and is at the same electrical potential as earth (zero volts). Recall from Section 3.3.1 that the earth is a conductor and that it can be considered electrically neutral (zero potential). Thus terminal *A* is called the *neutral* terminal.

Because terminal *A* is grounded, terminal *B* is electrically live or "hot" (120 V) with respect to terminal *A*. Wires connected to these terminals are called the *hot* and *neutral* wires.

Inside a building the hot and neutral wires enter a metal service (distribution) box, where a protective circuit breaker is placed in the hot wire line. The neutral wire is again grounded, as is the service entrance box. Both are connected to a ground rod, a cold-water pipe, or some other suitably grounded element. Sometimes a third wire is also connected to the grounded neutral. It is called the *equipment ground wire.*

The two or three wires are placed in a rigid thin-walled pipe, called a *conduit,* to protect the conductors on their way to metal wall-mounted receptacle boxes that hold the *receptacle outlets* (wall outlets). The conduit system is similar to a plumbing system without, of course, water. It should be noted that more often than not the equipment grounding conductor is not actually installed. Instead the continuous metal conduit system is used in place of this separate wire. For identification purposes, the hot-wire insulation may be any color except white, gray, or green. Black insulation is commonly used. White or gray is reserved for the neutral wire insulation. If a separate grounding conductor is present, its insulation must be green or green with a yellow stripe.

The ordinary energy distribution system is a *grounded* system because

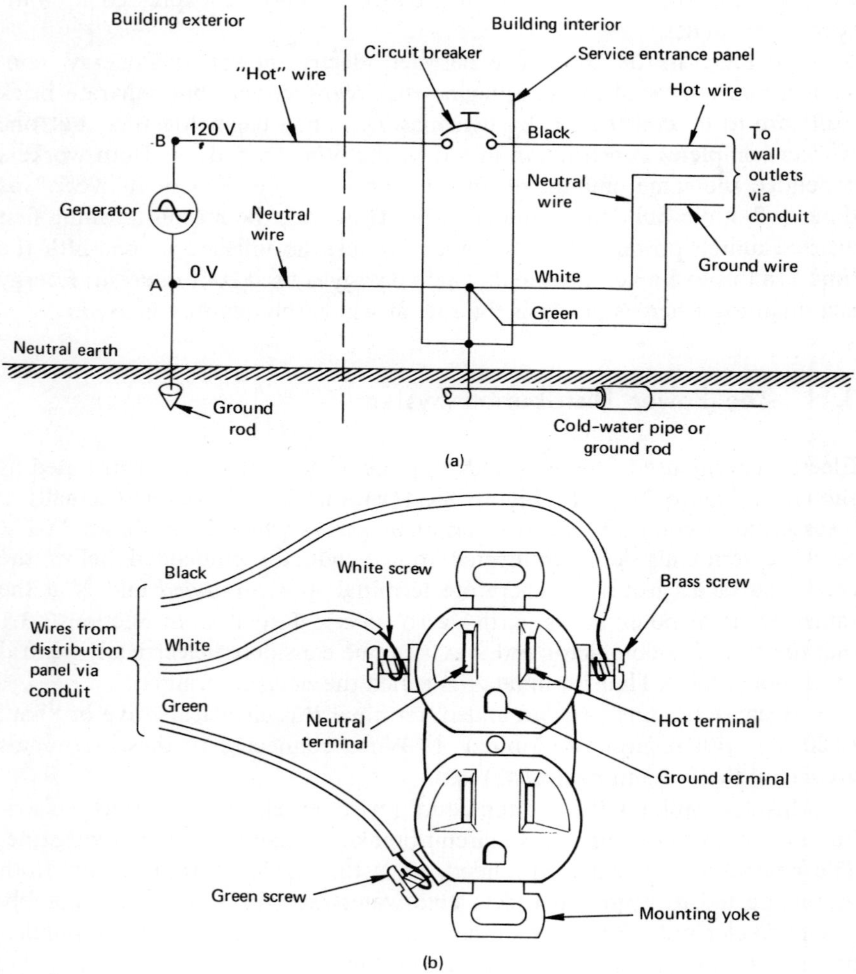

Fig. 3–34 Power distribution system: (a) layout from generator to building; (b) duplex receptacle outlet properly wired.

one side of the parallel electric circuit (called a *branch circuit*) it forms is at the earth's electric potential (zero volts); the other is live.

A receptacle outlet provides connection to the hot wire, the neutral wire, and, when it exists, the equipment ground wire, as shown in Figure 3-34(b). The receptacle outlet (sometimes called a *duplex*) has two parallel-connected sections. Wires are connected to three screw terminals. The white wire (neutral) must be connected to the white-colored (nickel-plated) terminal; the black wire (hot) must be connected to the brass terminal. The green wire must be connected to the green-colored terminal. If these color-wire combinations are not met, the receptacle is improperly wired and potentially hazardous when used. For example, inadvertent reversal of the black and neutral wires *reverse-polarizes* the outlet.

The two rectangular slots in the receptacle are of unequal length. The longer of the two is the neutral contact; the other is the hot contact. The round (U-shaped) hole is the equipment ground connection. When the receptacle is in place, a continuous path to ground exists from the equipment ground contact, through the conduit system, to the grounded neutral point at the distribution panel. In this way, even if a separate green-covered equipment ground wire is not present, the outlet nevertheless maintains a connection to ground. If the receptacle has a metal cover plate, the plate is also grounded.

As seen in Figure 3-34(a), the hot and neutral wires have 120 V ac between them. These wires carry current to operate the equipment. For example, if a monitor requires 3 A to operate, the 3 A are carried only by the hot and neutral wires. From the figure it can also be seen that 120 V ac exists between the hot wire and the equipment ground wire. The ground wire (or conduit, if a separate wire is not used) provides protection to anyone who might simultaneously touch the equipment and any grounded object. It is this wire that carries equipment fault current, leakage current, and other undesirable currents harmlessly to earth (see Section 3.12). It is important, especially in special care areas, that the resistance of this path to ground be as low as possible (less than one ohm). The installation of a proper separate ground wire undoubtedly provides a better path to ground than does the conduit, although conduit grounding may also be acceptable. The conduit is mechanically joined in sections. The joined parts tend to have more resistance than a continuous wire. A higher than normal grounding resistance (more than one ohm) means a poor quality ground and, in special care areas, may contribute to electrical hazards.

3.12 Equipment Leakage and Fault Current

Line-connected equipment uses operating current in order to perform assigned tasks. The user of equipment, particularly in special care areas, should be aware of two additional currents—*leakage* and *fault* currents.

As noted in Section 3.7.2, energized, insulated conductors have, inherently, stray capacitance. In addition, their insulation is imperfect. When they are required to conduct alternating current, some of the current leaks from the conductors. Because one side of the power distribution system is grounded, the leakage current naturally seeks ground, as shown in Figure 3-35.

Here the monitor is shown connected to an energized wall outlet via its

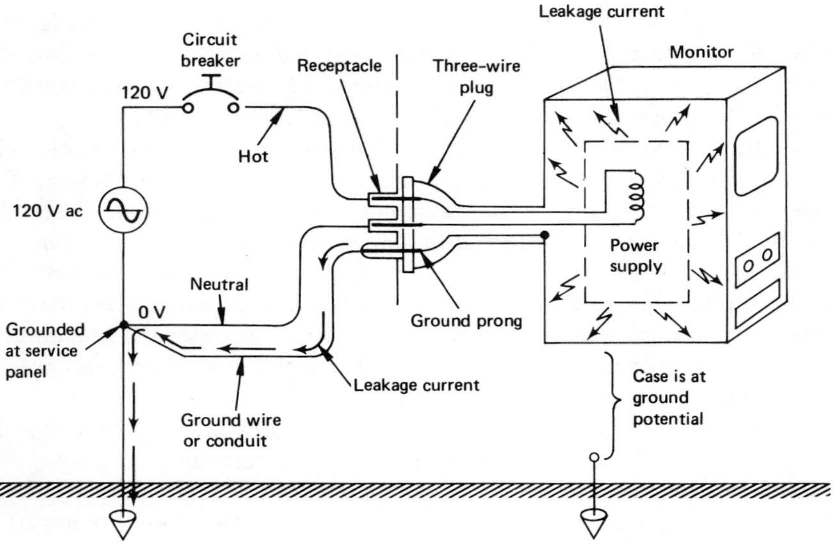

Fig. 3–35 Equipment grounding. Leakage current flows from case through line cord plug to ground rod; the case is grounded.

power cord and three-prong plug or *cap*. Whether turned on or not, inside the case of the monitor is 120 V ac. Its power supply contains a transformer (having many turns of insulated wire) needed for its operation. The monitor has a metal case that is properly grounded via the line cord. The combination of insulated conductors and alternating (changing) voltage gives rise to leakage current that passes to the case through stray capacitance. Because the three-wire plug has a ground prong in contact with the ground terminal of the receptacle, leakage current is able to flow harmlessly to ground. The equipment case is effectively at ground potential; it is not hot. If, on the other hand, the ground connection at the plug is broken through abuse, leakage current cannot escape to ground and the case will be hot (some value of voltage above ground). Also, if the resistance of the equipment's grounding conductor is high (more than 0.1 Ω), the case will be hot. Anyone now contacting the case and a grounded conductor will provide a path for the leakage current. Leakage current values may range from a few to several hundred microamperes. It is important to realize that the act of grounding an appliance does not preclude the existence of leakage current. It exists in all line-connected equipment whether they are turned on or not. (It follows that battery-powered equipment—an external pacer, for example—has no leakage current.) However, the proper grounding of an appliance provides a path whereby the leakage current and, if it occurs, fault current are able to exit to where they belong—to ground. Thus the appliance case is able to remain at ground potential.

When an equipment's case is not grounded, an electrical failure may precipitate a dangerous accident. For example, suppose that the monitor in Figure 3-35 were connected to the outlet through a two-wire extension cord or through a two-to-three-wire "cheater" adapter. (These items are commonplace in homes.) The monitor would operate but would not be grounded, since no path to ground exists. Now imagine that the hot wire accidentally contacts the monitor's case at the power cord's entry point (or inside). The wire's insulation may fail (a fault). The monitor will probably continue to operate, although considerable electrical interference or artifact may be present in its display. Nevertheless, its case will be hot (120 V with respect to ground). Anyone simultaneously touching the case and a grounded object will conduct a fault current, thereby receiving a shock.

Grounding the case allows the fault current to take the path of least resistance to ground through the low resistance value of the grounding conductor rather than through the human body. The fault current will trip the circuit breaker, thus alerting the staff to the problem. This is how the green ground wire (or grounding conduit) is used to protect personnel.

How electrical principles are applied in ensuring the safety of the patient is detailed in Chapter 18.

4

Electronics and Electronic Devices

A small battery-operated transistor radio, a heart-rate computer (called a cardiotachometer), a color-television receiver, and a multitrace patient monitor have something in common: all are *electronic devices*. Although each has its own purpose and function, all include components that incorporate the principles of electronics.

The term *electronics* is derived from the word *electron* and refers to the flow of electrons in a vacuum, a gas, or the semiconductor material in a transistor. In Chapter 3 electric current was defined as the flow or movement of electrons. Electronics is an application of electricity in which this electron flow is controlled in such a way as to produce certain desired results. For example, through control of electron flow it is possible to amplify the small electrical signal produced by a transducer (see Chapter 2) so that it can operate the display device in a medical instrument. In fact, the transducer itself may be an electronic device. Also, the presentation of an ECG pattern on a patient monitor is the direct result of a controlled beam of electrons striking the screen. From these examples it should be evident that electronics plays a vital role in modern medicine.

4.1 Basic Definitions

Regardless of its function, every electronic device has certain basic features. Some of these features, along with other pertinent terms, are illustrated in Figure 4-1.

The *input* of an electronic device is the location or connections to which incoming information is applied. If this information is in the form of a voltage that varies with time (perhaps representing a physiological variable), the varying voltage is called an electrical *signal* (see Chapter 2). A signal applied to the input is called the *input signal.* The connections to which the input signal is applied are called *input terminals.*

After a signal has been amplified or otherwise processed by the electronic device, it appears at the *output,* the location or connections from which the processed information can be obtained. In some electronic devices the processed information appears as an *output signal* that may be obtained from *output terminals.* In other cases, however, the output may be in a different form, such as sound from a loudspeaker or a pattern on a patient-monitor screen. Sometimes unwanted voltage variations appear at the output of an electronic device along with the signal. This undesirable companion of the output signal is called *noise* or *interference.* The most common source of interference is the 60-Hz power used by most electronic and electrical equipment in the home or hospital. Such interference is called *60-Hz interference* or simply *electrical interference.*

In any electronic device some point in the circuitry is considered as a reference for all voltages in the system. The equipment chassis or case often serves this purpose. In some devices one input terminal and one output terminal are both connected to the reference, and sometimes only one common reference terminal is provided for both input and output. In most instruments this reference is connected to ground (see Chapter 3) through a grounding wire in the power cord.

Every electronic device is composed of electronic components, such as *resistors, capacitors, transistors,* and *diodes,* which are organized into cir-

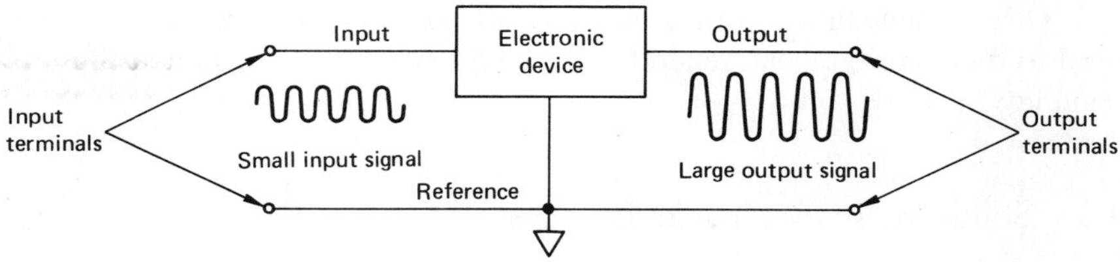

Fig. 4–1 General electronic device with basic terms.

cuits that serve as amplifiers, oscillators, and other parts of the equipment. Each part performs a designated role that contributes to the overall function of the device. Resistors and capacitors are defined and described in Chapter 3. Transistors and diodes are covered later in this chapter.

4.2 Vacuum Tubes

The most important application of electronic devices is *amplification,* a process by which an enlarged replica of an input signal is produced at the output. Without the ability to amplify small electrical signals, radios with loudspeakers, television receivers, and much of the instrumentation used in patient care would not be possible. In older equipment amplification was accomplished through the use of *vacuum tubes.* As the name implies, a vacuum tube is a glass tube (or, in some cases, metal or ceramic) from which all air is evacuated. Within the resulting vacuum are a number of metallic parts that are responsible for the operation of the tube. A typical vacuum tube is shown in Figure 4-2(a).

Operation of the vacuum tube requires that one of the internal elements, called the *cathode,* be heated. The heat is supplied by a heating element, called the *filament.* The cathode is coated with a special material which, when heated by the filament, gives off electrons that flow through the tube and create a current when proper operating voltages are applied. Because of the internal construction of the tube, a small input signal applied to a given set of connections is able to control the current flow through the tube. As a result, large voltage variations that correspond to the input signal appear at the output. Since the output signal is an enlarged replica of the input signal, amplification is achieved.

Although most vacuum tubes are used for amplification, some are designed for other purposes. Regardless of its use, however, a vacuum tube must be connected to a circuit composed of resistors and capacitors and must have proper voltages applied to its internal elements in order to function properly. Operating voltages of up to several hundred volts are required. Also, sufficient power must be available to heat the filament. Thus the power requirements for a vacuum tube amplifier are substantial.

Other disadvantages of the vacuum tube are its relatively large size, the need to dissipate the heat generated by its filament, and its limited life and reliability.

4.3 Solid-State Electronic Devices

In modern electronic instrumentation the vacuum tube has been replaced by *solid-state* electronic components that perform the same functions but have many advantages. Solid-state devices do not require heated filaments for their operation. Therefore they consume far less power than vacuum tubes and also generate less heat. Solid-state devices are also much smaller and more reliable, thus making it possible to build a complex electronic calculator in a pocket-sized package and equipment that enabled man to land on the moon.

The term *solid state* implies that in these devices current is controlled in a solid material instead of a vacuum. The most common materials used for this purpose are *silicon* and *germanium.* These materials are also called semiconductors because, as used in electronic circuits, their electrical resistance is somewhere between that of an insulator and a conductor.

4.3.1 Diodes

A *diode* is a two-element solid-state device capable of conducting current in one direction but not in the opposite direction. Although diodes are used in various types of electronic circuits, their principal application is in the conversion of alternating current (in which current flows in both directions) to direct current (in which current flows in one direction only). A circuit that converts ac to dc is called a *rectifier.* Power supplies in which rectifiers are utilized are described in Section 4.7.

4.3.2 The Transistor

The most prominent solid-state device is the *transistor,* which, like the vacuum tube, is primarily used for amplification. Its development in 1948 ushered in the era of solid-state electronics and made possible the transistor radio as well as other equipment that has since become a vital part of modern life. The transistor has also brought about drastic changes in medical instrumentation, resulting in smaller, safer, and more reliable equipment.

There are several different kinds of transistors, some of which vary considerably in their principles of operation. Nevertheless, all operate on the basis that a small input signal is able to control the current flow through the transistor and produce an output signal that is larger in magnitude but otherwise essentially identical to the input. Like the vacuum tube, a transistor requires other circuit elements—capacitors and resistors, for example—in order to perform its intended function. It must also be provided with a source of power from which it obtains the current to be controlled. A transistor circuit requires much lower voltages than a vacuum tube, however. A typical transistor circuit may use 5 to 15 V, whereas a vacuum tube circuit that performs the same function may require several hundred volts.

In addition to amplification, transistors can be used for a number of other purposes, including electronic switching and storage of data. Although certain kinds of transistors may be best suited for each function, the circuitry connected to the transistor usually determines its function.

4.3.3 Integrated Circuits

Modern manufacturing techniques have made it possible to form several transistors and all their associated resistors and capacitors on a single miniature silicon chip. Such multiple-component devices are called *integrated circuits.* Through their use complex circuitry can be greatly miniaturized and, because of their low power consumption, can be operated by very small batteries. They provide all the advantages of transistors but at a lower cost per circuit. To illustrate the degree of miniaturization that can be achieved with integrated circuits, a single chip of silicon slightly over 0.1 cm square may contain the equivalent of over 10,000 circuit components.

A comparison of the characteristics of the vacuum tube, transistor, and integrated circuits is given in Table 4-1. Their physical sizes are compared in Figure 4-2.

Table 4-1 Comparison Between Vacuum Tube, Transistor, and Integrated Circuit

Characteristics	*Vacuum Tube*	*Transistor*	*Integrated Circuit*
Physical size	Large	Small	Smaller
Power consumption	High	Low	Very low
Deterioration with time	Yes	No	No
Reliability	Good	Better	Best
Cost	Low	Low	Lowest
Suitable for use in medical equipment	Good	Very good	Excellent

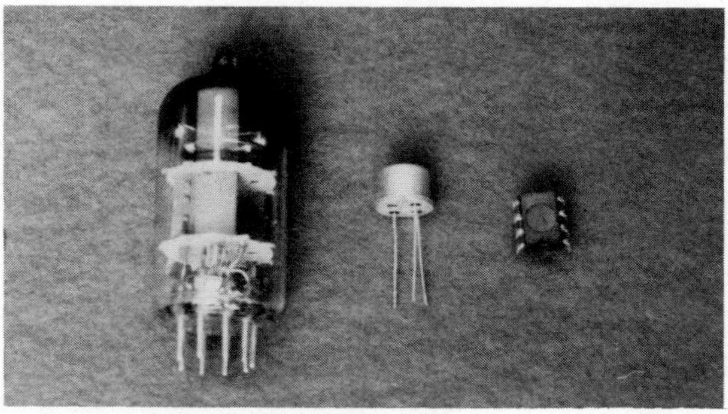

Fig. 4–2 Physical comparison between (a) a vacuum tube, (b) a transistor and (c) an integrated circuit. Note that although an integrated circuit may be larger than a transistor it may contain hundreds or thousands of components.

4.4 Amplifiers

Although a single transistor and its associated resistors and capacitors form an amplifier circuit, several such circuits are normally connected together in order to provide a required amount of amplification. The resulting unit is called an *amplifier*. Many different types of amplifiers are used in medical instrumentation, each with its own specific purpose. For example, a particular type of amplifier is used to amplify the small bioelectric potentials measured from the body (see Chapter 5).

A diagram of a simple amplifier is shown in Figure 4-3. The symbol for an amplifier is usually a triangle with the point indicating the output and the input connected to the opposite side. The amount by which the amplifier increases the magnitude of the input signal is its *gain*. The gain can be calculated as the *ratio* of the voltage of the output signal to the voltage at the input. Thus an amplifier with a gain of 1000 has an output signal that is 1000 times as large as the input signal. The amplifier shown in Figure 4-3 is defined as having a gain of 10. This means that a 1-V input signal results in an output signal of 10 V as shown. Also, it should be noted that some amplifiers *invert* the signal so that the output signal appears as an upside-down version of the input. Otherwise the output is a faithful reproduction of the input.

Amplifiers used in medical instruments commonly have gains ranging from 100 to 100,000. Some amplifiers have an adjustable gain with a "gain" or "sensitivity" control to permit the gain to be set to a desirable value. *Calibration* was defined in Chapter 2 as a procedure for adjusting an instrument so as to make its output reading correspond to the actual value of the variable being measured. Generally the calibration procedure includes adjustment of the amplifier gain setting.

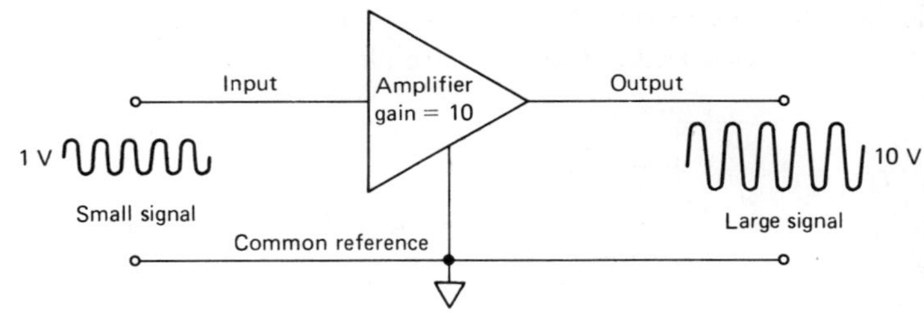

Fig. 4–3 Simple amplifier.

4.4.1 The Single-Ended Amplifier

The amplifier shown in Figure 4-3 is the simplest and most common type. It is called a *single-ended* amplifier because it has only one input terminal, one output terminal, and a common reference terminal, sometimes called "ground." Single-ended amplifiers are usually used where the signals to be amplified are relatively large and free of electrical interference. In general, however, they are unsuitable for amplifying the small voltages produced by biopotential electrodes or most transducers.

4.4.2 The Differential Amplifier

Where very small signals must be amplified in the presence of electrical interference, a special type of amplifier, called a *differential amplifier,* is required. A differential amplifier, as shown in Figure 4-4, has three inputs, one of which serves as the reference for the other two. An input signal can be applied between input 1 and the reference, and another signal can be applied between input 2 and the reference. The output is an enlarged replica of the *difference* between these two input signals, as the word differential implies.

To understand the use of the differential amplifier, assume that the voltage (a difference of potential) between two ECG electrodes is to be amplified. In Figure 4-5 electrodes *A* and *B* are connected to inputs 1 and 2 of the amplifier, respectively. A third electrode on the leg of the patient serves as a reference electrode and is connected to the common reference input of the amplifier. The signal that appears between electrode *A* and the reference electrode is applied to input 1, while the signal between electrode *B* and the reference electrode is applied to input 2. The desired ECG voltage, however, is the difference in potential between electrodes *A* and *B*. Since the output is an amplified reproduction of this difference, the desired signal is amplified, as shown in Figure 4-4. The interference voltages picked up by each of the two ECG electrodes are almost identical, however. When

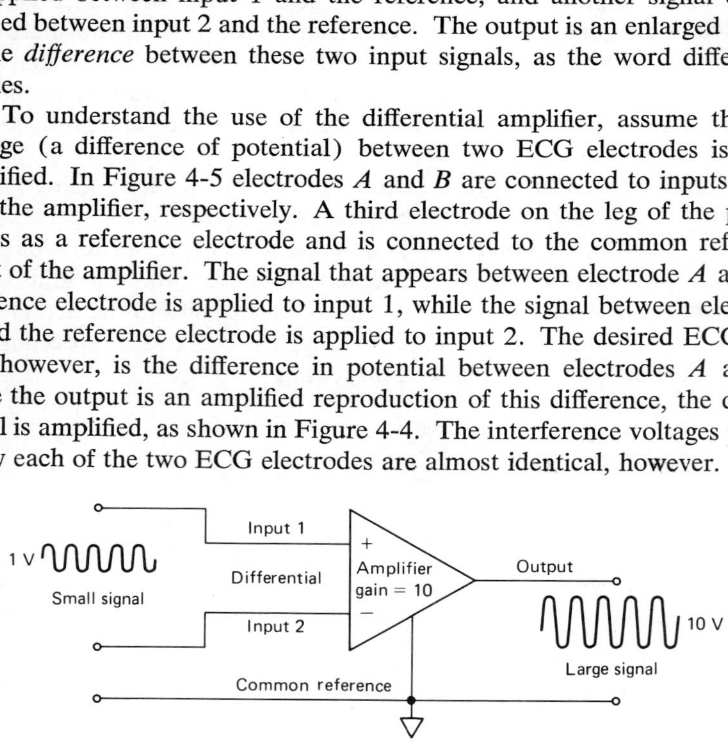

Fig. 4–4 Differential amplifier boosting a one volt differential signal.

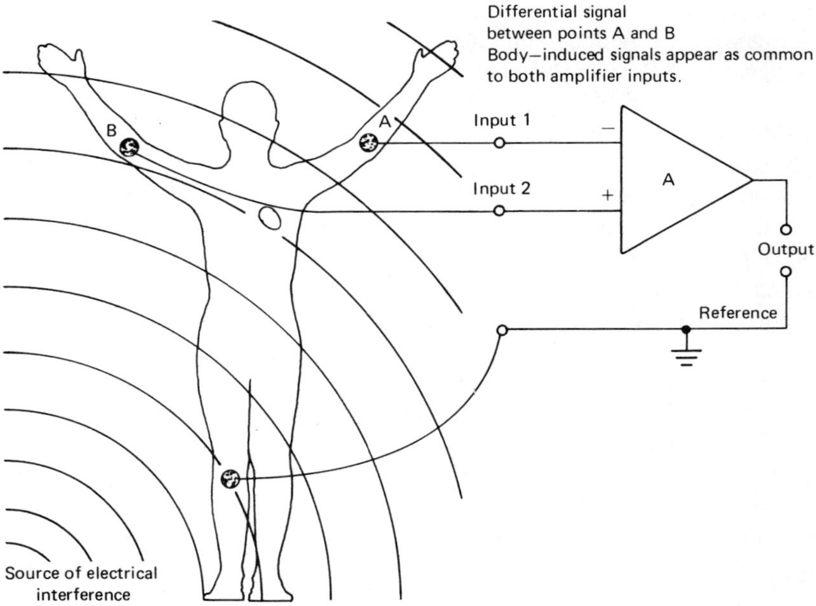

Fig. 4–5 Differential amplifier used for amplification of ECG signal.

they are applied to the two inputs of the differential amplifier, their *difference* is amplified. Since the difference between two nearly identical values is essentially zero, the interference voltages are effectively cancelled out and only the desired signal (the ECG voltage between electrodes *A* and *B*) is amplified, even though the interference voltages at the individual inputs may be much larger. In contrast, if the two ECG electrodes were simply connected to the input and reference of the single-ended amplifier shown in Figure 4-3, both the ECG signal *and* the interference voltage would be amplified. If the interference voltage were much larger, the desired ECG signal would be lost.

Since the interference voltage is *common* to both inputs 1 and 2, it is called a *common-mode* input. Figure 4-6 shows the cancellation of the common-mode interference. This characteristic of a differential amplifier to cancel common-mode voltage is called *common-mode rejection*. The amount by which the amplifier is able to reduce common-mode interference is called the *common-mode rejection ratio,* abbreviated *CMRR*. The higher this ratio, the better an amplifier is able to eliminate the interference. Typical CMRR values for medical amplifiers reach as high as several hundred thousand.

For example, an amplifier CMRR of 100,000 to 1 means that it will reject the common-mode signal better than one whose CMRR is only 1000 to 1. A typical CMRR for some medical amplifiers may be 50,000; however, high-quality medical amplifiers may have CMRRs as high as 500,000. Consider a typical ECG differential amplifier that has a gain of 1000 and a CMRR of 100,000 to 1. The differential signal applied to it will be amplified 1000 times, as it should be. Yet the common-mode signal will only be amplified by a factor of 1/100. If the CMRR were 200,000 to 1, the common-mode signal would be amplified by a factor of 1/200. In other words, the desired signal (the ECG) will be properly amplified and ultimately displayed; however, the undesired common noise, which may be much larger than the minute ECG signal, will be suppressed and not displayed. It is important to realize this basic difference—that the biopotential is amplified to the full extent of the capabilities of the amplifier, whereas the noise or common-mode signal is reduced by a factor of the CMRR. Theoretically, if a differential amplifier were perfect, the CMRR would be infinite and the noise signal would be zero. If the two input terminals of the differential amplifier are connected together and a signal is then applied between these two input terminals and the reference, the output from the amplifier will be zero. Figure 4-6 shows the operation of the perfect differential amplifier with a common-mode signal applied to it.

4.4.3 Isolation Amplifiers

Another special type of amplifier is the *isolation amplifier*. As the name implies, its purpose is to isolate its input connections from ground or any possible source of unwanted electric current. Thus, with this device, patients connected to line-powered electrical equipment are protected from receiving harmful electric currents through their bodies from the patient leads. Isolation amplifiers may be built into such equipment as ECG machines or patient monitors, or they may be obtained separately for use with older equipment that does not provide sufficient isolation. The need for isolation, together with other information on electrical safety, is described in Chapter 18.

Some isolation amplifiers do no more than isolate the input leads; they

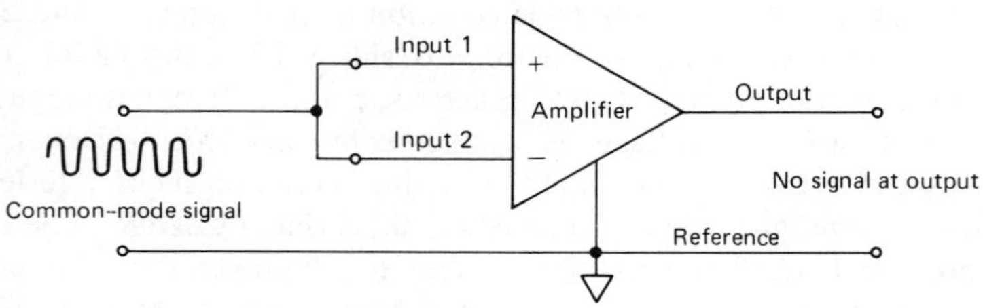

Fig. 4–6 Differential amplifier rejecting common-mode signal connected to its inputs.

have *unity gain,* which means that the output signal has the same value as the input. In this case, an additional amplifier is required to provide the necessary amplification. Other isolation amplifiers do provide some gain, but this gain seldom exceeds 100.

4.5 Electronic Filters

Without the word *electronic,* the term *filter* generally indicates some device capable of separation or selection. This same concept applies to an *electronic filter,* an electronic device used to separate electrical signals of different frequencies or to reject unwanted signals or interference by attenuating certain frequencies. Attenuation implies a sizable reduction in voltage. For example, 60-Hz interference from the electric power line can be removed from a signal that includes frequencies of from 0.01 to 30 Hz by attenuating all frequencies above 35 or 40 Hz. Also, an EEG signal can be separated into its different frequency bands (alpha, beta, etc.) by the use of filters.

Filters are classified according to the frequencies they pass and those they attenuate. The four basic types of filters are as follows:

1. *Lowpass filters,* which permit only frequencies below a designated frequency to pass. This designated frequency is called the *cutoff frequency.* All frequencies above cutoff are attenuated. Figure 4-7 shows the use of a lowpass filter in removing 60-Hz interference from an ECG signal. In this case, the cutoff frequency is around 40 or 50 Hz.
2. *Highpass filters,* which permit only frequencies above the cutoff frequency to pass. All lower frequencies are attenuated. Highpass filters are often used to reduce the effect of patient movements that tend to drive the pen of an ECG recorder off the paper.
3. *Bandpass filters,* which permit only a certain range or *band* of frequencies to pass and attenuate all frequencies both above and below the desired band. A bandpass filter has both an upper and

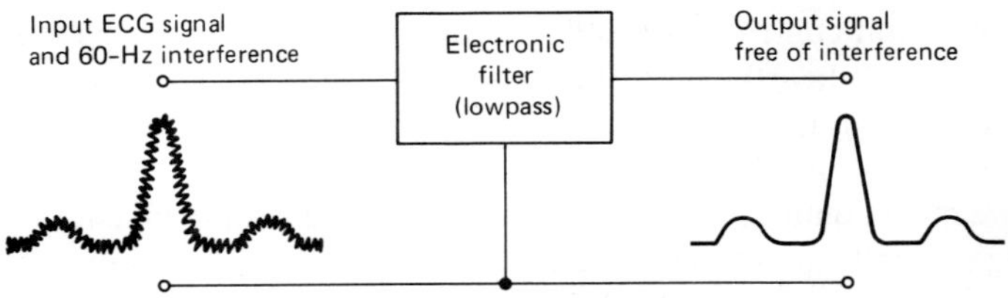

Fig. 4–7 Use of lowpass filter in removing 60-Hz. interference from an ECG signal.

a lower cutoff frequency. Proper selection of these frequencies permits the rejection of any interference or unwanted signals outside the frequency range required for the desired signal. Bandpass filters are used, for example, to separate the various frequency bands from an EEG signal.

4. *Band-rejection filters,* which attenuate all frequencies between the two cutoff frequencies. Usually band-rejection filters are used to reject a very narrow band of frequencies around 60 Hz to remove interference from a signal that contains frequencies both above and below 60 Hz.

Some amplifiers in medical instruments have built-in filters that pass the required bands of frequencies for their intended use. These filters are often adjustable so as to permit the user to select the upper or lower cutoff frequency (or both) that best meets the needs of a specific application. It should be noted that when a filter is adjusted to attenuate a certain range of frequencies, any signal information within the rejected frequency band will be eliminated along with the interference.

4.6 Electronic Display Devices

As indicated in Chapter 2, a *display device* is that portion of a medical instrument or instrumentation system in which the results of measurements are converted into a perceivable form and presented in a meaningful way to those using the instruments. The display can range in complexity from a simple indicator light to a complicated assortment of physiological waveforms on a special television screen type of presentation. Descriptions of several types of electronic display devices used in medical instrumentation follow.

4.6.1 Indicator Lights

The simplest type of display device is the indicator light. Such a light may be used to show that an instrument is turned on or to indicate the setting of a vital control. A flashing light is often used on a patient monitor to indicate each heartbeat of the patient. Lights are also used as warning devices or in conjunction with a warning buzzer to indicate which patient is in danger.

The most common type of indicator light is a simple *incandescent lamp.* Although usually much smaller, these lamps are of the same type as the familiar household light bulb. Lamps of this type glow when electric current flows through a fine internal wire, called the *filament.* Incandescent lamp indicators may be installed in the instrument behind a colored glass or plastic cover to provide light of an appropriate color, or they may be built into a lighted push-button type switch, which may also be colored. These lamps are available in a wide assortment of voltages ranging from less than 6 V to 120 V.

Another type of display lamp is a small *neon lamp,* which contains a neon gas that glows when a sufficient voltage is applied to it. Neon lamps, which usually produce an orange-colored glow, are smaller than most incandescent lamps and draw much less current.

A more recently developed source of light that can serve as an indicator is the *light-emitting diode (LED).* The LED consists of a small piece of special semiconductor material. When current flows through the diode in the proper direction, the LED glows. This device is much smaller than either type of lamp described above. In fact, in most cases, the LED produces just a dot of light. Nevertheless, they are small enough that the dots can be placed close together to form numerals or letters. (See Section 4.6.2.) A major advantage of the LED is extremely long life. Like transistors and other semiconductor devices, LEDs do not wear out. Thus they can be expected to last for many years without failure. Also, they draw very little current. Most LEDs emit a red glow; they are also available in yellow and green.

4.6.2 Numeric Displays

Many medical instruments provide information in the form of numerical values. These values may be displayed on a dial or a meter in which a pointer indicates the value, or they may be displayed in *digital* form. In a *digital display,* numerals indicating the displayed value light up or otherwise appear. In addition, letters of the alphabet are sometimes included.

In one common type of digital numeric display, each numeral is made up of a pattern of light-emitting diodes or lamps of some other type. Each lamp contributes either a dot of light or a short line segment. A commonly used numeric indicator utilizing seven line segments is shown in Figure 4-8.

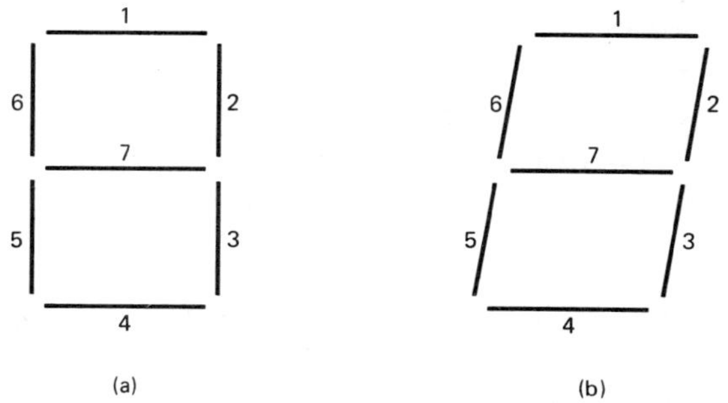

Fig. 4–8 Seven-segment digital numeric indicator: (a) straight; (b) slanted.

It can be obtained in either a straight or slanted version as shown. To produce a given numeral, voltage is applied to the appropriate segments. For example, if voltage is applied to segments 1, 2, 3, 4, and 7, the numeral "3" appears. On the other hand, if only segments 2 and 3 are lighted, a number "1" is displayed. In a similar manner, all numerals, 0 through 9, can be formed.

Another type of digital indicator, called a Nixie® tube, contains fine wires formed in the shape of numerals. These numerals are located one behind the other inside a glass tube filled with a gas. Only one of the numerals is lighted at a time, however, and the other numerals do not show. Connections to each wire permit the equipment to apply voltage directly to the appropriate numeral.

Several other types of digital numeric displays are also used in medical instruments. Regardless of the type, however, the total display must contain enough digits to display the necessary information. Where appropriate, a lighted decimal point is also included. A Nixie®-tube display in which body temperature is given to the nearest tenth of a degree Fahrenheit, for example, must contain at least four Nixie® tubes in addition to the decimal indicator in order to produce the four digits required.

4.6.3 Cathode-Ray Tube (CRT) Displays

In certain types of medical instruments, information that cannot be assessed in numerical form is required. In such cases, the actual physiological waveforms of such variables as the ECG, arterial blood pressure waveform, respiration patterns, and the phonocardiogram must be presented for observation. A special type of tube, called a *cathode-ray tube* (abbreviated *CRT*), is used to display such waveforms. This tube is similar to the picture tube in a television set. However, instead of displaying a television program, the CRT in a patient monitor or other medical instrument "writes out" the desired physiological waveforms.

The cathode-ray tube is actually a special type of vacuum tube. It contains an electron gun that "shoots" a steady stream of electrons focused toward the rear of the *viewing screen,* called the *faceplate.* This screen is coated with a special phosphor material that glows whenever it is struck by the electron beam, as shown in Figure 4-9. Two sets of deflection plates deflect the beam upward or downward and left or right, depending on the voltages applied to the plates. If no voltage is applied to any of the deflection plates, the electron beam produces a tiny spot of light at the center of the screen (point *B* in the figure). If a voltage is applied to the vertical deflection plates shown in Figure 4-9(a) with the upper plate positive with respect to the lower plate, the beam is deflected upward and produces a spot of light at point *A*. If, on the other hand, the upper

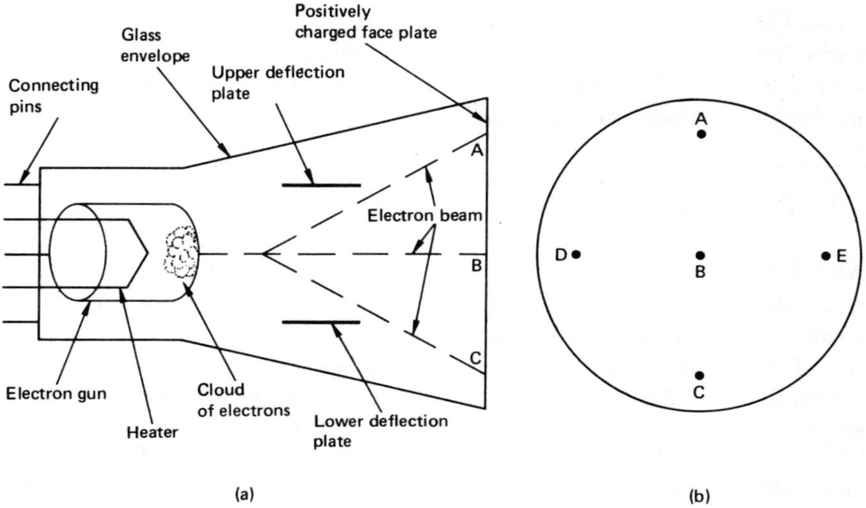

Fig. 4–9 Cathode-ray tube.

plate is negative with respect to the lower one, the beam is deflected downward and moves the spot to point *C*. If a voltage corresponding to a physiological variable, such as the amplified ECG voltage, is applied between the vertical deflection plates, the beam of electrons moves up and down in proportion to that voltage and follows the waveform. If, at the same time, another voltage pattern (corresponding to time) is applied to a pair of horizontal deflection plates (not shown in the figure) that causes the electron beam to move from left to right (from point *D* to point *E*) across the face of the tube, the physiological waveform is written on the face of the tube. This is the way in which most CRT displays operate. As soon as the electron beam has reached the right edge of the screen, it quickly returns back to the left to begin another sweep from left to right across the tube.

Some CRT displays present two or more waveforms simultaneously. Generally these CRTs do not contain more than one electron gun. However, special circuitry causes the electron beam to jump from waveform to wave form so rapidly that the jumps cannot be seen, and each waveform is presented without any apparent interruption.

After the electron beam has written a waveform on the CRT, the display remains for a short time and then fades out before the next sweep across the screen. In some cases, the display fades before the pattern can be observed as long as desired. To eliminate this problem, some patient monitors feature a *nonfading CRT display*. Although the same type of CRT is used, the waveform is not written on the screen in the manner described. Instead special circuitry in the monitor stores the information to be displayed and causes it to move slowly across the screen without fading. This type of monitor can also display letters and numerals on the screen along with the waveform.

4.7 Power Supplies

All electronic devices require electrical energy for their operation. Because such devices include transistors or vacuum tubes that require direct current, a source of dc power must be provided.

The simplest source of dc power is a battery that stores energy in chemical form. Nearly all portable electronic equipment, including transistor radios and pocket calculators, uses batteries. Batteries can either be nonrechargeable, like flashlight batteries, or rechargeable. Nonrechargeable batteries must be replaced periodically, whereas the chargeable type can be recharged when the stored energy has been used. Personnel using portable battery-operated equipment should be alert for signs that replacement or recharging is necessary. Some instruments include a built-in means of checking the condition of the battery.

Electronic equipment that is powered from the 115-V wall outlet must include a *power supply* to convert the alternating current obtained from the wall outlet to the direct current required by the equipment. A typical power supply consists of three basic components, as shown in Figure 4-10(a):

1. A *transformer* to step the line voltage up or down in order to provide the required voltage for the various circuits in the equipment. Figure 4-10(b) shows the 115-V ac line voltage. Figure 4-10(c) shows this voltage stepped down by the transformer for a particular application.
2. A *rectifier,* which is a device that converts the ac to dc. The output of the rectifier is not a smooth dc, however, as shown in Figure 4-10(d). Instead it fluctuates about an average dc value.
3. A *filter circuit* to remove the fluctuations and provide a smooth dc for operation of the various circuits in the equipment. The smooth dc output is shown in Figure 4-10(e).

In addition to these three basic components, many power supplies include circuitry to keep the dc voltage constant in spite of changes in the ac line voltage and regardless of how much current is being drawn from the power supply. This circuitry is called a *voltage regulator.*

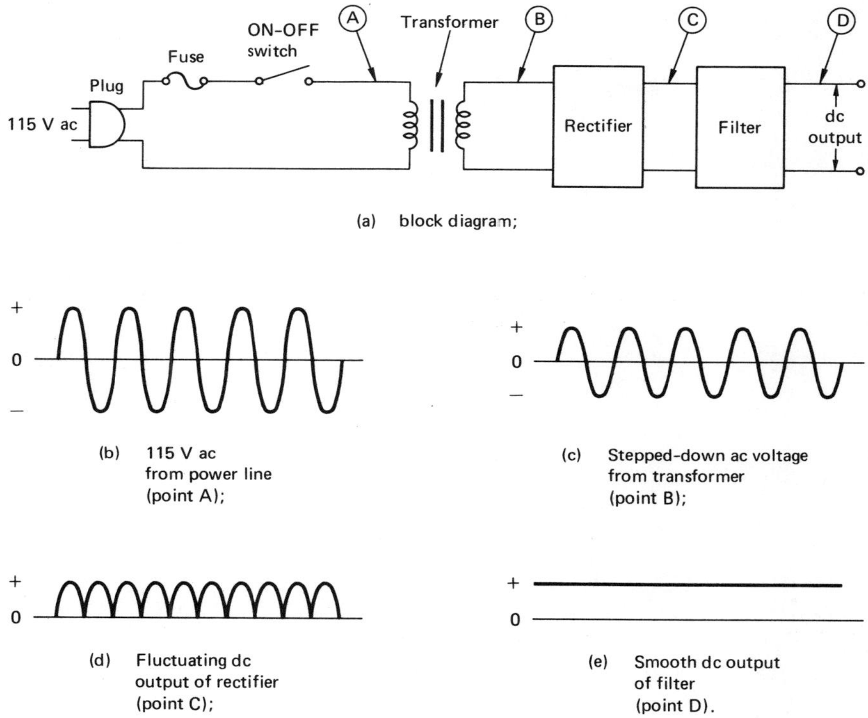

(a) block diagram;

(b) 115 V ac from power line (point A);

(c) Stepped-down ac voltage from transformer (point B);

(d) Fluctuating dc output of rectifier (point C);

(e) Smooth dc output of filter (point D).

Fig. 4–10 DC power supply—block diagram and voltage waveforms.

Note that an overcurrent fuse is inserted in the hot wire leading from the wall outlet to the transformer primary. Whenever the fuse melts or "blows," it signals a fault in the instrument. Once the fault is corrected, the same type and same value fuse must be used in replacement. The instrument case is usually grounded via the three-wire power cord.

Occasionally the component arrangement shown in Figure 4-10 along with the power cord is called the "power side" of the instrument. This situation contrasts with the actual amplifier circuits connected to a patient via a patient cable (with electrodes), called the "patient side" of the instrument. Thus, for simplicity, a patient-connected instrument is considered to have two sections—a power side and a patient side.

5

Physiological Variables

In Chapter 2 a *physiological variable* was defined as a measurable quantity associated with one or more functions and processes of the body. The bioelectric potentials (ECG, EEG, and EMG), blood pressures, volumes, and flow, respiratory pressures, volumes and flows, heart sounds, and body temperature are all physiological variables. The purpose of diagnostic medical instrumentation is to measure and display these variables in a meaningful way that aids the medical staff in diagnosing and treating disease.

An understanding of any biomedical instrument requires familiarity with the physiological variables to be measured by that instrument. The physiological sources of these variables and their relationship to associated body functions must also be understood. As a background for the various biomedical instruments to be described in this book, this chapter describes a number of important physiological variables and the way in which each is used. Because the book is written for nurses and other practitioners in patient care, a fundamental knowledge of physiology is assumed, although certain pertinent physiological processes are briefly reviewed. Emphasis is on the characteristics of those variables that must be considered in their measurement.

5.1 Bioelectric Potentials

In carrying out their various functions, certain systems of the body generate their own monitoring signals, which convey useful information about the functions they represent. These signals are the bioelectric potentials associated with nerve impulse conduction, brain activity, heartbeat, muscle activity, and so on. Bioelectric potentials are actually ionic voltages produced as a result of the electrochemical activity of certain special types of excitable cells. Through the use of *electrodes* (transducers that convert ionic potentials into electric voltages), these natural signals can be measured and displayed.

The idea that electricity is generated in the body goes back to the eighteenth century when an Italian anatomy professor, Luigi Galvani, claimed to have found electricity in the muscle of a frog's leg. In the century that followed several other scientists discovered electrical activity in various animals and in man. But it was not until 1903, when the Dutch physician William Einthoven first used the string galvanometer as a recording device, that electrocardiograms became practical. The advent of the vacuum tube, amplification, and solid-state devices has made possible better representation of bioelectric events. These developments, combined with a large amount of biological research activity, have opened many new avenues of knowledge in the application and interpretation of these important signals.

5.1.1 *The Resting Potential*

The human body has numerous tissues that are excitable, among them nerves and muscles. The cells from which they are made are encased in a selectively permeable (semipermeable) membrane that permits some substances to pass through it while others are effectively kept out. Although the membrane structure is reasonably well known, the exact mechanism by which its permeability is controlled is not. Nevertheless, the substances that are pertinent to the cell's bioelectric behavior have been identified by experimentation.

Bathing the cells is the body fluid, an electrolyte solution not unlike salt water that contains charged atoms called *ions*. The principal ions surrounding the cell are sodium (Na^+), potassium (K^+), and chloride (Cl^-). The protoplasm inside the cell also contains these ions. When the excitable cell is at rest (not stimulated), its membrane allows potassium and chloride ions to pass through with ease. However, because the membrane is only slightly permeable to sodium, sodium ions are effectively excluded. The sodium and potassium ions achieve a chemical balance between the inside and the outside of the cell by both passive and active processes. Diffusion of ions is largely passive and dependent on the existence of higher and lower ionic concentrations on opposite sides of the membrane. Active processes that maintain equilibrium include the sodium and potassium pumps. The sodium pump serves to move sodium from inside to outside the cell. This movement is against the higher concentration of sodium outside. Potassium is moved in a similar, although less important, mechanism from outside to inside the cell. The result is a high concentration of potassium inside the cell with a lower concentration in the surrounding fluids; the sodium concentration is higher outside the cell than inside. For each sodium ion inside the cell, there are approximately 10 sodium ions outside. Figure 5-1 illustrates this point.

Because both sodium and potassium ions are positive, the higher concentration of potassium inside the cell would tend to balance the excess sodium ions on the outside. However, potassium ions can pass freely through the cell membrane, whereas sodium cannot. As a result, the concentration gradient causes an outward diffusion of potassium ions. Because there is no corresponding inward diffusion of sodium, due to the impermeability of the membrane to that ion, the diffusion of potassium keeps the outside of the cell positive with respect to the inside. The inside is therefore negative with respect to the outside.

This membrane voltage is called the *resting potential* of the cell and

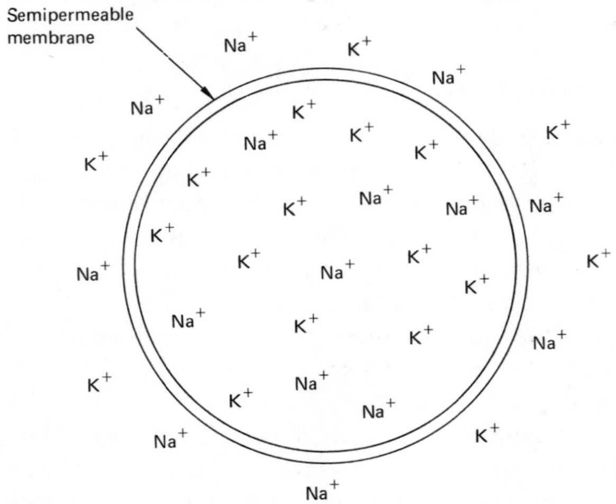

Fig. 5–1 Relative charge concentrations inside and outside an excitable cell at rest.

is maintained until some kind of disturbance or stimulus upsets the equilibrium. Since measurement of the membrane potential is made from the inside of the cell with respect to the body fluids, the resting potential is given as negative. The potential difference is similar to a battery's voltage. Thus an excitable cell at rest is charged or *polarized*. Research investigators have reported measuring membrane potentials in various cells ranging from —60 to —100 millivolts (mV). A cross section of a representative cell with its resting potential appears in Figure 5-2.

A voltage-indicating meter (*voltmeter*) is shown with its probes connected between the inside and outside of the cell. Experiments have shown that an ultrasmall probe can be inserted into certain large excitable cells without damaging their membranes. Upon membrane penetration, the voltmeter indicates that the inside of the cell is (nominally) 70 mV, negative with respect to the outside. The resting potential of a typical cardiac pacemaker cell is about —75 mV, whereas the resting potential of a ventricular or atrial muscle cell is approximately —90 mV.

5.1.2 The Action Potential

When a section of the cell membrane is stimulated by an electric current or another form of externally applied energy, the membrane changes its permeability to sodium and allows these ions to enter. This movement of sodium into the cell constitutes an ionic current flow that further reduces the membrane's barrier to sodium. The result is a large number of positively charged sodium ions quickly rushing into the cell, trying to reach a balance with the sodium ions outside. At the same time, potassium ions, which were in higher concentration inside the cell during the resting state, try to leave but are unable to move as rapidly as the sodium ions. As a result, the inside of the cell becomes slightly *positive* with respect to the outside, due to the imbalance of potassium ions. The

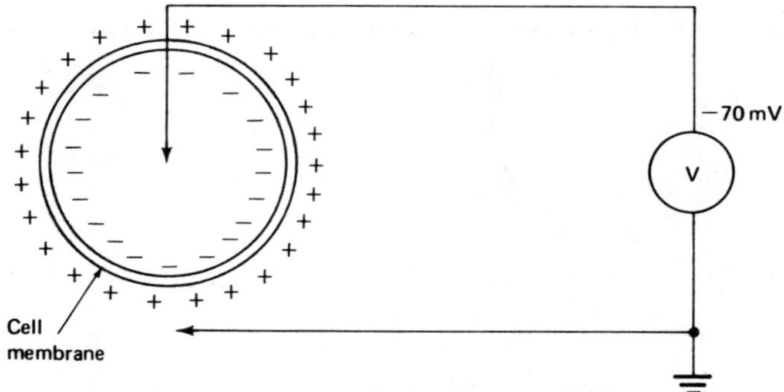

Fig. 5–2 Polarized cell with its resting potential.

resulting positive potential inside the cell (with respect to the outside) occurs momentarily and equals about 20 mV. A cell that has been excited and whose interior is positive with respect to its exterior is said to be *depolarized;* the process of changing from the resting state (with its resting potential) to a positive potential is called *depolarization.* Figure 5-3 shows the ionic movement associated with depolarization, and Figure 5-4 illustrates the cross section of a depolarized cell.

Once the rush of sodium ions through the cell membrane has stopped (a new state of equilibrium is reached), the ionic currents that lowered the barrier to sodium ions are no longer present and the membrane reverts to its original selectively permeable condition, in which the passage of sodium ions from the outside to the inside of the cell is again effectively blocked. Were this the only effect, however, it would take a long time for a resting potential to develop again. But such is not the case. Potassium

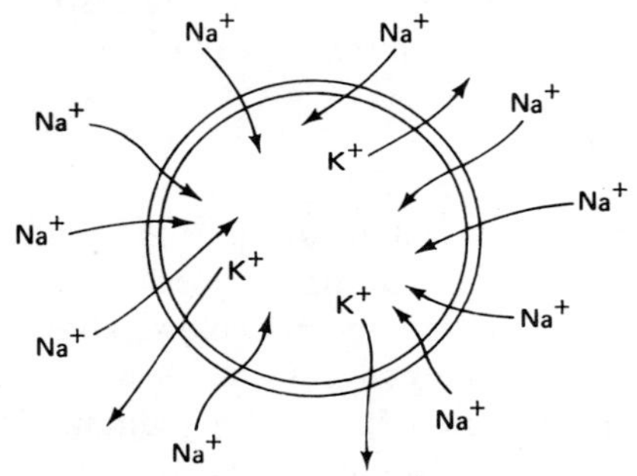

Fig. 5–3 Depolarization of a cell (Na+ ions rush into cell while K+ ions attempt to leave).

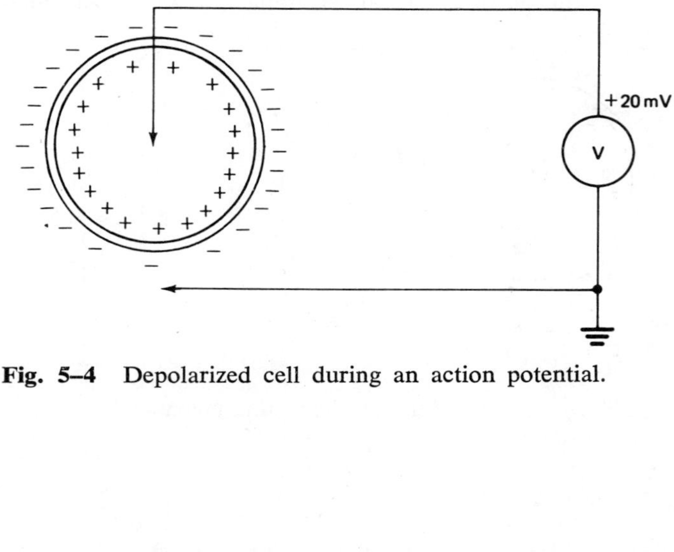

Fig. 5–4 Depolarized cell during an action potential.

ions now leave the cell at a rapid rate due to the large number of positive ions inside and the high concentration gradient. Meanwhile, the sodium pump provides transportation of sodium out of the cells. At this stage the cell again becomes polarized and assumes its resting potential, primarily because of the passive outward diffusion of potassium ions. This process is called *repolarization.* The length of time required for repolarization to occur is determined largely by the concentration of both sodium and potassium in the fluid. The sequential depolarization and repolarization actions of a stimulated excitable cell generate what is called the *action potential.*

Figure 5-5 shows the waveform of the action potential of a typical cardiac muscle cell as it reacts to an applied stimulating voltage. Important characteristics are noted along the time scale as time 1, 2, 3, and so on. At time 1, the cell is unstimulated (at rest) and polarized. Its interior is —90 mV with respect to its exterior. At time 2, an electric stimulus is abruptly applied with sufficient amplitude or strength to lower the membrane potential (the voltage inside the cell begins to decrease toward zero volts) and the cell begins to depolarize (discharge). Provided that

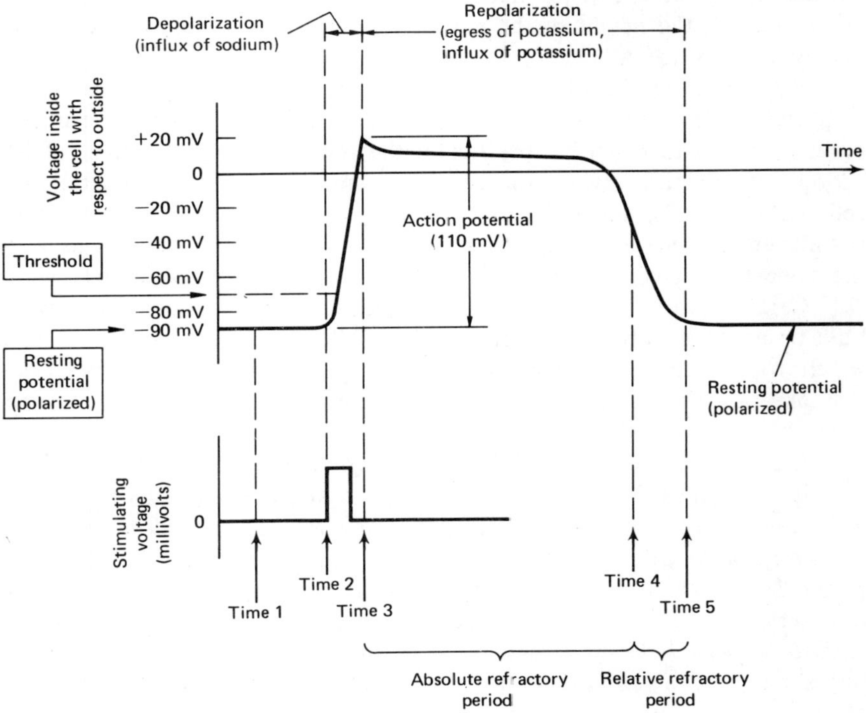

Fig. 5–5 Action potential waveform for a cardiac muscle cell.

the applied stimulus is of sufficient intensity to bring the membrane potential to its threshold value (about —70 mV for myofibrils), the cell quickly depolarizes to the point where its interior becomes positive (20 mV positive with respect to its exterior at time 3). At this time the cell is completely depolarized or discharged. Shortly thereafter potassium diffuses out of the cell and the cell begins to repolarize (recharge) as its membrane potential reverts to its resting value of —90 mV (time 4). The time interval during which heart muscle cells remain depolarized (from time 3 to time 5 in Figure 5-4) may last as long as 300 milliseconds (ms). In nerve and skeletal muscle cells, on the other hand, repolarization occurs so rapidly after depolarization that the waveform appears as a pulse or spike with as little as 1-ms total duration.

Another difference between heart muscle cells and nerve cells is in their mechanical response to excitation. Following depolarization, muscle cells contract or shorten. After repolarization, they relax. The length or size of a nerve cell, however, is not affected by an action potential. The height or value of an action potential is defined as the difference between the resting potential and the maximum positive potential. In the example in Figure 5-4, the height of the action potential is +20 mV minus —90 mV, or 110 mV (about 0.1 V).

Regardless of the method by which a resting cell is excited or the amplitude of the stimulus (provided that it is sufficient to cause the membrane potential to reach its threshold), the response and the height of its action potential are always the same for any given cell. Thus excitable cells obey what is called the *all-or-nothing law*. That is, if the stimulus is sufficient to generate an action potential, that action potential is usually the same for a given cell regardless of the intensity of the stimulus.

Certain heart cells are capable of producing action potentials with little or no externally applied stimulation. They are the *pacemaker cells,* which trigger each heartbeat by generating recurring action potentials that are largely attributable to special membrane characteristics of the cells.

Once an action potential has been generated, there is a period of time during which the cell will not respond to any new stimulus regardless of its amplitude. This period (from time 3 to time 4) is called the *absolute refractory period,* during which the cell resists all excitation attempts. This period equals about 250 ms for cardiac cells and lasts only about 0.5 ms in a nerve cell. Following the absolute refractory period there is a *relative refractory period* during which another action potential can be evoked, but a much stronger (than normal) stimulus is required. The duration of the relative refractory period is about 50 ms for cardiac cells and approximately 0.1 ms for a nerve cell.

5.1.3 *Propagation of the Action Potential*

When an action potential is evoked and ionic currents flow, as already described, the process can, in turn, excite neighboring cells or adjacent areas of the same cell. This process is called *propagation*. In the heart muscle, propagation is from one heart muscle fiber (myofibril) to another, whereas in a neuron the propagation travels along the axon from the cell body to the axon terminals.

The rate at which an action potential travels along a fiber or is propagated from cell to cell is called the *propagation rate*. In heart muscle cells, the average rate is from 0.2 to 0.4 meter per second (m/s), although in special time-delay fibers between the atria and ventricles (the AV node) the action potentials are propagated at even slower rates (0.03 to 0.05 m/s). In nerve fibers, the propagation rate (also called the nerve conduction rate or conduction velocity) varies widely, depending on the type and diameter of the nerve fiber. The usual velocity in nerve fibers ranges from 20 to 140 m/s. Thus, in an adult of average height, the time required for an action potential to travel from the brain to a leg muscle may be as little as 15 ms.

5.1.4 *Measurement of Bioelectric Potentials*

In measuring bioelectric potentials, a pair of *electrodes* is needed to convert the ionic potentials and currents in the body into electric voltages and currents. Electrodes are described in Chapter 6.

Although measurement of individual action potentials can be made in some types of cells, such measurements are difficult because they require precise placement of an electrode inside or adjacent to a specific cell. The more common form of measured biopotentials results from the combined effect of a large number of action potentials as they appear at the surface of the body or at one or more electrodes inserted into a muscle, nerve, or some part of the brain.

The exact method by which these potentials reach the surface of the body is not known. A number of theories seem to explain most of the observed phenomena fairly well, but none exactly fits the situation. Many attempts have been made, for example, to explain the biopotentials from the heart as they appear at the surface of the body. Despite the method by which these patterns of potentials reach the surface of the body or implanted measuring electrodes, they can be measured as specific bioelectric signal patterns that have been studied extensively and can be defined quite well.

The next four sections describe the more significant bioelectric potential waveforms. The designation of the waveform itself generally ends in the suffix *gram,* whereas the name of the instrument used to measure the potentials and graphically reproduce the waveform ends in the suffix *graph.* For example, the electrocardiogram (the name of the waveform resulting from the heart's electrical activity) is measured on an electrocardiograph (the instrument). The waveform may also be displayed on a patient monitor, as mentioned in Chapter 4.

5.1.5 The Electrocardiogram

As noted, the biopotentials generated by the muscles of the heart result in the *electrocardiogram,* abbreviated *ECG* (sometimes *EKG,* from the German *elektrokardiogramm*). In order to understand the origin and significance of the ECG, it is necessary to consider the anatomy of the heart and its performance in the cardiovascular system. Figure 5-6 shows a cross section of the interior of the heart.

The four chambers of the heart act as two synchronized two-stage pumps. The right heart supplies blood to the lungs for oxygenation (*pulmonary circulation*), whereas the left heart supplies blood to the rest of the system (*systemic circulation*). The incoming blood fills the *right atrium.* When filled, the right atrium contracts and forces blood through the *tricuspid valve* into the *right ventricle,* which then contracts to pump the blood into the pulmonary circulation system. From the pulmonary system the oxygenated blood enters the *left atrium.* From there it is pumped through the *mitral,* or *bicuspid valve,* into the *left ventricle.* When the left ventricular muscles contract, the blood is pumped into the systemic circulatory system. The two atria are synchronized to pump together, after which the two ventricles act together.

Excitation of the heart does not proceed directly from the central nervous system like most other muscle innervations but is initiated in the *sinoatrial (SA)* node, or *pacemaker,* a special group of excitable cells. The pacemaker spontaneously generates action potentials at a regular rate, although the rate is influenced by nerves that accelerate or inhibit its value. To initiate the heartbeat, the action potential generated by the pacemaker propagates (from the SA node) in all directions along the surface of both atria towards the junction of the atria and ventricles, the AV node. At this point, special nerve fibers act to delay the propagation so as to provide proper timing between the pumping action of the atria and the ventricles. During this delay time, the atria complete their contraction, forcing blood into the ventricles in order to complete their filling. Afterward the AV node initiates an impulse into the ventricles through the *bundle of His* and thence into the bundle branches that connect to *Purkinje fibers* in the myocardium. The wavefront in the ventricles, however, does

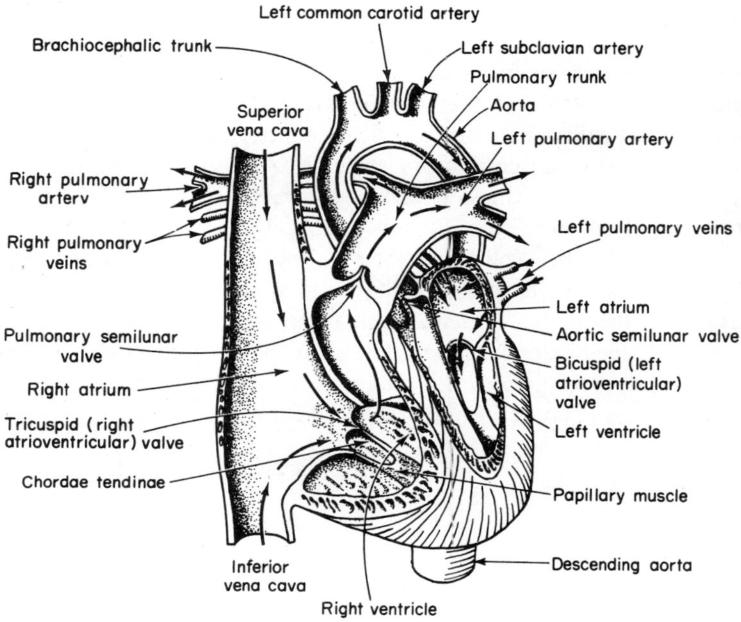

(a)

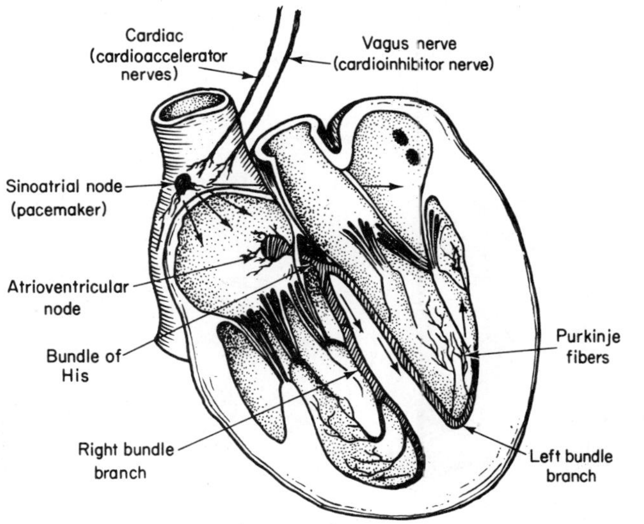

(b)

Fig. 5–6 The heart: (a) internal structure; (b) conducting system (from W. F. Evans, *Anatomy and Physiology, The Basic Principles,* Englewood Cliffs, N.J., Prentice-Hall, Inc., 1971, by permission).

not follow along the surface but is perpendicular to it and moves from the inside to the outside of the ventricular wall, until the entire ventricle becomes depolarized. Then the ventricles contract, forcing blood into the pulmonary and systemic circulatory systems. As indicated earlier, a wave of repolarization follows the depolarization wave (by about 0.2 to 0.4 s). This repolarization, however, is not initiated from neighboring muscle cells but occurs as each cell returns to its resting potential independently.

Figure 5-7 shows a typical ECG as it appears when recorded from the surface of the body. Letter designations have been arbitrarily given to each of the prominent features. They can be correlated with events of action potential propagation. To facilitate recognition and analysis, the horizontal segment (baseline) of this waveform is referred to as the

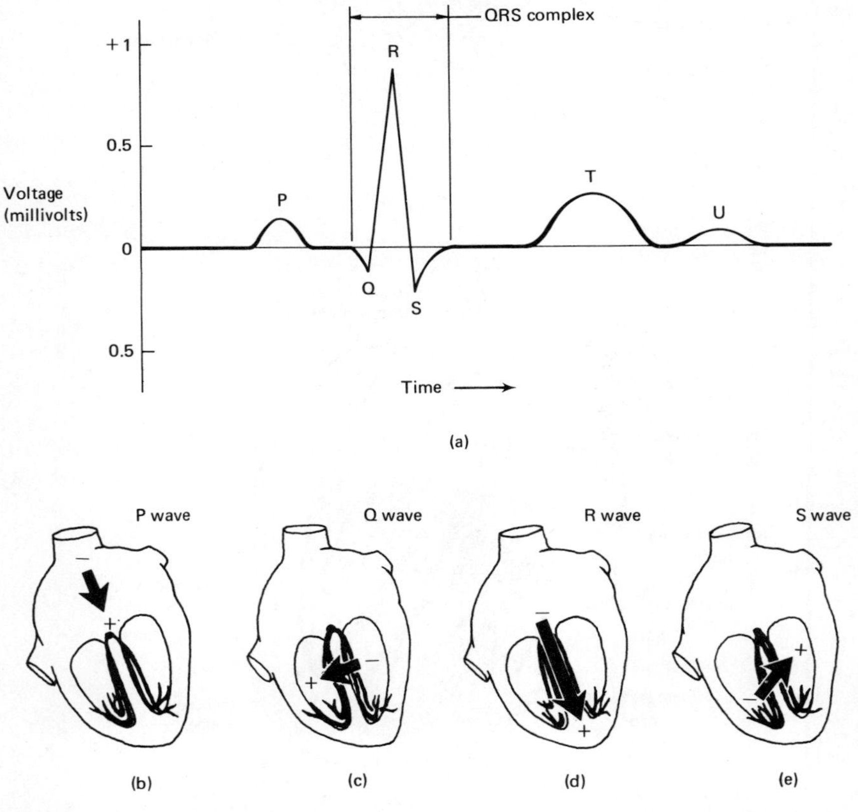

Fig. 5–7 The electrocardiogram: (a) typical wave form; (b) P wave vector illustrates atrial depolarization; (c) Q wave vector; (d) R wave vector; (e) S wave vector.

isopotential or *isoelectric line.* The *P wave* represents the electrical activity associated with depolarization of atrial musculature as action potentials (forming a wave of positivity) travel from the SA node, where they originate, toward the AV node. In Figure 5-7(b) the depolarizing wave is represented by a vector with polarity signs added to indicate the general direction of wave travel and the resulting potential difference that occurs across the atrial musculature. Thus the P wave vector represents a depolarizing wave with a certain strength traveling from the SA node toward the AV node. As the wave propagates, the area around the AV node becomes electrically positive while the area near the pacemaker becomes negative. Because the resulting electric field manifests itself at the body's surface, the lower chest area becomes positive and the area of the upper chest becomes negative during atrial excitation. When an electrocardiograph, used to measure the ECG, is properly attached through electrodes to these areas, the resulting P wave appears positive (above baseline), as shown in Figure 5-7(a).

Whereas atrial depolarization occurs in one general direction, the ventricles depolarize in three directions. Immediately after the impulse delay period, initial depolarization of the ventricles begins in the septal area just below the AV node, as shown in Figure 5-7(c). Because the walls of the left ventricle are thicker than the walls of the right ventricle, the depolarizing wave travels from left to right, causing the left side of the body to become negative while the right side becomes positive. This is recorded as the *Q wave,* which appears below the baseline (negative) in Figure 5-7(a). Normally the amplitude of the Q wave is less than the amplitude of the P wave and is not seen in some tracings.

Figure 5-7(d) shows the R wave vector representing the depolarization of most (but not quite all) of the remaining ventricular musculature. Because the ventricular muscle is massive (compared to the atrial muscle), the R wave vector is shown longer than the vector illustrating atrial depolarization. However, their directions are nearly the same (from the top of the heart toward the apex). Therefore in Figure 5-7(a) the recorded R wave, like the P wave, appears above the baseline, but its peak amplitude value is much greater than the value of the P wave. The R wave is usually the most prominent feature in the ECG. The normal peak value of the R wave is approximately 1 mV (from baseline to peak) when measured at the surface of the body and about 40 mV when measured inside the heart.

The *S wave* vector shown in Figure 5-7(e) represents the depolarization of the remaining portion of the ventricles. Since, for this wave, the apex becomes negative while the AV node area becomes positive, the recorded S wave appears below the baseline in Figure 5-7(a). In general, the amplitude of the S wave is greater than the amplitude of the Q wave. However, for some patients, the S wave amplitude is so small that it is not recorded.

The *QRS complex* is the combined result of the depolarization of the ventricles that occurs as described. Prior to this time interval, the atria are repolarizing. However, because of its small amplitude, the repolarizing wave pattern of the atria is not obtainable at the body's surface. Thus the baseline normally remains flat between the end of the P wave and the start of the QRS complex.

As the ventricles begin to depolarize, they contract. Later they repolarize. Ventricular repolarization is represented by the *T wave.* The *U wave,* if present, is generally believed to be the result of afterpotentials in the ventricular muscle. The U wave is more frequently seen in tracings from infants than from adults, but it may also be seen in tracings from patients with a potassium imbalance or an enlarged heart. Following repolarization, the ventricles relax.

Typical peak amplitude values for a normal ECG (measured at the surface of the body) are as follows:

P wave	0.2 mV
Q wave (if present)	0.1 mV
R wave	0.5 to 1.5 mV
S wave (if present)	0.2 mV
T wave	0.1 to 0.5 mV

Other important characteristics of the ECG are its various intervals and segments identified in Figure 5-8. Typical values for a normal adult with a heart rate of 60 beats per minute (one beat per second) are as follows:

Intervals

P-R	0.12 to 0.20 s
QRS	0.06 to 0.10 s
S-T	0.18 to 0.30 s
Q-T	0.35 to 0.40 s

Segments

P-R	0.04 to 0.80 s
S-T	0.12 to 0.16 s

Typically, the total time needed for one complete cycle of the heart's electrical activity ranges from approximately 0.4 to 0.6 second. During the Q-T interval, the ventricles are refractory. Thus from the onset of the QRS complex to the start of the T wave, the ventricles will not respond to any stimulus. However, during the period of the T wave, some of the ventricular

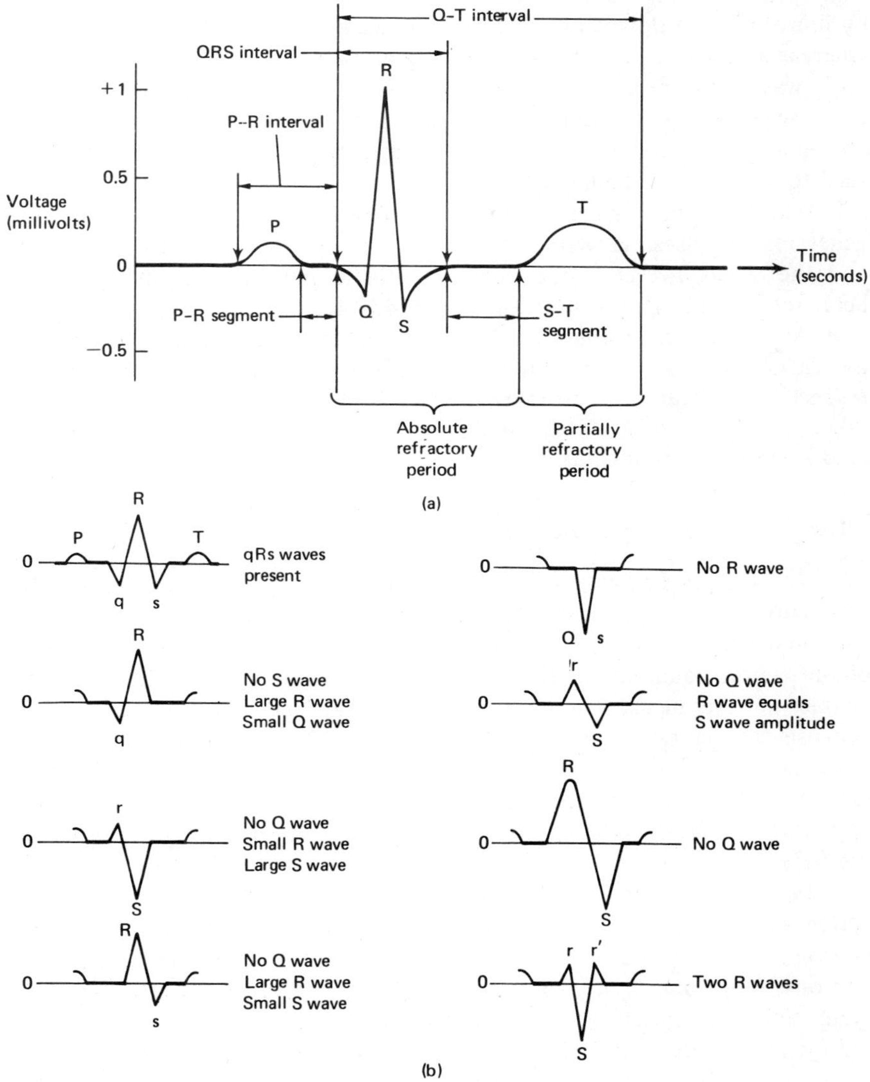

Fig. 5–8 ECG intervals, segments and refractory periods.

cells will respond to a normal stimulus while others remain in their refractory state. This is known as the heart's vulnerable period.

It should be noted that any upward excursion appearing during the QRS interval is, by definition, called an R wave. If a second positive excursion appears during the interval, it is called an R-prime (R′) wave. Also, by convention, a downward deflection preceding an R wave is a Q wave, whereas a downward deflection following an R wave is called an S wave. If no R wave appears in the QRS interval, any downward deflection is called a QS wave. Some examples of the notation applied to waves that occur during the QRS interval are shown in Figure 5-7(b). Lowercase letters are used to signify the smaller deflections.

The heart rate is controlled by the frequency at which the SA node generates impulses. However, nerves of the sympathetic nervous system and the vagus nerve of the parasympathetic nervous system cause the heart rate to quicken or slow down, respectively.

As suggested in Figure 5-8(b), the shape and polarity of each of the ECG features vary with the location of the measuring electrodes with respect to the heart. A cardiologist normally bases a diagnosis on readings taken from several electrode locations. Measurement of the ECG is covered in more detail in Chapter 7.

5.1.6 The Electroencephalogram (EEG)

The recorded representation of the bioelectric potentials generated by the neuronal activity of the brain is called the *electroencephalogram,* abbreviated *EEG.* It was once thought that the EEG is the combined effect of the action potentials in the various cell bodies and nerve fibers in the vicinity of the measuring electrodes. It is now believed, however, that because the pathways and time relationships of action potentials in the brain are almost random in nature, the action potentials contribute very little to the EEG. Instead it is theorized that the bioelectric potentials appearing on the surface of the scalp represent the effect of synchronized *graded potentials* in various combinations of neurons within the brain.

In order to define graded potentials and show their relationship to action potentials, it is necessary to describe briefly the manner in which neurons communicate with each other. Figure 5-9 shows three types of neurons. The *neuron* is the basic unit of the nervous system. In each type, action potentials are initiated in either the cell body or the axon hillock immediately adjacent to the cell body. From there they are propagated down the axon to the axon terminals, where they either initiate contraction of a muscle fiber or communicate with other neurons. In the brain, the axon terminals generally interact with dendrites or cell bodies of other neurons. An interconnection between two neurons is called a *synapse.* There are literally billions of synapses within the brain.

The arrival of an action potential at an axon terminal causes release of a chemical transmitter substance that quickly crosses the narrow gap

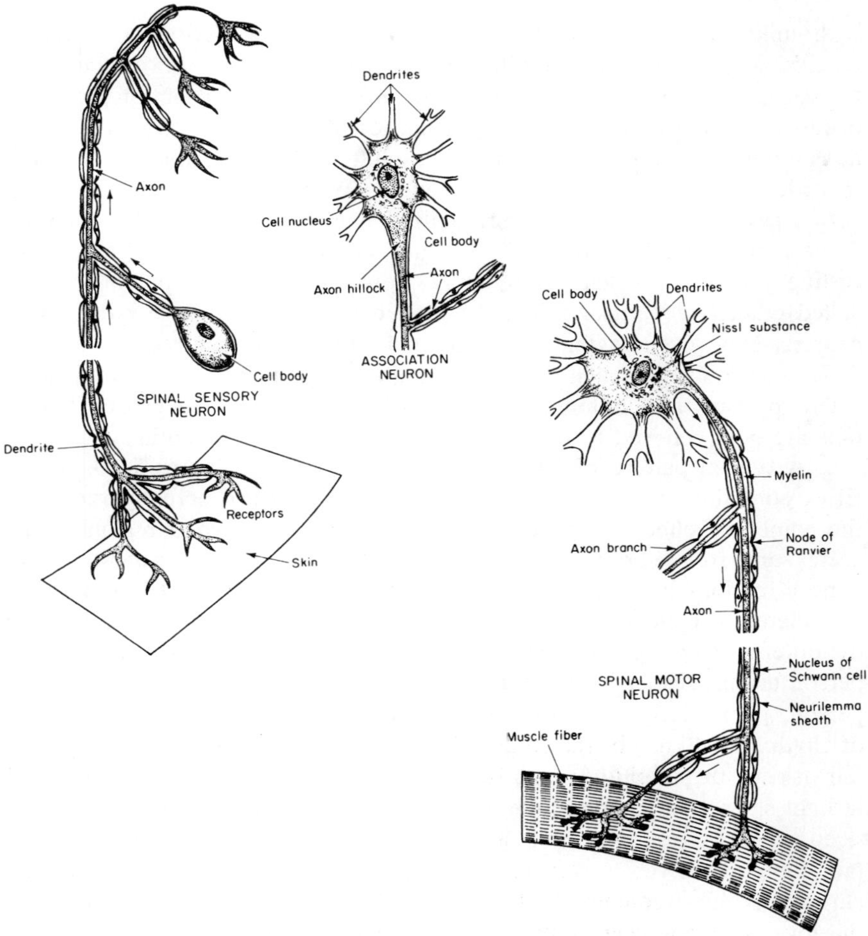

Fig. 5–9 Schematic drawings: Three different types of neurons (from W. F. Evans, *Anatomy and Physiology, The Basic Principles,* Englewood Cliffs, N.J., Prentice-Hall, Inc., 1971, by permission).

of the synapse to act on the membrane of the receiving dendrite or cell body. In an *excitatory synapse,* the effect of the chemical is to reduce the negative resting potential on the inside of the cell a slight amount in order to bring that potential nearer the threshold that would generate an action potential. In an *inhibitory synapse,* the chemical causes the resting potential to become more negative, thus pulling that potential farther away from the threshold. Any given neuron is acted on by a large number of other neurons, some with excitatory synapses and others with inhibitory synapses. If a sufficient number of excitatory synapses receive action potentials simultaneously, the negative resting potential of the receiving neuron is reduced to the threshold and an action potential occurs. If some of the inhibitory synapses also receive action potentials at the same time, a greater number of excitatory synapses must be actuated in order to generate the action potential. With the continual arrival of action potentials at the axon terminals that affect it, the resting potential of each neuron in the brain is changing continuously. These changes in resting potential, which occur more slowly than action potentials, are called *graded potentials*. Often the graded potentials of large numbers of neurons in a given region of the brain become synchronized for a time. This synchronization then breaks up, and other patterns of synchronization occur, perhaps at a different frequency. Such synchronized graded potentials are now believed to be the major source of EEG potentials.

A typical pattern of EEG waveforms appears in Figure 5-10. These EEG potentials, measured at the surface of the scalp, actually represent the combined effect of graded potentials over a fairly wide region of the cortex and from various points beneath. In general, these potentials are almost random in nature. However, certain characteristic EEG patterns are related to epileptic seizures and sleep. The waveforms associated with the different stages of sleep are shown in Figure 5-11. An alert, wideawake person usually displays an unsynchronized high-frequency EEG. A drowsy person, particularly with his eyes closed, often produces a large amount of rhythmic activity in the range of 8 to 13 Hz. As the person begins to fall asleep, the amplitude and frequency of the waveform decrease; and in light sleep a large-amplitude, low-frequency waveform emerges. Deeper sleep generally results in even slower and higher-amplitude waves. At certain times, however, a person, still sound asleep, breaks into an unsynchronized high-frequency EEG pattern for a time and then returns to the low-frequency sleep pattern. The period of high-frequency EEG that occurs during sleep is called *paradoxical sleep* because the EEG is more like that of an awake, alert person than of one who is asleep. Another name is *rapid eye movement* (REM) sleep, for associated with the high-frequency EEG is a large amount of rapid eye movement beneath the closed eyelids. This phenomenon is often associated with dreaming, although it has not been shown conclusively that dreaming is related to REM sleep.

Experiments have shown that the frequency of the EEG seems to be affected by the mental activity of a person. Still, the wide variation among individuals and the lack of repeatability in a given person from one occasion to the next make the establishment of specific relationships difficult.

The various frequency ranges of the EEG have arbitrarily been given Greek-letter designations because frequency seems to be the most promi-

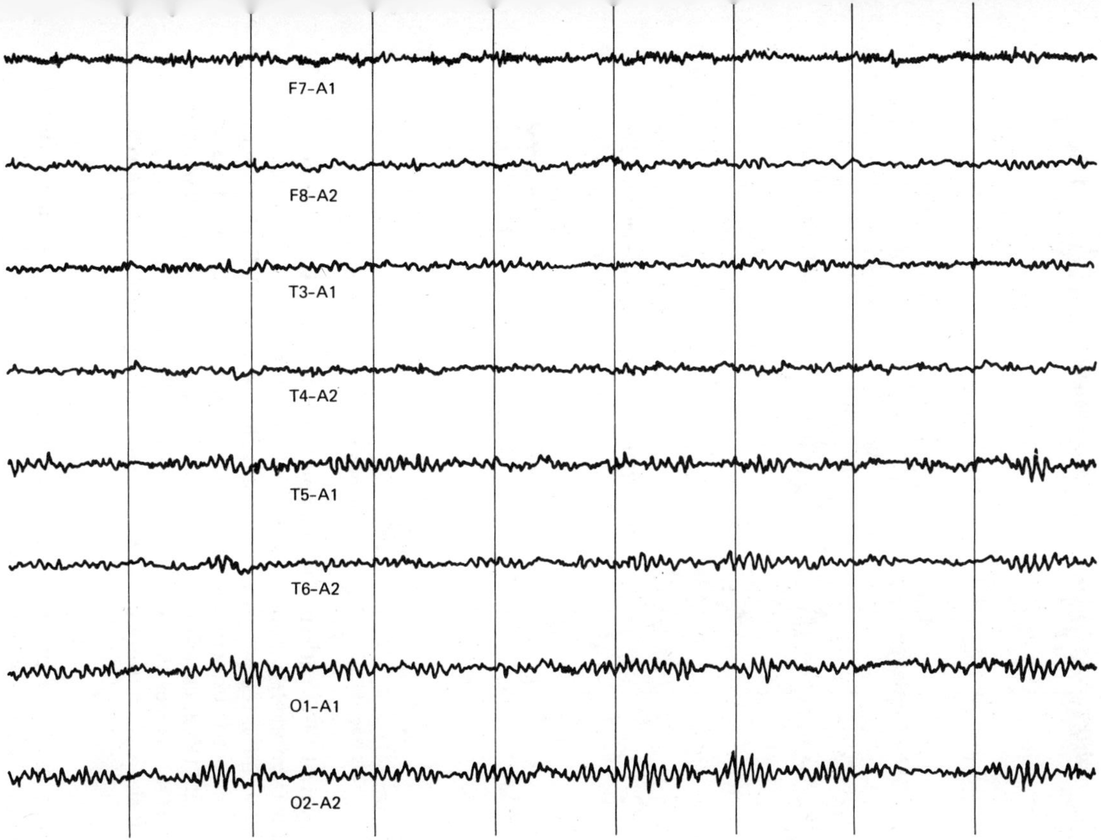

Fig. 5–10 Typical human electroencephalogram. The eight tracings indicate regions of scalp from which each channel of EEG was measured with respect to one of two reference ear electrodes (A1 and A2). (Figure 10–12 shows the layout of the electrodes.) (*Courtesy Veterans Administration Hospital, Sepulveda, California.*)

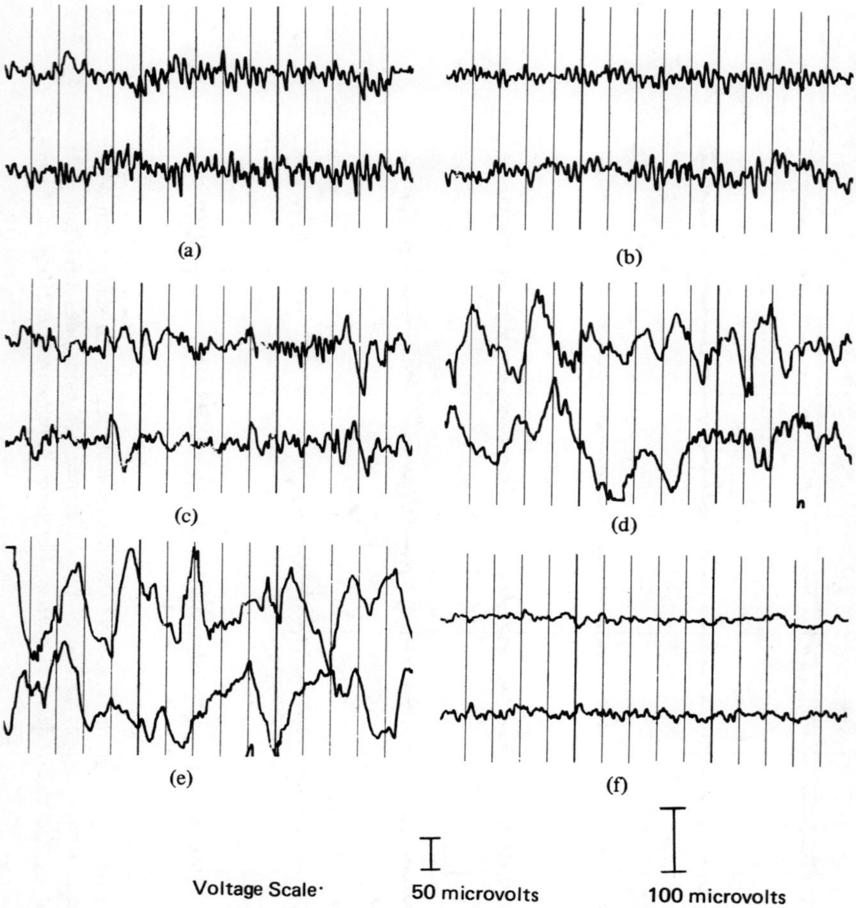

Fig. 5–11 Typical EEG patterns for different stages of sleep. In each case the upper record is from the left frontal region of the brain and the lower tracing is from the right occipital region. (a) Awake and alert—mixed EEG frequencies; (b) Stage 1—subject is drowsy and produces a large amount of alpha waves; (c) Stage 2—light sleep, occasional slow waves appear; (d) Stage 3—slow-wave sleep; (e) Stage 4—deeper slow-wave sleep; (f) Paradoxical or rapid eye movement (REM) sleep. (*Courtesy Veterans Administration Hospital, Sepulveda, California.*)

nent feature of an EEG pattern. Electroencephalographers do not agree on the exact ranges, but most classify the EEG frequency bands or rhythms approximately as follows:

Below 3½ Hz	delta waves
From 3½ Hz to about 8 Hz	theta waves

From about 8 Hz to about 13 Hz	alpha waves
Above 13 Hz	beta waves

The EEG is one of the principal physiological variables used in *biofeedback,* a technique in which information about some seemingly involuntary body process is fed back to a person so that he can learn to control it. In a typical biofeedback experiment with EEG, the brightness of a light or some other indication of the amount of alpha wave activity being received by the measuring electrodes is given a patient. He then learns which physical, mental, or emotional conditions seem to produce the greatest amount of alpha and is able to control these conditions to some extent.

5.1.7 The Electromyogram (EMG)

The bioelectric potentials associated with muscle activity constitute the *electromyogram* (EMG). These potentials may be measured at the surface of the body near a muscle of interest or directly from the muscle by penetrating the skin with needle electrodes. Since the purpose of most EMG measurements is to obtain an indication of the amount of activity of a given muscle, or group of muscles, rather than of an individual muscle fiber, the pattern is usually a summation of the individual action potentials from the fibers constituting the muscle or muscles being measured. As with the EEG, EMG electrodes pick up potentials from all muscles within the range of the electrodes. Consequently, potentials from nearby large muscles may interfere with attempts to measure the EMG from smaller muscles, even though the electrodes are placed directly over the small muscles. Where this is a problem, needle electrodes inserted directly into the muscle are required.

As stated in Section 5.1.2, the action potential of a given muscle (or nerve fiber) has a fixed magnitude regardless of the intensity of the stimulus that generates the response. Thus, in a muscle, the intensity with which the muscle acts does not increase the net height of the action potential pulse but does increase the rate with which each muscle fiber fires and the number of fibers that are activated at any given time. The amplitude of the measured EMG waveform is the instantaneous sum of all the action potentials generated at any given time. Because these action potentials occur in both positive and negative polarities at a given pair of electrodes, they sometimes add and sometimes cancel. Thus the EMG waveform appears very much like a random noise waveform with the energy of the signal a function of the amount of muscle activity and electrode placement. A typical EMG waveform is shown in Figure 5-12. Methods and instrumentation for measuring EMG are described in Chapter 17.

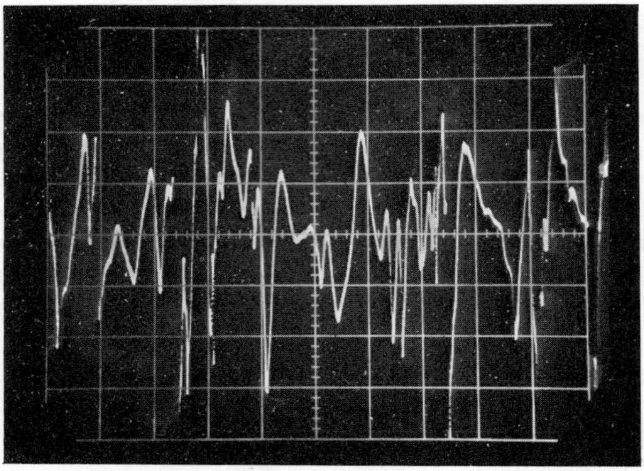

Fig. 5–12 Typical electromyogram waveform. EMG of normal "interference pattern" with full strength muscle contraction producing obliteration of the baseline. Sweep speed is 10 milliseconds per cm; amplitude is 1 millivolt per cm. (*Courtesy of the Veterans Administration Hospital, Portland, Oregon.*)

5.2 Blood Pressure and Flow

Although the electrocardiogram described in Section 5.1.5 reflects the electrical activity of the heart, it does not in any way indicate the effectiveness with which the heart is able to pump blood.

The average adult heart at rest pumps about 5 to 6 liters of blood per minute; and since the volume of blood, on the average, is about 5 liters, a complete circulation takes place every minute during rest. With heavy exercise, the circulation rate is increased considerably. At any given time about 75 to 80% of the blood volume is in the veins, about 20% in the arteries, and the remainder in the microcirculation.

The systemic circulation of blood is the result of pressures developed by the contraction of the musculature of the left ventricle. Figure 5-13 shows the typical values of pressure in the left atrium, left ventricle, and the aorta. The electrocardiogram and heart sounds are included for reference purposes.

In examining the aortic wave, it can be seen that during systole the ejection of blood from the left ventricle is rapid at first. As the rate of pressure change decreases, the rounded maximum of the curve is obtained. The peak aortic pressure during systole is a function of left ventricular stroke volume, the peak rate of ejection, and the distensibility of the walls

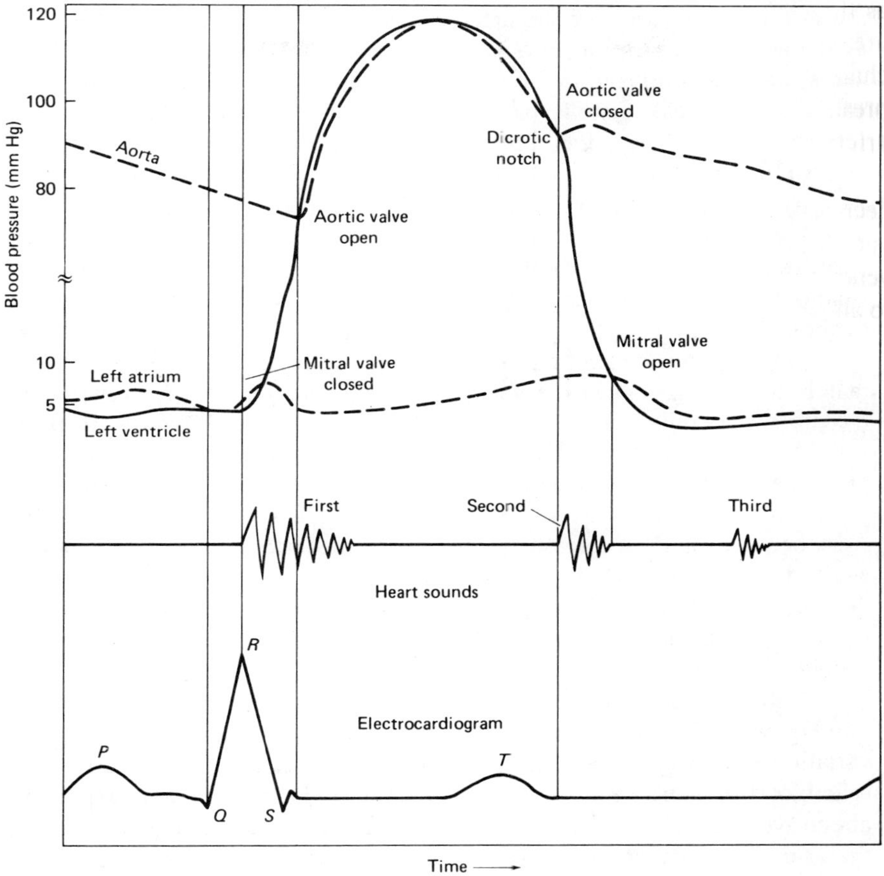

Fig. 5–13 Relationship of heart sounds to function of the cardiovascular system.

of the aorta. In a diseased heart, ventricular contractability and rigid atherosclerotic arteries produce unwanted rises in blood pressure.

When the systolic period is completed, the aortic valve is closed by the back pressure of blood (against the valve). This effect can be seen on the pressure pulse waveform as the *dicrotic notch*. When the valve is closed completely, the arterial pressure gradually decreases as blood pours into the countless peripheral vascular networks. The rate at which the pressure falls is determined by the pressure achieved during the systolic interval, the rate of outflow through the peripheral resistances, and the diastolic interval.

The form of the arterial pressure pulse changes as it passes through the arteries. The walls of the arteries cause damping and reflections; and as the arteries branch out into smaller arteries with smaller cross-sectional areas, the pressures and volumes change, and hence the rate of flow also changes. The peak systolic pressure gets a little higher and the diastolic pressure flatter. The mean pressure in some arteries (e.g., the brachial artery) can be as much as 20 mm Hg higher than that in the aorta.

As the blood flows into the smaller arteries and arterioles, the pressure decreases and loses its oscillatory character. Pressure in the arterioles can vary from about 60 mm Hg down to 30 mm Hg. As the blood enters the venous system after flowing through the capillaries, the pressure is down to about 15 mm Hg.

In the venous system, the pressure in the venules decreases to approximately 8 mm Hg, and in the veins to about 5 mm Hg. In the vena cava, the pressure is only about 2 mm Hg. Because of these differences in pressure, measurement of arterial blood pressure is quite different from that of venous pressure. For example, a 2-mm Hg error in systolic pressure is only of the order of 1.5%. In a vein, however, this would be a 100% error. Also because of these pressure differences, the arteries have thick walls, while the veins have thin walls. Moreover, the veins have larger internal diameters. Since about 75 to 80% of the blood volume is contained in the venous system, the veins tend to serve as a reservoir for the body's blood supply.

Systolic blood pressure in the normal adult is in the range of 95 to 140 mm Hg, with 120 mm Hg being average. These figures are subject to much variation with age, climate, eating habits, and other factors. Normal diastolic blood pressure ranges from 60 to 90 mm Hg, with 80 mm Hg being about average. This pressure is usually measured in the brachial artery in the arm. For comparison purposes, pressures of 130/75 can be expected in the aorta and in the left ventricle, 9/5 in the left atrium, 25/0 in the right ventricle, 3/0 in the right atrium, and 25/12 in the pulmonary artery.

In the hospital, blood pressure is measured within the various chambers of the heart and throughout the circulatory system. Methods of indirect and direct measurement of blood pressure are described in detail in Chapters 8 and 9, respectively.

A summary of typical dimensions, blood flow velocities, and blood pressures at major points in the cardiovascular system is shown in Table 5-1.

The blood flow at any point in the circulatory system is the volume of blood that passes that point during a unit of time. It is normally measured in milliliters per minute or liters per minute. Blood flow is highest in the pulmonary artery and the aorta where these blood vessels leave the heart. The flow at these points, called *cardiac output,* is between 3.5 and 5 l/m in a normal adult at rest. In the capillaries, on the other hand, the blood flow

Table 5-1 Cardiovascular System—Typical Values

Vessel	*Number in Thousands*	*Diameter (mm)*	*Length (mm)*	*Mean Velocity (cm/s)*	*Pressures (mm Hg)*
Aorta	–	10.50	400	40.0	100
Terminal arteries	1.8	0.60	10	$<$10.0	40
Arterioles	40,000	0.02	2	0.5	40–25
Capillaries	$>$million	0.008	1	$<$0.1	25–12
Venules	80,000	0.03	2	$<$0.3	12–8
Terminal veins	1.8	1.50	100	1.0	$<$8
Vena cava	–	12.50	400	20.0	3–2

can be so slow that the travel of individual blood cells can be observed under a microscope.

From the cardiac output or the blood flow in a given vessel, a number of other characteristic variables can be calculated. The cardiac output divided by the number of heartbeats per minute gives the amount of blood ejected during each heartbeat, or the *stroke volume.* If the total amount of blood in circulation is known, and this volume is divided by the cardiac output, the *mean circulation time* is obtained. By dividing the blood flow through a vessel by the cross–sectional area of the vessel, the *mean velocity* of the blood at the point of measurement can be calculated.

In the arteries, blood flow is pulsatile. In fact, in some blood vessels a reversal of the flow can occur during certain parts of the heartbeat cycle. Because of the elasticity of their walls, the blood vessels tend to smooth out the pulsations of blood flow and blood pressure.

Blood flow depends on the blood pressure and the flow resistance of the blood vessels in the same way as electric current flow depends on voltage and resistance. The flow resistance of the capillary bed, however, can vary over a wide range. For instance, when exposed to low temperatures or under the influence of certain drugs (e.g., nicotine), the body reduces the blood flow through the skin by *vasoconstriction* (narrowing) of the capillaries. Heat, excitement, or local inflammation, among other factors, can cause *vasodilation* (widening) of the capillaries, which increases the blood flow, at least locally. Because of the wide variations that are possible in the flow resistance, the determination of blood pressure alone is not sufficient to assess the status of the circulatory system.

The velocity of blood flowing through a vessel is not constant throughout the cross section of the vessel but is a function of the distance from the wall surfaces. The velocity is zero at the wall, with the highest velocity occurring at the center of the vessel. Some blood flow meters measure the mean velocity of the blood instead of the blood flow. If, however, the cross-sectional area of the blood vessel is known, these devices can be calibrated directly in terms of blood flow.

If the local blood velocity exceeds a certain limit (as may happen when a blood vessel is constricted), small eddies can occur, and the *laminar flow* changes to a *turbulent flow* pattern for which the flow rate is more difficult to determine.

Direct quantitative measurement of blood flow in specific vessels is seldom done clinically, since presently available methods require exposure of the vessel. Qualitative procedures, however, can be used to indicate the existence of significant blood flow in a vessel or region of the body. Cardiac output, stroke volume, total blood volume, and mean circulation time are measured routinely. Other variables and parameters related to cardiac output and the flow of blood include variations in the size of the ventricles through the complete cardiac cycle, *pulse wave velocity* (the rate at which the arterial pulse travels from the heart to some point in the arterial system), and estimates of regional blood flow. Instrumentation and techniques for measuring these variables are described in Chapter 12.

5.3 Heart Sounds

For centuries the medical profession has been helped in its diagnosis of certain types of heart disorders by the sounds and vibrations associated with the beating of the heart and the pumping of blood. The technique of listening to sounds produced by the organs and vessels of the body is called *auscultation,* and it is still in common use today. During training the physician or practitioner learns to recognize sounds or changes in sounds that can be associated with various types of disorders.

In spite of its widespread use, however, auscultation is rather subjective, and the amount of information that can be obtained by listening to the sounds of the heart depends largely on the skill, experience, and hearing ability of the physician or nurse. Thus different people may hear the same sounds differently and perhaps interpret them differently.

The heart sounds occur at the time of closure of major valves in the heart. This timing could easily lead to the false assumption that the sounds are primarily caused by the snapping together of the vanes of these valves. In reality, this snapping action produces almost no sound because of the cushioning effect of the blood. The principal cause of heart sounds seems to be vibrations set up in the blood inside the heart by the sudden closure of the valves. These vibrations, together with eddy currents induced in the blood as it is forced through the closing valves, produce vibrations in the walls of the heart chambers and in the adjoining blood vessels.

A graphic representation of the heart sounds is included in Figure 5-13.

The first heart sound is caused by the closure of the atrioventricular valves and occurs approximately at the time of the QRS complex of the ECG. The second heart sound is caused by closure of the semilunar valves, which release blood into the systemic and pulmonary circulation systems. These valves close at the end of systole, just before the atrioventricular valves reopen. The second heart sound occurs about the time of the end of the T wave of the ECG.

A third heart sound is sometimes heard, especially in young adults. This sound, which occurs from 0.1 to 0.2 seconds after the second heart sound, is attributed to the rush of blood from the atria into the ventricles, which causes turbulence and some vibration of the ventricular walls. The sound actually precedes atrial contraction, which means that the inrush of blood to the ventricles causing this sound is passive, pushed only by the venous pressure at the inlets to the atria and pulled by the force of gravity into the ventricles. Actually, about 70% of blood flow into the ventricles occurs before atrial contraction.

A so-called atrial heart sound, which is not audible but may be visible on a graphic recording, occurs when the atria actually do contract, squeezing the remainder of the blood into the ventricles. The inaudibility of this heart sound is a result of low amplitude and low frequency of the vibrations.

In abnormal hearts, additional sounds called *murmurs* may be heard between the normal heart sounds. Murmurs are generally caused either by improper opening of the valves (which requires the blood to be forced through a small aperture) or by regurgitation, which results when the valves do not close completely and allow some backward flow of blood. In either case, the sound is due to high-velocity blood flow through a small opening. Another cause of murmurs can be a small opening in the septum, which separates the left and right sides of the heart. In this case, pressure differences between the two sides of the heart force blood through the opening, usually from the left ventricle into the right ventricle, bypassing the systemic circulation.

Normal heart sounds are quite short in duration, approximately one-tenth of a second for each, while murmurs usually extend between the normal sounds. There is also a difference in frequency range between normal and abnormal heart sounds. The first heart sound is composed primarily of energy in the 30– to 45–Hz range, with much of the sound below the threshold of audibility. The second heart sound is usually higher in pitch than the first, with maximum energy in the 50– to 70–Hz range. The third heart sound is an extremely weak vibration, with most of its energy at or below 30 Hz. Murmurs, on the other hand, often produce much higher pitched sounds. One particular type of regurgitation, for example, causes a murmur in the 100– to 600–Hz range.

Although auscultation is still the principal method of detecting and analyzing heart sounds, other techniques are often employed. For example, a graphic recording of heart sounds, such as shown in Figure 5-13, is called a *phonocardiogram*. Even though the phonocardiogram is a graphic record, like the electrocardiogram, it extends to a much higher frequency range.

An entirely different waveform is produced by the vibrations of the heart against the thoracic cavity. The vibrations of the side of the heart as it thumps against the chest wall form the *vibrocardiogram,* whereas the tip or apex of the heart hitting the rib cage produces the *apex cardiogram*.

Sounds and pulsations can also be detected and measured at various locations in the systemic arterial circulation system where major arteries approach the surface of the body. The most common one is the *pulse,* which can be felt with the fingertips at certain points on major arteries. The waveform of this pulse can also be measured and recorded. In addition, when an artery is partially occluded so that the blood velocity through the constriction is increased sufficiently, identifiable sounds can be heard downstream through a stethoscope. These sounds, called the *Korotkoff sounds,* are used in the common method of blood pressure measurements and are discussed in detail in Chapter 8.

Another cardiovascular measurement worthy of note is the *ballistocardiogram*. Although not a heart sound or vibration measurement of the type described earlier, the ballistocardiogram is related to these measurements in that it is a direct result of the dynamic forces of the heart as it beats and pumps blood into the major arteries. The beating heart exerts certain forces on the body as it goes through its sequence of motions. As in any situation involving forces, the body responds, but because of the greater mass of the body, these responses are generally not noticeable. However, when a person is placed on a platform that is free to move with these small dynamic responses, the motions of the body due to the beating of the heart and the corresponding blood ejection can be measured and recorded to produce the ballistocardiogram. Like the vibrocardiogram and the apex cardiogram, the ballistocardiogram provides information about the heart that cannot be obtained by any other measurement.

5.4 Temperature Measurement

Body temperature is one of the oldest known indicators of the general well-being of a person. Techniques and instruments for the measurement of temperature have been commonplace in the home for years and throughout all kinds of industry, as well as in the hospital. Except for the narrow range required for physiological temperature measurements and the size and shape of the sensing element, instrumentation for measurement of temperature in the human body differs very little from that found in various industrial applications.

Two basic types of temperature measurements can be obtained from the human body: systemic and skin surface measurements. Both provide valuable diagnostic information, although the systemic temperature measurement is much more commonly used.

Systemic temperature is the temperature of the internal regions of the body. This temperature is maintained through a carefully controlled balance between the heat generated by the active tissues of the body, mainly the muscles and the liver, and the heat lost by the body to the environment. Measurement of systemic temperature is accomplished by temperature-sensing devices placed in the mouth, under the armpits, or in the rectum. The normal oral (mouth) temperature of a healthy person is about 98.6°F (37°C). The underarm temperature is about one degree lower, and the rectal temperature is about one degree higher than the oral reading. The systemic body temperature can be measured most accurately at the tympanic membrane in the ear, which is believed to approximate the temperature at the "inaccessible" temperature control center in the brain.

Surface or skin temperature is also a result of a balance, but here the balance is between the heat supplied by blood circulation in a local area and the cooling of that area by conduction, radiation, convection, and evaporation. Thus skin temperature is a function of the surface circulation, environmental temperature, and air circulation around the area from which the measurement is to be taken. In order to obtain a meaningful skin temperature measurement, it is usually necessary to have the subject remain with no clothing covering the region of measurement in a fairly cool ambient temperature (around 70°F). Care must be taken, however, to avoid chilling and the reactions relative to chilling. If a surface measurement is to include the reaction to the cooling of a local region, it should be recognized that the cooling of the skin increases surface circulation, which in turn causes some local warming of adjacent areas. Heat transferred into the site of measurement from adjacent areas of the body must also be taken into account.

5.5 Variables in the Respiratory System

The exchange of gases in any biological process is termed *respiration.* To sustain life, the human body must take in oxygen, which combines with carbon, hydrogen, and other elements furnished by food material to produce heat and energy for the performance of work. As a result of this process of *metabolism,* which takes place in the cells, a certain amount of water is produced along with the principal waste product, carbon dioxide (CO_2). The entire process of taking in oxygen from the environment, transporting the oxygen to the cells, removing the carbon dioxide from the cells, and exhausting this waste product into the atmosphere must be considered within the definition of respiration.

In the human body, the tissue cells generally are not in direct contact with their external environment. Instead the cells are bathed in fluid. This tissue fluid can be considered as the *internal environment* of the body. The cells absorb oxygen from this fluid and discharge waste materials, including carbon dioxide, into the fluid. The circulatory blood is the medium by which oxygen is brought to the internal environment. Carbon dioxide is carried from the tissue fluids by the same mechanism. The exchange of gases between the blood and the external environment takes place in the *lungs* and is termed *external respiration.*

The function of the lungs is to oxygenate the blood and to eliminate carbon dioxide in a controlled manner. During inspiration fresh air enters the respiratory tract, becomes humidified and heated to body temperature, and is mixed with the gases already present in the region comprising the trachea and bronchi. This gas is then mixed further with the gas residing in the alveoli as it enters these small sacs in the wall of the lungs. Oxygen diffuses from the alveoli to the pulmonary capillary blood supply, whereas carbon dioxide diffuses from the blood to the alveoli. The oxygen is carried from the lungs and distributed among the various cells of the body by the blood circulation system, which also returns the carbon dioxide to the lungs. The entire process of inspiring and expiring air, exchange of gases, distribution of oxygen to the cells, and collection of CO_2 from the cells forms what is known as the *pulmonary function.* Tests for assessing the various components of the process are called *pulmonary function tests.*

The field of instrumentation for obtaining pulmonary measurements is quite complex. However, tests and instrumentation for the measurement of respiration can be divided into two categories. The first includes tests designed to measure the mechanics of breathing and the physical characteristics of the lungs; the second category concerns the diffusion of gases in the lungs, the distribution of oxygen, and the collection of carbon dioxide.

Breathing is accomplished by musculature that literally changes the volume of the thoracic cavity and, in so doing, creates negative and positive pressures that move air into and out of the lungs. Two sets of muscles are involved: those in and near the diaphragm that cause the diaphragm to move up and down, changing the size of the thoracic cavity in the vertical direction, and those that move the rib cage up and down to change the lateral diameter of the thorax.

The *diaphragm* is a special dome- or bell-shaped muscle located at the bottom of the thoracic cavity, which, when contracted, pulls downward to enlarge the thorax. This action is the principal force involved in inspiration. At the same time as the diaphragm moves downward, a group of external intercostal muscles lifts the rib cage and sternum. Because of the shape of the rib cage, this lifting action also increases the effective diameter of the thoracic cavity. The resulting increase in thoracic volume creates a negative pressure (vacuum) in the thorax. Since the thorax is a closed chamber and the only opening to the outside is from the inside of the lungs, the negative pressure is relieved by air entering the lungs. The lungs themselves are passive and expand only because of the internal pressure of air in the lungs, which is greater than the pressure in the thorax outside the lungs.

Normal expiration is essentially passive, for, on release of the inspiratory muscles, the elasticity of the lungs and the rib cage, combined with the tone of the diaphragm, reduces the volume of the thorax, thereby developing a positive pressure that forces air out of the lungs. In forced expiration a set of abdominal muscles pushes the diaphragm upward very powerfully while the internal intercostal muscles pull the rib cage downward and apply pressure against the lungs to help force air out.

During normal inspiration the pressure inside the lungs, the *intra-alveolar pressure,* is about —3 mm Hg, whereas during expiration the pressure becomes about +3 mm Hg. The ability of the lungs and thorax to expand during breathing is called the *compliance,* which is expressed as the volume increase in the lungs per unit increase in intra-alveolar pressure. The resistance to the flow of air into and out of the lungs is called *airway resistance.*

Assessment of the physical characteristics of the lungs consists primarily of measuring a number of lung volumes and capacities. Often these measurements are made during special breathing tests. These volumes and capacities and the various tests involved are described in detail in Chapter 14, along with the required instrumentation. Other tests concerned with the mechanics of breathing require measurement of intra-alveolar and intra-thoracic pressures and instantaneous airflow. These variables and associated instrumentation are also included in Chapter 14, as are methods of assessing the diffusion of gases in the lungs and measuring the concentrations of oxygen and carbon dioxide in the expired air and the blood.

5.6 Other Physiological Variables

The preceding sections of this chapter describe a number of physiological variables commonly used in clinical medicine. Instrumentation and techniques for measuring these variables are discussed in subsequent chapters.

Although an attempt was made to include those variables of most significance to the nurse or paramedical practitioner, an exhaustive coverage of all physiological variables of clinical interest is not claimed. In addition, there are many physiological variables that may be involved in research but that are not generally used in the clinical setting.

6

Electrodes

In observing the measurement of an electrocardiogram (ECG) or some other form of bioelectric potential, as discussed in Chapter 5, one could conclude that the measuring electrodes are simply terminals or contact points with which voltages can be obtained at the surface of the body. This conclusion, however, is incorrect and does not satisfy the theory that explains the origin of these bioelectric potentials. It must be realized that the bioelectric potentials generated in the body are ionic potentials, produced by ionic current flow. In order to measure these ionic potentials efficiently, they must be converted into electronic potentials before they can be measured by conventional methods. Realization of this fact led to the development of the modern noise-free, stable measuring devices now available.

As noted in Chapter 5, devices that convert ionic potentials into electronic potentials are called *electrodes*. The theory of electrodes and the principles governing their design and performance are inherent in an understanding of the measurement of bioelectric potentials. This same theory also applies to electrodes found in chemical transducers, such as those used to measure pH, P_{O_2}, and P_{CO_2} of the blood. Electrodes for blood gas analysis are discussed in Chapter 14. This chapter describes electrodes used in measuring bioelectric potentials, dealing first with the basic theory of electrodes and then with the various types used in medical instrumentation.

6.1 Electrode Theory and Characteristics

In their simplest form, electrodes used to measure biopotentials are pieces of metal that may be placed on or inside the body, whose fluids, as noted in Chapter 3, may be considered as electrolytes. When a metal comes in contact with an electrolytic solution, an electrochemical reaction produces a difference of potential (a voltage) between the metal and the solution. The chemical reactions that occur between metals and electrolytes influence the performance of physiological electrodes. They also form the basis of the ordinary battery, or voltaic cell. Therefore the chemical principles of the simple voltaic cell shown in Figure 6-1 can be used to explain electrode theory.

In Figure 6-1(a) a silver electrode is shown in a salt solution, the electrolyte. Because silver is a good conductor of electricity, it has an abundance of loosely held or relatively free valence electrons (see Chapter 3). When silver is placed in an electrolyte, some of its valence electrons enter the solution, causing the previously electrically neutral electrode to become positively charged with respect to the electrolyte. The resulting potential difference is called a *half-cell potential,* one of two potentials associated with a voltaic cell or battery. For silver placed in an electrolyte, the half-cell voltage is approximately 0.8 V, so that the electrode is positive with respect to the electrolyte. When a copper electrode is placed in the electrolyte, as shown in Figure 6-1(b), some of its valence electrons also enter the solution, causing the copper electrode to become positively charged with respect to the electrolyte. The value of this half-cell potential is approximately 0.3 V, so that the copper electrode is also positive with respect to the electrolyte. Figure 6-1(c) shows both metals placed in the electrolyte. Since the half-cell potentials for the silver and copper electrodes are 0.8V and 0.3V respectively, and both electrodes are positive with respect to the electrolyte, the difference of potential between the electrodes equals 0.5 V (+0.8 V minus +0.3 V = 0.5 V). The silver electrode is positive with respect to the copper electrode. In this way, two dissimilar metals in contact with a common electrolyte produce a dc voltage between their terminals and may be used to form a battery. From the foregoing it follows that two *similar* metals in contact with a common electrolyte should produce no difference of potential between them, as illustrated in Figure 6-2.

Figure 6-2(a) shows a cross section of two silver plates used as biopotential electrodes in contact with the surface of the skin, which acts as an

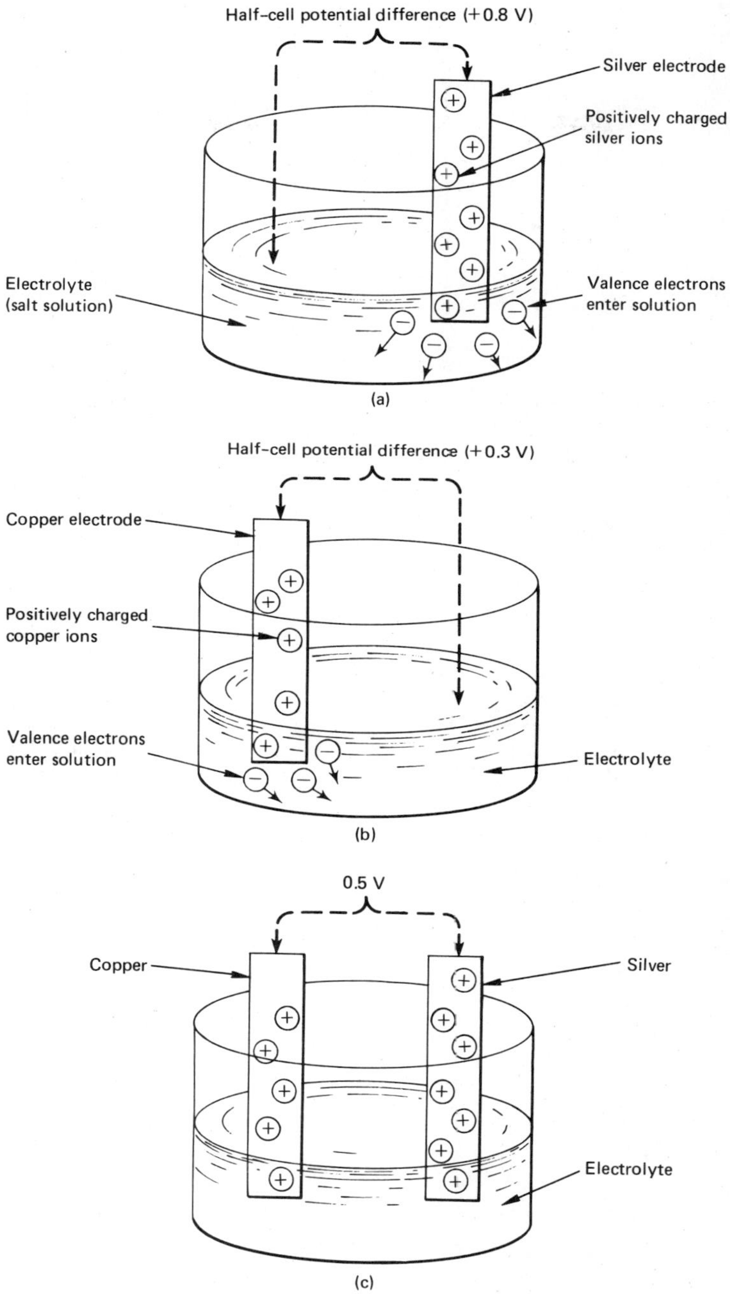

Fig. 6–1 Metal-electrolyte chemical reactions: (a) silver electrode half-cell potential; (b) copper electrode half-cell potential; (c) resulting terminal voltage.

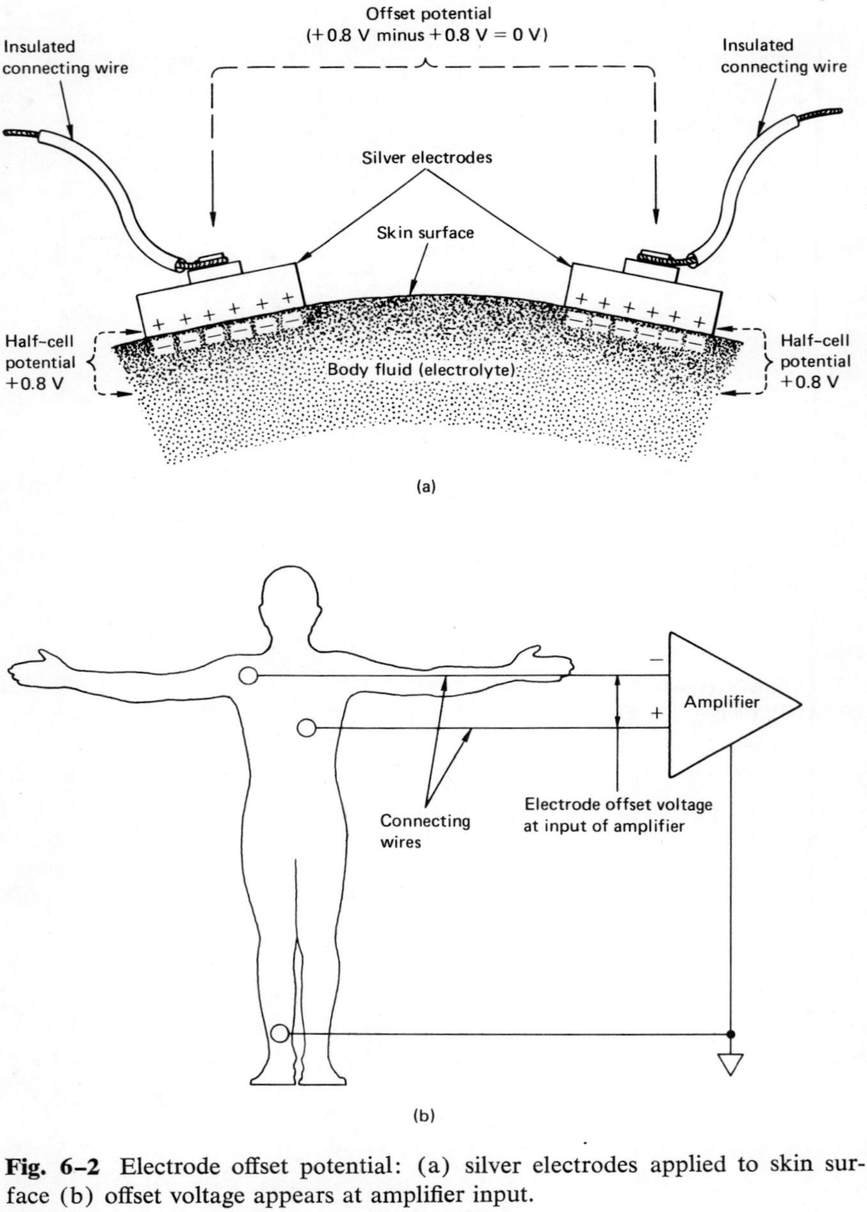

Fig. 6–2 Electrode offset potential: (a) silver electrodes applied to skin surface (b) offset voltage appears at amplifier input.

electrolyte. If chemically identical, the metals will each develop equal half-cell potentials, and the resulting voltage between the electrodes will equal zero.

The difference of potential between the terminals of physiological electrodes in contact with the body is called the *electrode offset voltage.* If the electrodes shown in Figure 6-2(a) were chemically identical (an ideal supposition), the value of offset voltage would equal zero. In practice, even matched electrodes have some chemical differences. Thus some value of offset voltage usually occurs between the terminals of applied physiological electrodes. When, as shown in Figure 6-2(b), the electrodes are connected through wires to the input of an amplifier, the amplifier will respond to the resulting dc offset voltage as well as to the physiological variable obtained from the body.

The values and polarities of electrode half-cell potentials depend largely on the types of materials used. As shown in Figure 6-2(a), the silver electrode in contact with an electrolyte produces a +0.8 V half-cell potential, which is approximately 800 times greater than the value of the ECG that may be measured at the surface of the body. Even when closely matched electrodes are used, the resulting dc offset voltage may still greatly exceed the value of the physiological variable to be measured. A large offset voltage may interfere with or influence the desired measurement and cause undesired artifacts.

Experiments have shown that the chemical activity that takes place within an electrode can cause voltage fluctuations (noise) to appear without any physiological input. Such variations may also appear as artifacts. Both the half-cell potential and noise can be reduced by proper choice of electrode materials or, in some cases, by special treatment. It has been found that the *silver-silver chloride (Ag-AgCl) electrode* is the most stable type of electrode and that its electrode potential is low in value. This type of electrode is prepared by chemically coating a piece of nearly pure silver with silver chloride, a salt. The coating is normally done by placing a cleaned piece of silver in a sodium-chloride solution. A second piece of silver is also placed in the solution, and the two are connected to a dc voltage source such that the electrode to be chlorided is made positive with respect to the other. The silver ions then combine with chloride ions from the salt solution to produce a thin film of neutral silver chloride molecules that coats the silver electrode. When this type of electrode is cleaned after use, care must be taken not to damage the silver chloride coating. These electrodes may be cleaned with a soft cotton-tipped swab and isopropyl alcohol or lukewarm water.

When an electrode contacts the skin surface, a certain amount of electrical resistance exists at the electrode-skin interface. Reliable artifact-free physiological recordings require that the electrodes make good (low-resistance) contact with the skin. Since the top layer of skin consists largely of dead cells, along with a certain amount of oil and grime, the skin's natural electrical resistance is high compared to the resistance of the body's fluids.

Thus in applying skin-surface electrodes, the electrode site is usually prepared or treated in order to lower the skin resistance. The layer of dead cells may be removed from the electrode site with alcohol or some other suitable cleansing agent. A commercially available conductive (electrolytic) jelly or paste should then be applied between the electrode and the skin so as to form a bridge between the ions in the body and the electrode surface and to ensure a low value of electrode-skin interface resistance. Some pastes contain very fine abrasive particles in the electrolyte. These pastes may be used both to prepare the electrode site and to lower the contact resistance.

The size and type of electrodes to be used are also important in determining the electrode resistance. Larger electrodes tend to have lower resistance. Surface electrodes generally have resistances of 2000 to 10,000 Ω, whereas small needle electrodes have much higher resistances.

6.2 Biopotential Electrodes

Electrodes used to obtain bioelectric potentials from the body are found in many sizes and forms. Although any type of electrode can be used to sense ECG, EEG, or EMG potentials, the larger electrodes are usually associated with ECG, since localization of the measurement is not important. Smaller electrodes are used in EEG and EMG measurements and in fetal monitoring.

The earliest bioelectric potential measurements used *immersion electrodes,* which were simply buckets of saline solution into which the subject placed his hands and feet, one bucket for each extremity. As might be expected, this type of electrode (Figure 6-3) presented many difficulties, such as restricted position of the subject and danger of electrolyte spillage.

A great improvement over the immersion electrodes were the *plate electrodes* (Figure 6-4), first introduced about 1917. Originally these electrodes were separated from the subject's skin by cotton or felt pads soaked in a saline solution. Later, conductive jelly replaced the soaked pads and the metal was allowed to contact the skin. Plate electrodes of this type are still in use today, as well as saline-soaked gauze pads.

Another fairly old type of electrode still in use is the *suction-cup electrode* shown in Figure 6-5. In this type, only the rim actually contacts the skin. Suction-cup electrodes are available in two sizes. The size usually applied to adults has a cup diameter of approximately 30 mm; a smaller size (15-mm diameter cup) is designed for infant use. Ordinarily, suction-cup electrodes are used for the chest lead for the ECG (see Chapter 7).

One of the difficulties in using plate electrodes is the possibility of electrode slippage or movement. This problem also occurs with the suction-

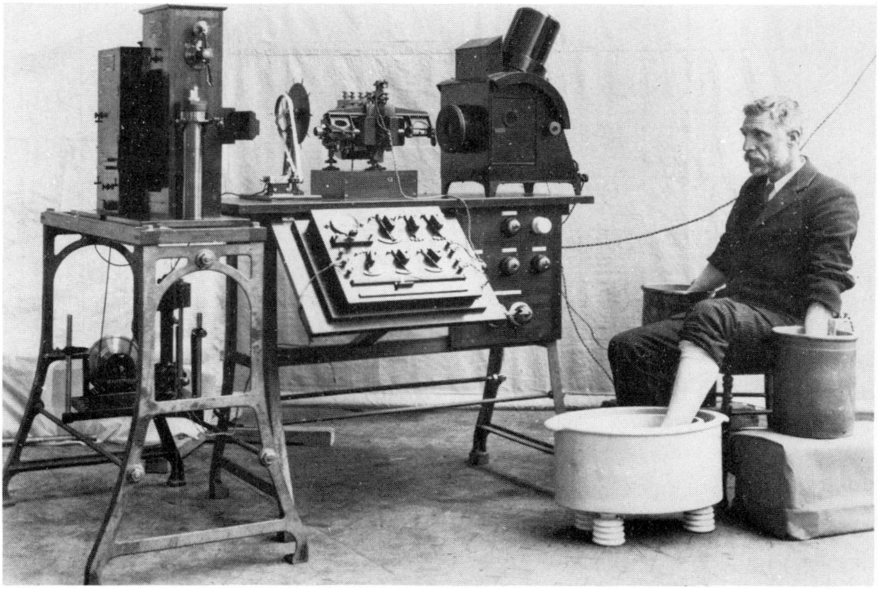

Fig. 6–3 ECG measurement using immersion electrodes. Original Cambridge electrocardiograph (1912) produced under agreement with Prof. Willem Einthoven, the father of electrocardiography. (*Courtesy of Cambridge Instruments, Cambridge, Massachusetts.*)

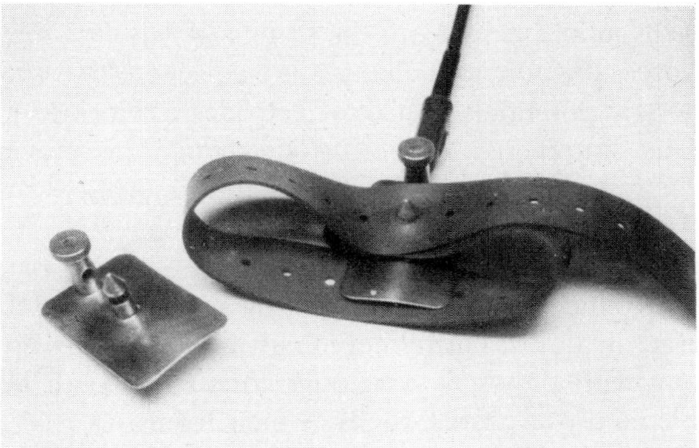

Fig. 6–4 Metal plate electrodes. These are usually made of or plated with, silver, nickel, or some similar alloy.

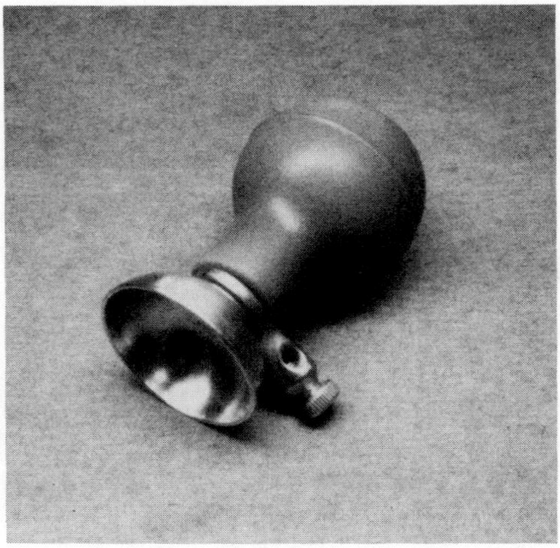

Fig. 6–5 Suction cup electrode.

cup electrode after a sufficient length of time. A number of solutions were sought, including the use of adhesive backing and a surface resembling a nutmeg grater that penetrates the skin to lower the contact resistance and reduce the likelihood of slippage.

All the preceding electrodes suffer from a common problem. All are sensitive to movement, some to a greater degree than others. Even the slightest movement changes the thickness of the thin film of electrolyte between metal and skin and thus causes changes in the offset potential and contact resistance. These changes appear as motion artifacts on ECG tracings or patient monitors and are the source of *baseline drift* or *wandering*. In many cases, the potential changes are so severe that they completely block the bioelectric potentials that the electrodes attempt to measure. The adhesive tape and "nutmeg grater" electrode reduce this movement artifact by limiting electrode movement and reducing interface resistance, but neither is satisfactorily insensitive to movement.

More recently, a new type of electrode, the *floating or fluid column electrode,* was introduced in varying forms by several manufacturers. Here movement artifact is almost entirely eliminated by avoiding any direct contact of the metal with the skin. The only conductive path between metal and skin is the column of paste or jelly, which forms an electrolyte bridge. Even with the electrode surface held at a right angle with the skin surface, performance is not impaired as long as the electrolyte bridge maintains contact with both the skin and the electrode. Figure 6-6 illustrates a cross section of a floating electrode and Figure 6-7 shows a typical floating electrode. It can be seen that the electrode's metal surface is recessed and cannot directly contact the skin.

Floating electrodes are generally attached to the skin by means of two-

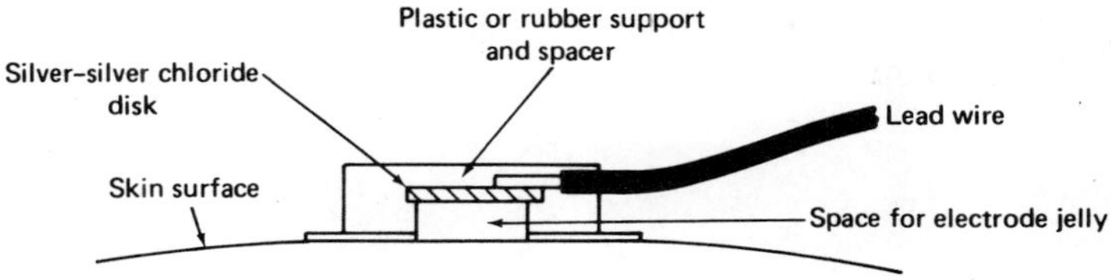

Fig. 6–6 Diagram of a floating skin-surface electrode.

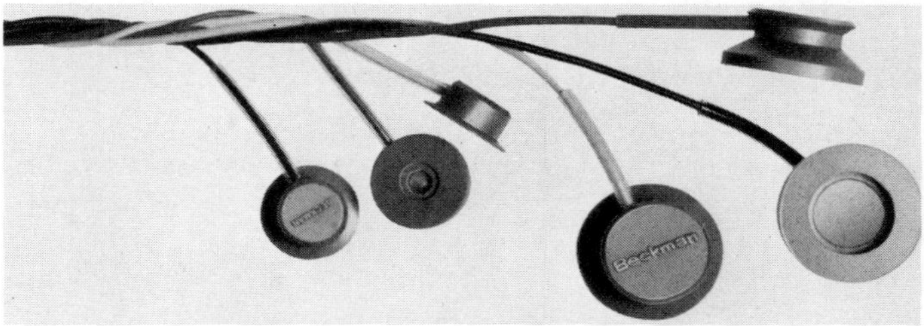

Fig. 6–7 Side, bottom, and top views of a floating skin-surface electrode. *(Courtesy of Beckman Instruments, Inc., Fullerton, California.)*

sided adhesive collars (or rings), which adhere to the plastic surface of the electrode and the skin.

Various types of *disposable electrodes* have been introduced within the last few years to eliminate the usual requirement for cleaning and care after each use and to facilitate application. Primarily intended for ECG monitoring, these electrodes can also be used for EEG and EMG measurements. In general, disposable electrodes are of the floating type with simple snap connectors by which the connecting wires (which are reusable) are attached. Some disposable electrodes are prejelled by the manufacturer to eliminate the need to apply jelly between the electrode and the prepared skin surface.

One of the new developments is a disposable electrode that requires neither conductive jelly nor skin preparation. This pasteless electrode contains a column of electrolytic fluid and a thin-film permeable membrane used to contact the skin. When applied to the skin, the microporous membrane allows the electrolyte to keep the skin's surface moist, thus eliminating the need to prepare the electrode site.

Through recent improvements, disposable electrodes can be used for extended periods of time in continuous patient-monitoring applications with little discomfort to the patient. Flexible plastic electrode supports or cups and soft foam-plastic adhesive rings allow these electrodes to conform to the body's contour. Also, when applied to the skin, the foam-plastic rings tend to prevent air from reaching the electrode and drying the jelly. Thus low skin resistance is maintained for relatively long periods of time. Some typical disposable electrodes are shown in Figure 6-8.

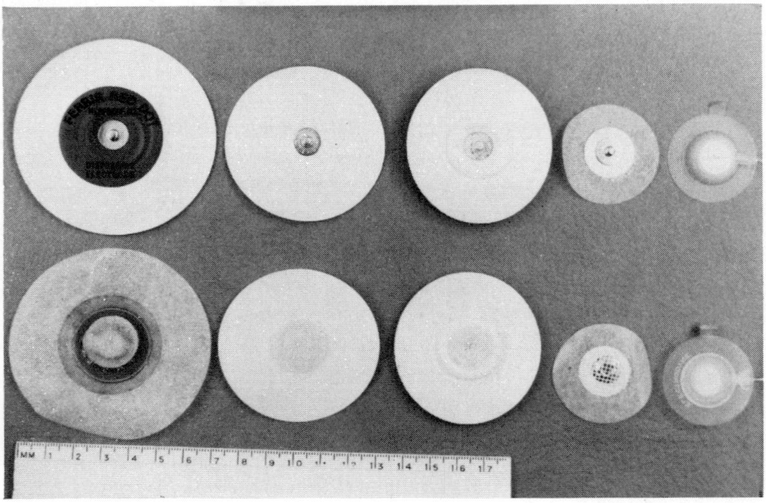

Fig. 6–8 Typical disposable electrodes (top and bottom views).

All skin electrodes used for continuous monitoring should be periodically repositioned to nearby sites on the patient's skin because of the high incidence of skin irritation that the electrolyte medium and adhesive may cause. Some special care units have a policy of repositioning and changing the electrodes (if disposable) every 8 hours; others do so at least once every 24 hours, depending on the sensitivity of the patient's skin.

Special types of surface electrodes have been developed for other applications. For example, an *ear clip electrode* (Figure 6-9) was de-

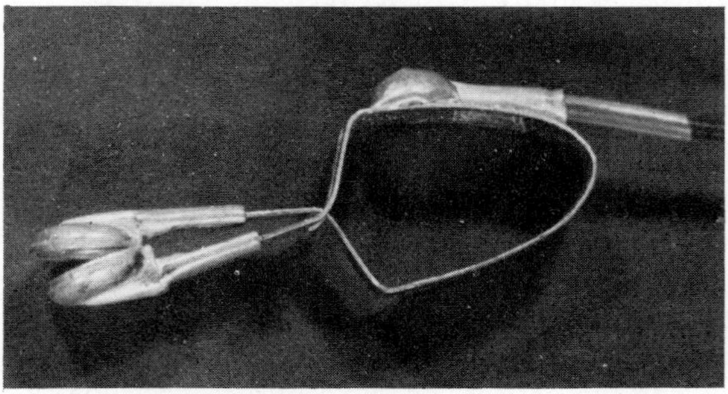

Fig. 6–9 Ear clip electrodes. (*Courtesy of Veterans Administration Hospital, Sepulveda, California.*)

veloped for use as a reference electrode for EEG measurements. *Scalp surface electrodes* for the measurement of EEG are usually small disks about 7 mm in diameter or small solder pellets that are placed on the cleaned scalp via an electrolyte paste. This type of electrode is shown in Figure 6-10.

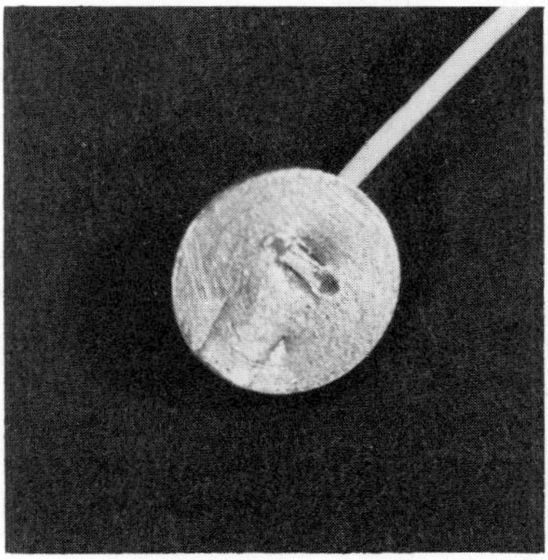

Fig. 6–10 EEG scalp surface electrode. *(Courtesy of Veterans Administration Hospital, Sepulveda, California.)*

In order to reduce movement artifact, some electroencephalographers use small subdermal needles to penetrate the scalp for EEG measurements. These *needle electrodes* (Figure 6-11) are not inserted into the brain; instead they merely penetrate the skin. They are simply inserted through a small section of the skin just beneath the surface and parallel to it.

Occasionally longer needles are actually inserted into the brain in order to obtain localized measurement of potentials from a specific part of the brain. Such electrodes must be very precisely located in order to identify the origin of the measured potential.

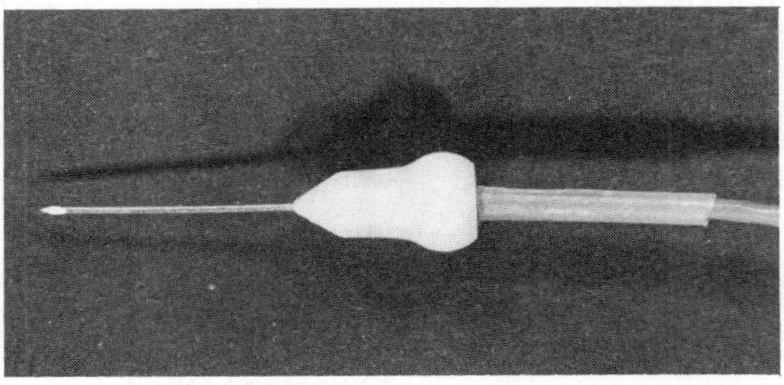

Fig. 6–11 Subdermal needle electrode for EEG. *(Courtesy of Veterans Administration Hospital, Sepulveda, California.)*

Simultaneous measurement from various depths in the brain along a certain axis can be accomplished with special multiple-depth electrodes. This type of electrode usually consists of a bundle of fine wires, each terminating at a different depth or each having an exposed conductive surface at a specific, but different, depth.

Some needle electrodes consist merely of fine insulated wires, placed so that their tips, which are bare, are in contact with the nerve, muscle, or other tissue from which the measurement is made. The remainder of the wire is covered with some form of insulation to prevent shorting. Wire electrodes of copper or platinum are often used for EMG pickup from specific muscles. The wires are either surgically implanted or introduced by means of a hypodermic needle that is later withdrawn, leaving the wire electrode in place. With this type of electrode, the metal-electrolyte interface takes place between the uninsulated tip of the wire and the electrolytes of the body, although the wire is dipped into an electrolyte paste before insertion in some cases.

In some applications, the hypodermic needle is part of the electrode configuration and is not withdrawn. Instead the wires forming the electrodes are carried inside the needle, which creates the hole necessary for insertion and protects the wires. A single wire inside the needle serves as a *unipolar electrode,* which measures the potentials at the point of contact with respect to some indifferent or reference potential obtained by placing an electrode some distance from the muscle of interest. If two wires are placed inside the needle, the measurement is called *bipolar* and provides a very localized measurement between the two wire tips.

Electrodes for measurement of potentials from beneath the skin need not actually take the form of needles, however. Conductive catheters containing electrodes and wires permit the recording of the ECG from within the chambers of the heart itself.

Appropriate types of electrodes have been developed for direct fetal heart rate and fetal ECG-monitoring applications. They are illustrated in Figure 6-12.

Figure 6-12(a) shows a silver-silver chloride *clip electrode,* which actually consists of two (bipolar) electrodes in a single unit for bipolar measurement. During a delivery procedure, the insulated silver-silver chloride clip is attached to the fetal presenting part by means of special forceps. The silver-silver chloride loop electrode then makes electrical contact with the maternal electrolytic fluids. The connecting lead wires are attached to a suitable fetal monitor. *A spiral electrode* is shown in Figure 6-12(b). This bipolar electrode is applied through a sterilized guide (tube) until its retaining spring contacts the fetal presenting part. A slight clockwise rotation of a drive assembly (not shown) then allows the spring and the silver-silver chloride tip to penetrate the fetus. Figure 6-12(c) illustrates a disposable

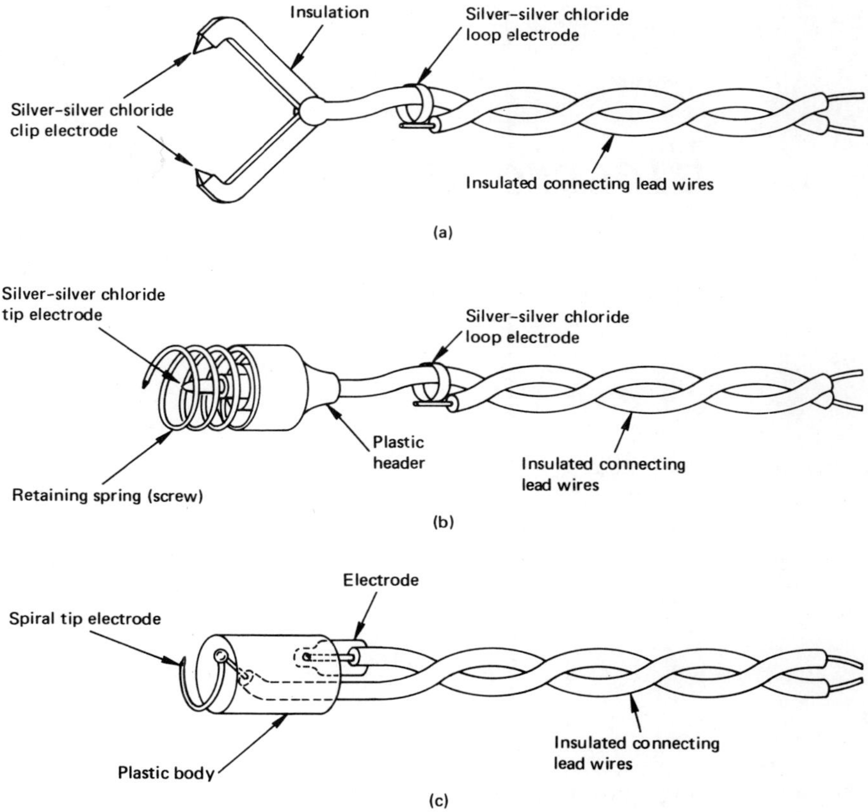

Fig. 6–12 Fetal monitoring, silver-silver chloride electrodes: (a) bipolar clip-on type; (b) bipolar spiral (screw) type; (c) spiral-tip disposable electrode.

fetal spiral electrode. Although not a silver-silver chloride type, the electrode is nevertheless bipolar. In applying fetal electrodes, care must be taken that the sharp tips do not penetrate the fetal face or fontanels.

7

Electrocardiography

The electrocardiograph was the first electrical device to find widespread use in medical diagnostics, and it still remains the most important tool for the diagnosis of cardiac disorders. Although it provides invaluable diagnostic information, especially in the case of arrhythmias and myocardial infarction, certain disorders—for instance, those involving the heart valves—cannot be diagnosed from the electrocardiogram. Other diagnostic techniques, however, such as angiography (Chapter 15) and echocardiography (Chapter 17), can provide the information not available in the electrocardiogram. The first electrocardiographs appeared in hospitals around 1910, and while ECG machines have benefited from technological innovations over the years, little has actually changed in the basic technique. Most of the terminology and several of the methods still employed date back to the early days of electrocardiography and can be understood best in a historical context.

7.1 History

As noted earlier, the discovery that muscle contractions involve electrical processes dates back to the eighteenth century. At that time, however, the technology was not advanced enough to allow a quantitative study of the electrical voltages generated by the contracting heart muscle. It was not until 1887 that the first electrocardiogram was recorded by Waller. The device used for the recording, the so-called *capillary electrometer,* was fragile and difficult to adjust, which limited use of the technique. The *string galvanometer,* which Einthoven introduced to electrocardiography in 1903, was a considerable improvement. Einthoven's contribution to electrocardiography, however, was not limited to the introduction of this device. He also explained the relationship between the various phases of the heart contraction and the excursions of the recorded trace and suggested locations for electrode placement that are still used today. For this reason, Einthoven can rightfully be considered the father of electrocardiography. A string-galvanometer electrocardiograph similar to the one used by Einthoven is shown in Figure 6-3 of Chapter 6.

Such devices lacked electronic amplification, and the current to deflect the galvanometer had to be provided by the electrodes. Consequently, immersion electrodes with a very low impedance were necessary. The ECG trace was recorded on a photographic film that had to be processed before the ECG could be read. Because the sensitivity depended on the adjustment of the galvanometer and on the resistance of the electrodes, a calibration voltage of 1 mV was inserted before each electrocardiogram was taken in order to *standardize* the recording. Around 1920, electrocardiographs with electronic amplifiers became available. The increased sensitivity of these devices made it possible to replace the immersion electrodes with the more convenient small plate electrodes still in use today. It also allowed the use of more rugged galvanometer types instead of the delicate string galvanometer. Despite these improvements, the electrocardiographs still used photographic film or photographic paper as a recording medium. This disadvantage was overcome with the introduction of direct-writing recorders (about 1946), which used ink or the transfer of pigment from a ribbon to record the ECG trace on a moving paper strip, where it was immediately visible without processing. Later, a special heat-sensitive paper was developed. This type of paper is now used almost exclusively as a recording medium for electrocardiograms. Early direct-writing recorders were not able to reproduce fine details as well as the photographic recorders did. Despite their inconvenience, therefore, photographic recorders continued to be used by some physicians. Technical improvements over the past years, however, have made available direct-recording electrocardiograph machines that show all details of the ECG signal that are necessary for medical diagnosis.

7.2 Electrodes and Leads

In order to record an electrocardiogram, a number of electrodes, usually five, are affixed to the body of the patient. The electrodes are connected to the ECG machine by the same number of electrical wires. These wires and, in a more general sense, the electrodes to which they are connected are usually called *leads*. The electrode applied to the right leg of the patient, for example, is called the RL lead. For the recording of the electrocardiogram, two electrodes or one electrode and an interconnected group of electrodes are selected and connected to the input of the recording amplifier. It is somewhat confusing that the particular electrodes selected and the way in which they are connected are also referred to as a lead. In order to avoid this ambiguity, in this book the term *lead* will be used only to indicate a particular group of electrodes and the way in which they are connected to the amplifier. For the individual lead wire, as well as the physical connection to the body of the patient, the term *electrode* will be used. The reader, however, should be aware of the double meaning that the term lead can have in normal usage.

As described in Section 5.1.5, the voltage generated by the pumping action of the heart is actually a vector whose magnitude, as well as spatial orientation, changes with time. Because the ECG signal is measured from electrodes applied to the surface of the body, the waveform of this signal is very dependent on the placement of the electrodes. Figure 5-7(a) shows a typical ECG waveform. Some of the segments of this trace however may almost disappear for certain electrode placements, whereas others may show up clearly on the recording. For this reason, in a normal electrocardiographic examination, the electrocardiogram is recorded from a number of different leads, usually 12, to ensure that no important detail of the waveform is missed. Placement of electrodes and names and configurations of the leads have become standardized and are used the same way throughout the world.

7.2.1 *Electrodes*

The placement of the electrodes, as well as the color code used to identify each electrode, is shown in Figure 7-1. In his experiments Einthoven had found it advantageous to record the electrocardiogram from electrodes placed vertically as well as horizontally on the body. As shown

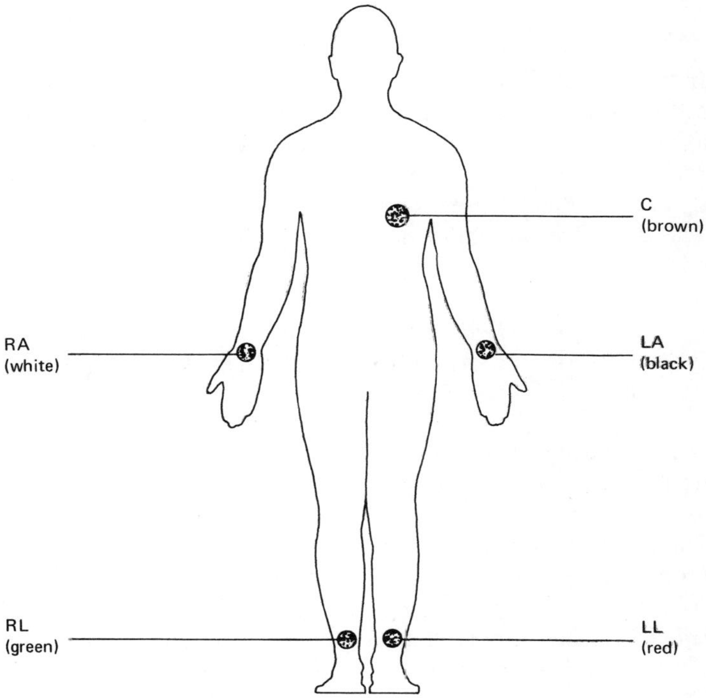

Fig. 7–1 Abbreviations and color codes used for ECG electrodes.

in Figure 6-3 he had his patients place not only both arms but also one leg into the earthenware crocks used as immersion electrodes. The leg selected was the left one, probably because it terminates vertically below the heart. The early electrocardiograph machines thus employed three electrodes, of which only two were used at one time. With the introduction of the electronic amplifier, an additional connection to the body was needed as a ground reference. Although an electrode could have been positioned almost anywhere on the body for this purpose, it became a convention to use the "free" right leg.

The *chest* or *precordial electrodes* were introduced later. Although plate electrodes are normally used for the electrodes at the extremities, the chest electrode is often the suction type shown in Figure 6-5. It should be noted that abbreviations referring to the extremities are used to identify the electrodes even when they are actually placed on the chest, as in the case of the patient-monitoring applications described in Chapter 11.

7.2.2 Leads

In the normal electrode placement shown in Figure 7-1, four electrodes are used to record the electrocardiogram; the electrode on the right leg is only for ground reference. Because the input of the ECG recorder has only two terminals, a selection must be made among the available active electrodes. The 12 standard leads used most frequently are shown in Figure 7-2. The three *bipolar limb lead* selections first introduced by Einthoven, shown in the top row of the figure, are as follows:

Lead I	Left Arm (LA) and Right Arm (RA)
Lead II	Left Leg (LL) and Right Arm (RA)
Lead III	Left Leg (LL) and Left Arm (LA)

These three leads are called *bipolar* because for each lead the electrocardiogram is recorded from two electrodes and the third electrode is not connected.

The other leads shown in Figure 7-2 are of the *unipolar* type, which was introduced by Wilson in 1944. For unipolar leads, the electrocardiogram is recorded between a single *exploratory electrode* and the *central terminal,* which has a potential corresponding to the center of the body. This central terminal is obtained by connecting the three active limb electrodes together through resistors of equal size. The potential at the connection point of the resistors corresponds to the mean or average of the potentials at the three electrodes. In the *unipolar limb leads,* one of the limb electrodes is used as an exploratory electrode as well as contributing to the central terminal. This double use results in an ECG signal that has a very small amplitude. In the *augmented unipolar limb leads,* the limb electrode used as an exploratory electrode is not used for the central terminal, thereby increasing the amplitude of the ECG signal without changing its waveform appreciably. These leads are designated aVR, aVL, and aVF (F as in foot).

For the *unipolar chest leads,* all three active limb electrodes are used to obtain the central terminal, while a separate chest electrode is used as an exploratory electrode.

The electrocardiograms recorded from these 12 lead selections are shown in Figure 7-3. It can be seen that the trace from lead selection I or II resembles most closely the idealized waveform of Figure 5-9; some of the other traces are quite different in appearance.

In addition to the lead systems already discussed, there are certain additional lead modifications that are of considerable use in the coronary care unit. The most widely used modification for ongoing ECG monitoring

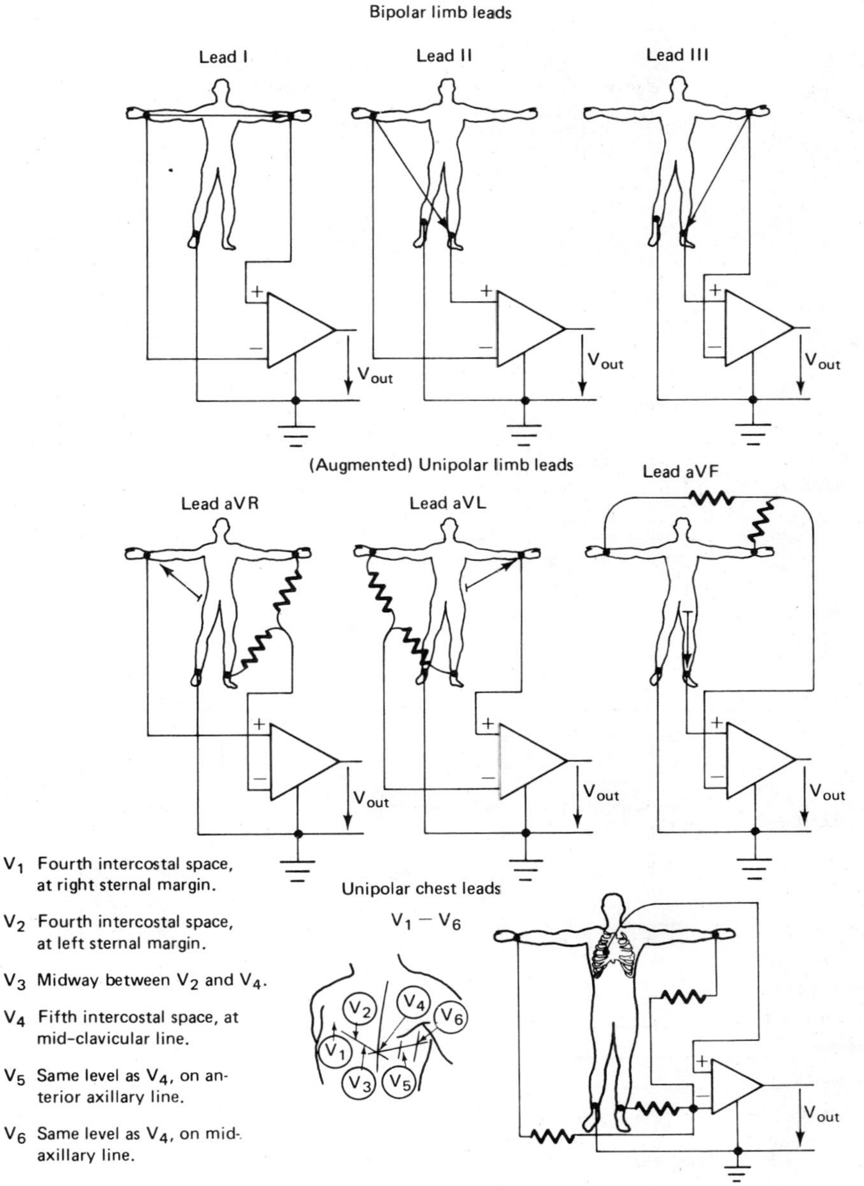

Fig. 7–2 The 12 standard ECG lead configurations.

is the *Modified Chest Lead I (MCL_1)* also called the *Marriott Lead,* after its inventor. This lead system simulates the V_1 position with electrode place-

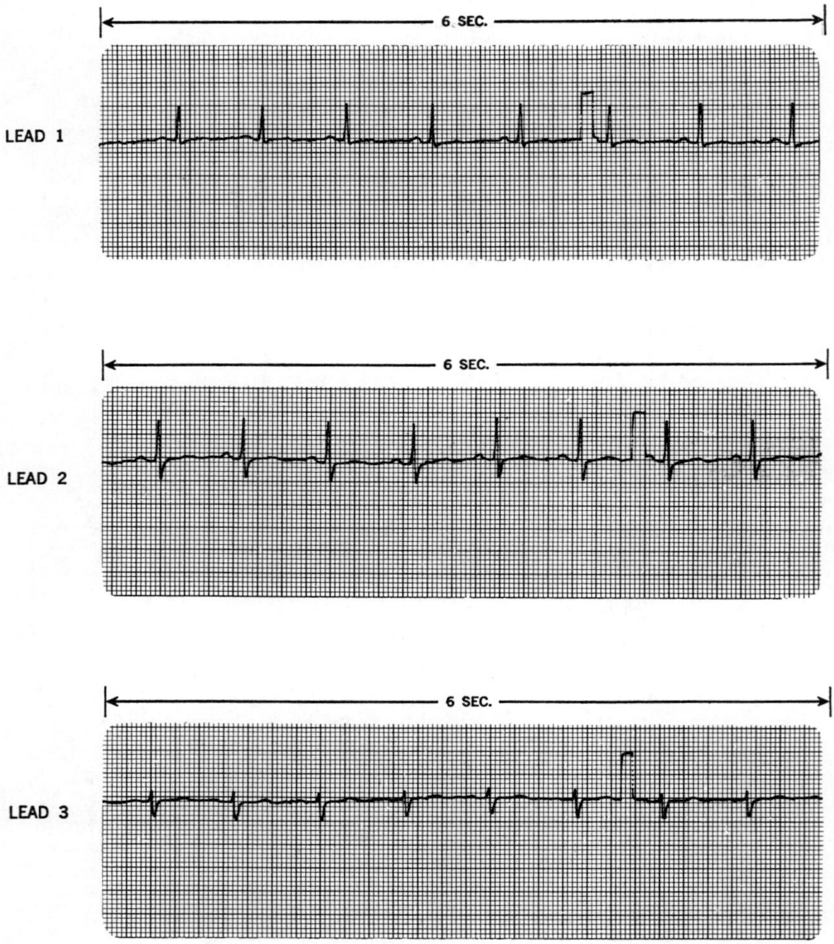

ATRIAL RATE ______ P-R INTERVAL ______ PATIENT POSITION ______
VENTRICULAR RATE ______ QRS INTERVAL ______ ELECTRICAL AXIS ______
RHYTHM ______ Q-T INTERVAL ______ S-T SEGMENT ______
P WAVES ______ T WAVES ______
REMARKS

Fig. 7–3 12-lead electrocardiogram mounted for filing.

ment as follows: positive electrode, fourth intercostal space, right sternal border; negative electrode just below the outer portion of the left clavicle, with ground just about anywhere, but usually below the right clavicle. The monitor is set on lead I for this bipolar tracing. Recordings obtained in this

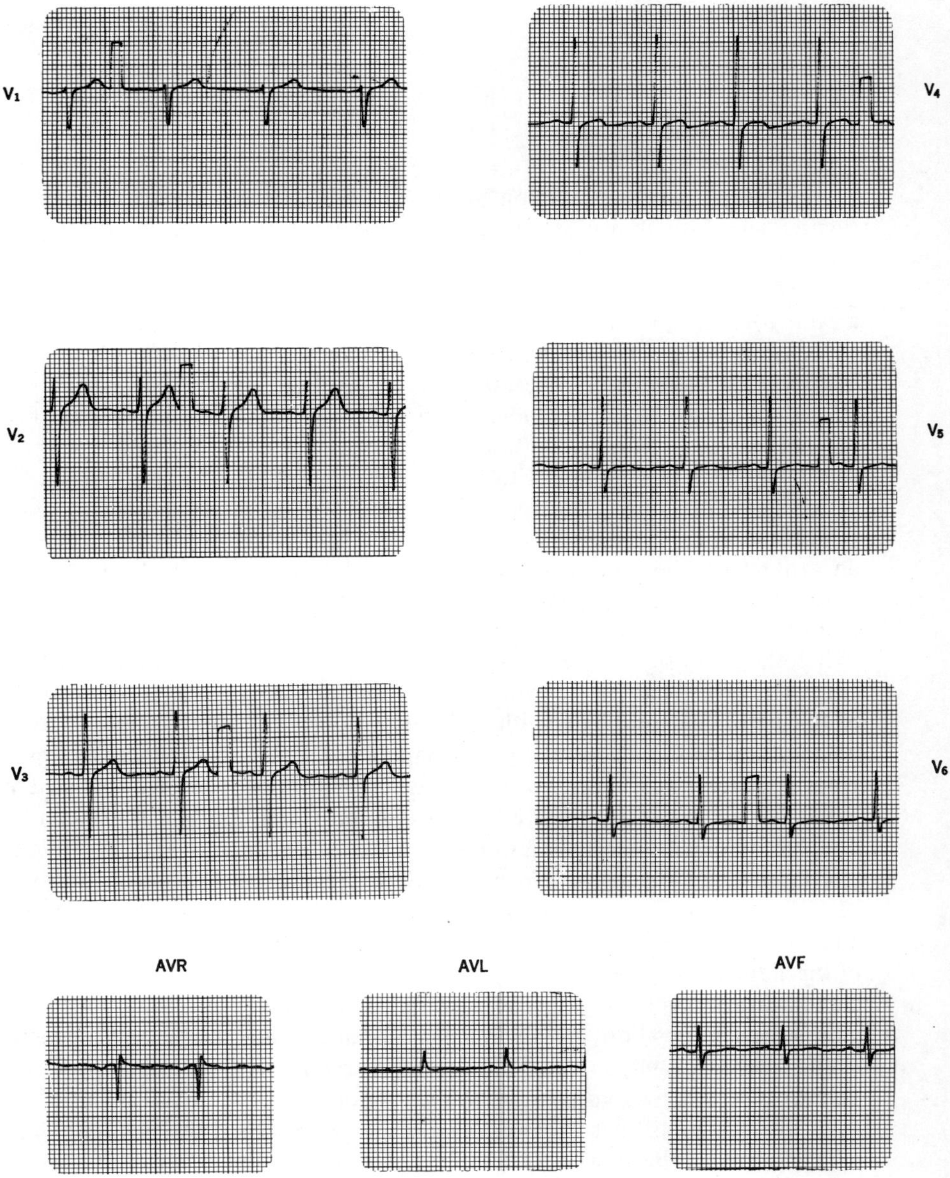

Fig. 7–3 (Continued.)

way are very useful in differentiating left ventricular ectopic rhythms from aberrant right ventricular or supraventricular rhythms. The former situation usually necessitates prompt therapeutic action; the latter is of less clinical significance.

7.3 ECG Recorders

The principal parts or building blocks of an ECG recorder are shown in Figure 7-4. Also shown are the controls usually found on ECG recorders; the dotted lines indicate the building block with which each control interacts.

The connecting wires for the patient electrodes originate at the end of a *patient cable,* the other end of which plugs into the ECG recorder. The wires from the electrodes connect to the *lead selector switch,* which also incorporates the resistors necessary for the unipolar leads. A push button allows the insertion of a *standardization* voltage of 1 mV to standardize or calibrate the recorder. Although modern recorders are stable and their sensitivity does not change with time, the ritual of inserting the standardization pulse before or after each recording when recording a 12-lead ECG is still followed. Changing the setting of the lead selector switch introduces an artifact on the recorded trace. A special contact on the lead selector switch turns off the amplifier momentarily whenever this switch is moved and turns it on again after the artifact has passed. From the lead selector switch the ECG signal goes to a *preamplifier.* This amplifier is a differential amplifier (see Chapter 4) with a high common-mode rejection. It is ac coupled to avoid problems with small dc voltages that may originate from polarization of the electrodes (see Chapter 6). The preamplifier also provides a switch to set the *sensitivity* or *gain.* With most patients, this switch is left in position "1." If the ECG trace is too small, the sensitivity can be doubled by placing the switch in position "2." For patients with exceptionally large ECG signals, it can be halved by placing the switch in position "1/2." Older ECG machines also have a continuously variable sensitivity adjustment, sometimes marked *standardization adjustment.* With the help of this adjustment, the sensitivity of the ECG recorder can be set so that the standardization voltage of 1 mV causes a pen deflection of 10 mm (with the gain switch in position 1). In modern amplifiers the gain usually remains stable once adjusted, so the continuously variable gain control is now frequently a screwdriver adjustment at the side or rear of the ECG recorder.

The preamplifier is followed by a dc amplifier called the *pen amplifier,* which provides the power to drive the *pen motor* that records the actual ECG trace. The input of the pen amplifier is usually accessible separately, with a special *auxiliary input* jack at the rear or side of the ECG recorder. Thus the ECG recorder can be used to record the output of other devices, such as the *electromotograph,* which records the Achilles Reflex. A *position* control on the pen amplifier makes it possible to center the pen on the recording paper. All modern ECG recorders use heat-sensitive paper, and the pen is actually an electrically heated *stylus,* the temperature of which

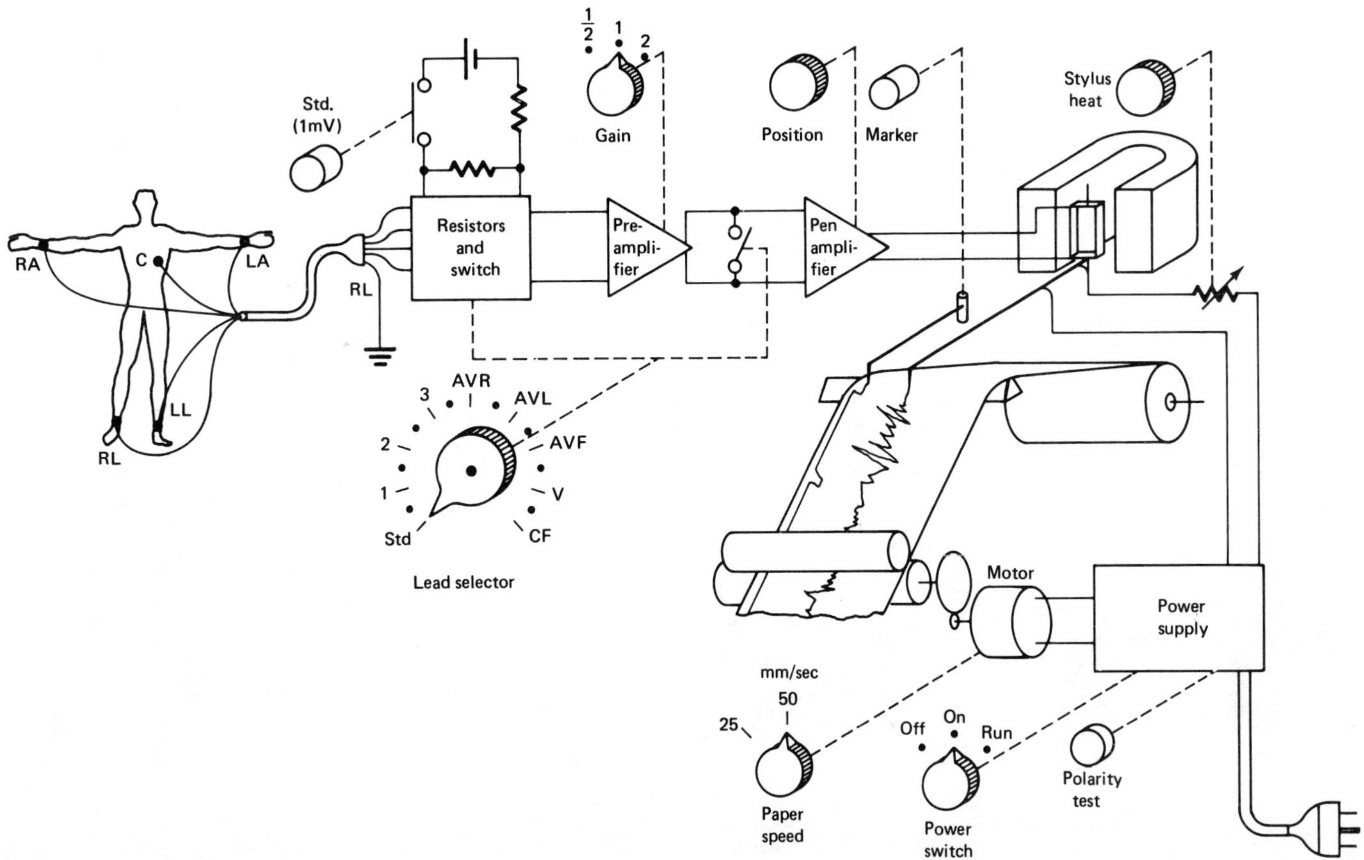

Fig. 7–4 Building blocks and controls of a modern ECG machine.

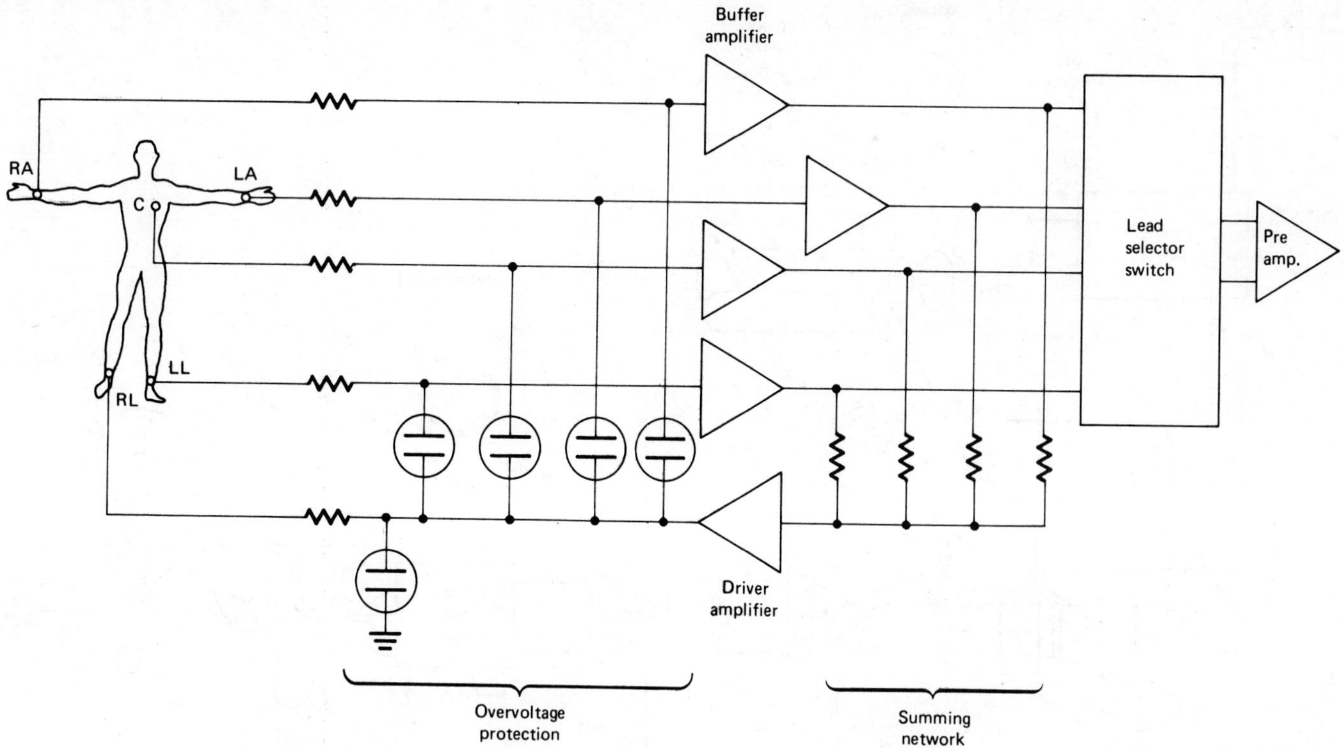

Fig. 7–4 (Continued.)

can be adjusted with a *stylus heat* control for optimal recording trace. Beside the recording stylus, there is a *marker* stylus that can be actuated by a push button and that allows the operator to mark a coded indication of the lead being recorded at the margin of the electrocardiogram. Normally electrocardiograms are recorded at a paper speed of *25 mm/s,* but a faster speed of *50 mm/s* is provided to allow better resolution of the QRS complex at very high heart rates or when a particular waveform detail is desired.

The *power switch* of an ECG recorder has three positions. In the *ON* position the power to the amplifier is turned on, but the paper drive is not running. In order to start the paper drive, the switch must be placed in the *RUN* position. In some ECG machines the lead selector switch has auxiliary positions (between the lead positions) in which the paper drive is stopped. In older ECG machines a push button or metal "finger contact" allows the operator to check whether the recorder is connected to the power line with the right polarity. Because the improper connection of older machines can create a shock hazard for the patient, this test must be performed prior to connecting the electrodes to the patient. Modern ECG machines, which have line plugs with grounding pins, do not require such a polarity test. The front plate of a modern ECG machine, including the controls described, is shown in Figure 7-5.

The building blocks shown in Figure 7-4 are typical for an older ECG machine. Modern devices, however, are more complicated and contain additional elements. For example, the figure shows the RL lead as being connected to ground. Modern machines frequently use the so-called *driven RL lead,* a feature that reduces the sensitivity to ac interference (see next section). Instead of connecting the central terminal resistors directly to the electrodes, modern ECG machines have isolation amplifiers in all active patient connections. Consequently, the input resistance of the amplifier is increased and the preparation of the electrode sites becomes less critical because a higher electrode impedance can be tolerated. The preamplifier in a modern ECG machine is frequently *isolated from ground* with the power and signal connections being provided by light beams or transformers. The *isolated patient leads* reduce the electrical shock hazard in certain applications (see Chapter 18).

7.4 Practical Considerations for ECG Recording

The previous sections described the basic principle of ECG recording, but several practical aspects must be observed in order to obtain diagnostically useful electrocardiograms.

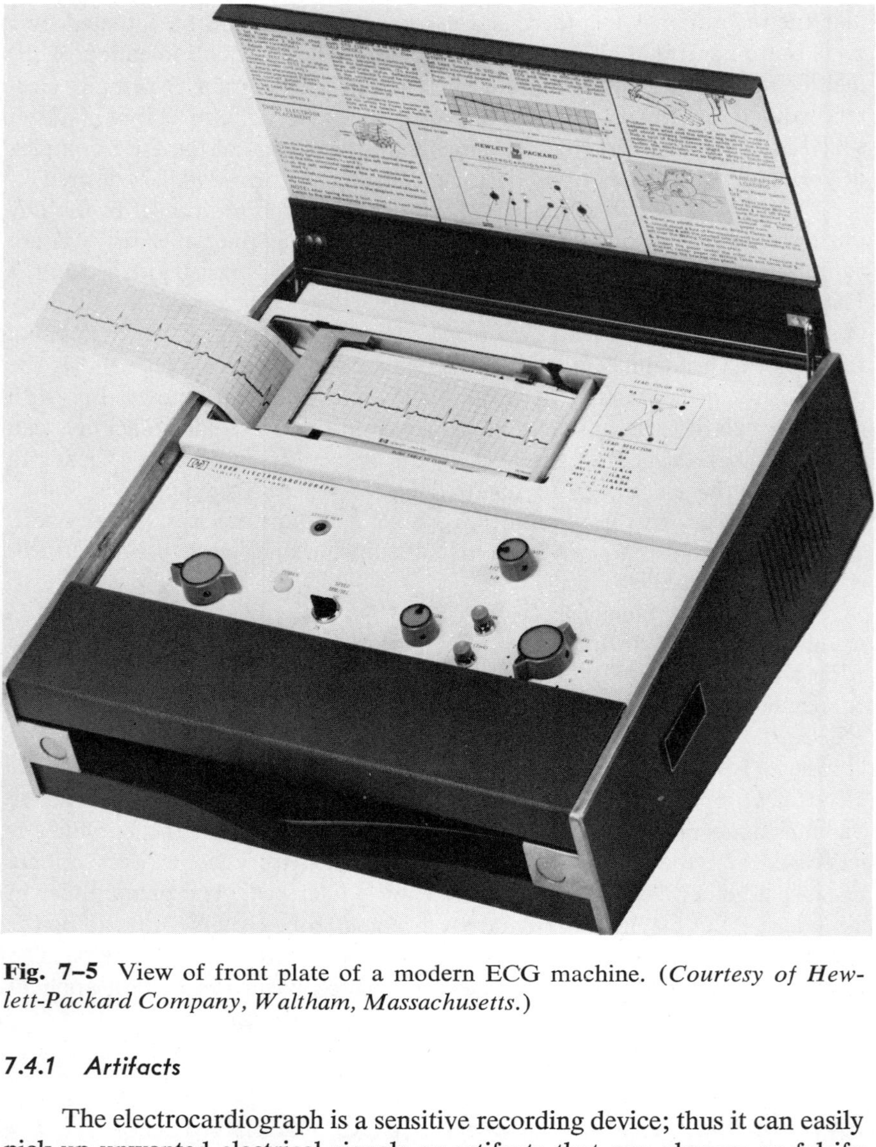

Fig. 7–5 View of front plate of a modern ECG machine. (*Courtesy of Hewlett-Packard Company, Waltham, Massachusetts.*)

7.4.1 Artifacts

The electrocardiograph is a sensitive recording device; thus it can easily pick up unwanted electrical signals or artifacts that can obscure or falsify the actual ECG signal. Sometimes it may require all the skills of an experienced ECG operator to locate the source of such artifacts and correct the situation. The most frequent types and their causes will be discussed briefly below.

Alternating current interference is caused by a small part of the power-line voltage being coupled to the input of the ECG recorder. It is manifested by a widening of the baseline, which can be resolved to a regular wave of constant amplitude by switching to a paper speed of 50 mm/s. This interference can have several different causes, and the following conditions should be checked.

1. Be sure that the patient does not touch or make contact with any metal object, such as a bed rail, bed stand, or piece of metal furniture.
2. Remove or unplug any other electrical appliances, such as clocks, radios, and lamps, in the vicinity of the patient.
3. If older ECG machines are used, make sure that the polarity test has been performed properly before connecting the cable to the patient.
4. Be sure that all electrodes have been applied with the right amount of electrode paste or jelly and that all electrode straps are tight enough.
5. Severe ac interference which occurs consistently in one particular location or when the ECG recorder is connected to one particular receptacle could indicate faulty wiring or a faulty receptacle. This situation should be checked by an electrician to avoid possible danger to staff and patient.

Muscle potentials can cause an unsteady trace if the patient is not completely relaxed. They can be distinguished from ac interference because they do not have a regular pattern. Therefore it is important that the patient be comfortable and relaxed while the electrocardiogram is recorded. In patients with parkinsonism or palsy, however, it may be difficult to get a satisfactory recording.

Wandering of the baseline can result from gross movements of the patient or from mechanical strain on the electrode wires, which causes a sudden change of electrode potentials.

An *indistinct trace,* which either has an overly wide but solid baseline or a fuzzy baseline or which disappears during the excursions of the R wave, can be caused by improper adjustment of the stylus temperature or by a buildup of waxy residue on the heated stylus. If adjusting the stylus temperature does not help, the residue can be burned off by putting the lead selector switch in the "Standard" position and gently lifting the stylus off the paper while the stylus temperature is set to maximum for about 10 seconds.

Regarding other possible sources of artifacts and remedies, the reader is referred to the operation manuals of the manufacturers.

7.4.2 Placement of Electrodes

The normal placement of electrodes is shown in Figure 7-1. Sometimes the question arises as to where to place the limb electrodes if the extremities cannot be used because of casts or an amputation. When this problem arises, it should be kept in mind that the extremities were originally chosen for electrode placement mainly to duplicate the immersion electrodes first used. If the wrist or ankle area of a limb is not accessible, identical ECG traces can be obtained by placing the electrode on the same limb closer to the trunk or, if necessary, at the shoulder or hip from which the inaccessible limb originates. Because the right leg electrode serves only as a reference, it can be placed anywhere on the trunk or on another limb if the right leg is not accessible. However, it should not be placed immediately adjacent to one of the other electrodes.

The six chest electrode positions are relatively close to each other. When moving the electrode from position to position, great care should be taken not to smear the electrode paste or jelly because doing so could result in erroneous ECG characteristics. The same precaution is even more important if separate electrodes are used for all chest positions, as in the case of the automatic multichannel recorders described in Section 7.5.

7.4.3 Coding and Mounting of Electrocardiograms

If the electrocardiogram of a patient is recorded in the 12 standard lead configurations, the resulting paper strip is from 3 to 6 ft long. Even if folded in accordion fashion, the strip is still inconvenient to read and store. Therefore it is usually cut up, and sections of the recordings from the 12 leads are mounted as shown in Figure 7-3. Because it is easy to mix up the cut sections, the leads from which each trace was recorded are encoded at the margin of the paper, using the marker pen. The code markers consist of short marks (dots) and long marks (dashes) and look similar to Morse code. No standard code has been established for this purpose, however, and three of the more commonly used code combinations are shown in Figure 7-6.

The cut sections of the electrocardiogram can be mounted by inserting them in pockets of a special folder with cutouts to make the trace visible. This is the way in which the electrocardiogram in Figure 7-3 was mounted. It should be noted that the recordings from the three limb leads are longer than those from the other lead selections in order to show several QRS complexes; they are called *rhythm strips*. Commercial systems are available to simplify the mounting by die-cutting the paper strip and using mounting cards with adhesive pads. With the automatic three-channel recorders described in the next section, the mounting is greatly simplified.

Lead	Code 1	Code 2	Code 3
I	•	•	–
II	• •	• •	– –
III	• • •	• • •	– – –
AVR	• –	–	– •
AVL	• • –	– –	– • •
AVF	• • • –	– – –	– • • •
V1	– •	– •	•
V2	– • •	– • •	• •
V3	– • • •	– • • •	• • •
V4	– • • • •	– • • • •	• • • •
V5	– • • • • •	– • • • • •	• • • • •
V6	– • • • • • •	– • • • • • •	• • • • • •

Fig. 7–6 Examples of codes used to identify the various leads on the ECG recording.

7.5 Special Types of ECG Recorders

Although very little has changed over the past three decades in the appearance and operation of the basic single-channel ECG recorder, new and radically different types of electrocardiographs have found increasing use over the past few years.

7.5.1 Automatic Three-Channel Recorders

Where large numbers of electrocardiograms are recorded and mounted daily, substantial savings in personnel can be achieved by the use of *automatic three-channel recorders.* These devices not only record three leads simultaneously on a three-channel recorder, but they also switch automatically to the next group of three leads. An electrocardiogram with the 12 standard leads, therefore, can be recorded automatically as a sequence of four groups of three traces. The time required for the actual recording is only about 10 seconds. The groups of leads recorded and the time at which the switching occurs are automatically identified by code markings at the margin of the recording paper. At the end of the recording, standardization pulses are inserted in all three recording channels. Although the actual recording time is reduced substantially compared to single-channel recorders, more time is required to apply the electrodes to the patient because separate electrodes must necessarily be used for each chest position. The mounting of the electrocardiogram, however, is simplified substantially, for no cutting or mounting of the individual lead selections is required. A modern recorder of this type is shown in Figure 7-7.

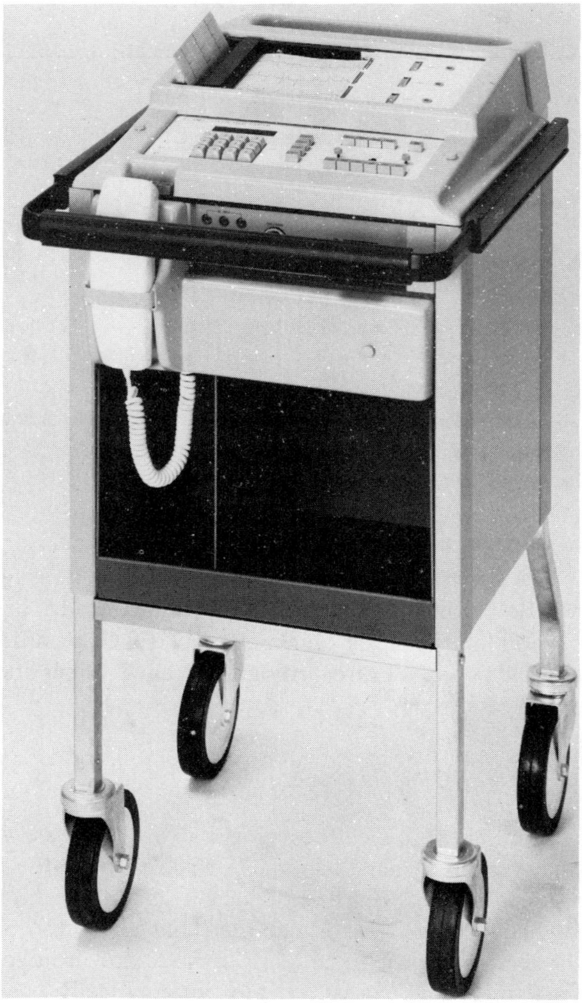

Fig. 7–7 Automatic three-channel ECG recorder with keyboard for entering patient data and telephone coupler to send ECG and data to a remote computer via telephone lines. *(Courtesy of Hewlett-Packard Company, Waltham, Massachusetts.)*

7.5.2 Electrocardiographs for Computer Processing

The automatic analysis of electrocardiograms by computers is used increasingly (see Chapter 19). This technique requires that the ECG signal from the standard leads be transmitted sequentially to the computer by some suitable means, together with additional information on the patient. The automatic three-channel recorders can frequently be adapted for this purpose. The ECG signals can either be recorded on a tape for later computer entry or can be directly transmitted to the computer through special lines or regular telephone lines using a special acoustical coupler (see Chapter 19). Information regarding the patient is entered with thumbwheel switches or from a keyboard and is transmitted along with the ECG signal. During the transmission of the signal, the electrocardiogram is simultaneously recorded to verify that the transmitted signals are free of artifacts.

7.5.3 Vector Electrocardiographs

As noted in Section 5.1.5, the voltage generated by the activity of the heart can be described as a vector whose magnitude and spatial orientation change with time. In the type of electrocardiography described thus far, only the magnitude of the voltage is recorded. *Vectorcardiography,* on the other hand, presents an image of both the magnitude and the spatial orientation of the heart vector. The heart vector, however, is a three-dimensional variable, and three "views" or projections on orthogonal planes are necessary to describe the variable fully in two-dimensional figures. In order to pick up the ECG signals for vector electrocardiograms, special lead placement systems must be used, with the so-called *Frank system* being the one most frequently employed. The vectorcardiogram is usually displayed on a cathode-ray tube, similar to those used for patient monitors. Each QRS complex is displayed as a sequence of "loops" on this screen, which is then photographed with a Polaroid® camera. Vectorcardiographs that use computer techniques to slow down the ECG signals and allow the recording of the vectorcardiogram with a mechanical X-Y recorder are also available.

7.5.4 Electrocardiograph Systems for Stress Testing

Coronary insufficiency frequently does not manifest itself in the electrocardiogram if the recording is taken during rest. In the *Masters test* or *two-step exercise test,* a physiological stress is imposed on the cardiovascular system by letting the patient repeatedly walk up and down a special pair of 9-inch-high steps prior to recording his electrocardiogram. Based on the same principle is the *exercise stress test* in which the patient walks at a specified speed on a treadmill whose inclination can be changed. While the Masters test is normally conducted using a regular single-channel electrocardiograph, special systems are available for the exercise stress test. These systems, however, are usually made up of a number of individual instruments which are described in this book.

An exercise stress test system typically consists of the following parts:

1. A treadmill which may incorporate an automatic programmer to change the speed and inclination in order to apply a specific physiological stress.
2. An ECG radiotelemetry system to allow recording of the ECG without artifacts while the patient is on the treadmill.
3. An ECG monitor with a cathode-ray-tube display and heart rate meter.
4. An ECG recorder.
5. An automatic or semi-automatic sphygmomanometer for the indirect measurement of blood pressure.

Because the exercise stress test involves a certain risk for patients with known or suspected cardiac disorders, a dc defibrillator is usually kept available while the test is performed.

7.5.5 *Continuous ECG Recording (Holter Recording)*

Because a normal electrocardiogram represents only a brief sample of cardiac activity, arrhythmias which occur intermittently or only under certain conditions, such as emotional stress, are frequently missed. The technique of continuous ECG recording, which was introduced by Norman Holter, makes it possible to capture these kinds of arrhythmias. To obtain a continuous ECG, the electrocardiogram of a patient is recorded during his normal daily activity by means of a special magnetic tape recorder. The smallest device of this type can actually be worn in a shirt pocket and allows recordings of the ECG for four hours. Other recorders, about the size of a camera case, are worn over the shoulder and can record the electrocardiogram for up to 24 hours. The recorded tape is analyzed using a special scanning device which plays back the tape at a higher speed than that used for recording. By this method, a 24-hour tape can be reviewed in as little as 12 minutes. During the playback, the beat-to-beat interval of the electrocardiogram is displayed on a cathode-ray tube as a picket-fence-like pattern in which arrhythmia epsiodes are clearly visible. Once such an epsiode has been discovered, the tape is backed up and slowed down to obtain a normal electrocardiogram strip for the time interval during which the arrhythmias occured. A special time clock is synchronized by the tape drive to correlate the onset of the epsiode with the activity of the patient.

8

Indirect Measurement of Blood Pressure

As noted, myocardial infarction is the cause of well over half a million deaths annually in the United States. One of the critical measurements in the prediction of possible heart problems and the monitoring of patients with such problems or after attacks is that of blood pressure. There are two parallel systems in the circulation of blood. The right half of the heart is the pump that supplies blood to the lungs for oxygenation; the left side of the heart supplies blood to the rest of the system. The circulatory path for blood flow through the lungs is called *pulmonary circulation,* and the circulatory system that supplies oxygen and nutrients to the cells of the body is called the *systemic circulation.* The pumping action itself is performed by contraction of the heart muscles surrounding each chamber of the heart. These muscles receive their own blood supply from the *coronary arteries,* which surround the heart like a crown (corona). The *coronary arterial system* is a special branch of the systemic circulation.

The overall functions of the cardiovascular system can be measured by considering three parameters. The *systemic arterial blood pressure* is a force that results in blood flow through arteries, capillaries and veins. The flow is controlled by the resistance it encounters in the arteries due to their size, shape, any deposits on the walls (e.g., atherosclerosis), and the flexibility or rigidity of the walls (e.g., arterial sclerosis). This controlling factor is known as the *peripheral vascular resistance.* The flow from the heart itself is measured as the *cardiac output.* The topics of blood flow, volume, and cardiac output are discussed in Chapter 11.

A nurse is primarily concerned with the measurement of the systemic arterial blood pressure as a routine procedure. This procedure occurs daily or hourly or at whatever time intervals are indicated by the state of the patient and is usually done as an indirect measurement, as defined later in the chapter. In critical care areas, measurements are frequently direct and may involve the pulmonary vasculature as well as central venous and arterial systems.

This chapter is concerned with blood pressure characteristics, with indirect measurements and methods, and, finally, with some practical clinical considerations.

8.1 Blood Pressure

Although it is not the intent of this book to present the detailed physiology of the body systems to be measured, a little background is necessary in order to develop an overall understanding of what really goes on in the blood pressure system.

The heart's pumping cycle is divided into two major parts: systole and diastole. *Systole* (sĭs′tō·lē) is defined as the period of contraction of the heart muscles, specifically the ventricular muscle, at which time blood is pumped into the pulmonary artery and the aorta. *Diastole* (dī·ăs′tō·lē) is the period of dilation of the heart cavities as they fill with blood.

Once the blood has been pumped into the arterial system, the heart relaxes, the pressure in the chambers decreases, the outlet valves close, and in a short time the inlet valves open again to restart the diastole and initiate a new cycle in the heart. The mechanism of this cycle and its control will be discussed later.

After passing through many bifurcations of the arteries, the blood reaches the vital organs, the brain, and the extremities. The last stage of the arterial system is the gradual decrease in cross section and the increase in the number of arteries until the smallest type (arterioles) is reached. These arteries feed into the capillaries, where oxygen is supplied to the cells and carbon dioxide is received from the cells. In turn, the capillaries join into venules, which become small veins, then larger veins, and ultimately form the superior and inferior vena cavae. The blood supply to the heart itself is from the aorta through the coronary arteries into a similar capillary system to the cardiac veins. This blood returns to the heart chambers by way of the coronary sinus.

The heart beats at an average rate of about 75 beats per minute in a normal adult, although this figure can vary considerably. The heart rate increases when a person stands up and decreases when he sits down, the range being from about 60 to 85. On the average, it is higher in women and generally decreases with age. In an infant, the heart rate may be as high as 140 beats per minute under normal conditions. The heart rate also increases with heat exposure and other physiological and psychological factors.

The heart pumps about 5 liters of blood per minute, and since the volume of blood in the average adult is about 5 to 6 liters, the result is a complete turnover every minute during rest. With heavy exercise, the circulation rate is increased considerably. At any given time, about 75 to 80% of the blood volume is in the veins, about 20% in the arteries, and the remainder in the capillaries.

Systolic (maximum) blood pressure in the normal adult is in the range of 95 to 140 mm Hg, with 120 mm Hg being average. These figures are subject to much variation with age, climate, eating habits, and other factors. Normal diastolic blood pressure (lowest pressure between beats) ranges from 60 to 90 mm Hg, with 80 mm Hg being about average under most circumstances. This pressure is measured in the brachial artery in the arm. For comparison purposes with pressures of 130/75 in the aorta, 130/5 can be expected in the left ventricle, 9/5 in the left atrium, 25/0 in the right ventricle, 3/0 in the right atrium, and 25/12 in the pulmonary artery. These values are given as

Systolic pressure/Diastolic pressure.

Figure 8-1 is a schematic representation of the normal pressures.

With regard to measurements, the events in the heart that relate to the blood pressure as a function of time should be understood. Figure 8-2 illustrates this point. The two basic stages of diastole and systole are shown with a more detailed time scale of phases of operation below. The blood pressure waves for the aorta, the left atrium, and the left ventricle are drawn to show time and magnitude relationships. Also, the correlated electrical events are shown at the bottom in the form of the electrocardiogram.

Examining the aortic wave, it can be seen that, during systole, the ejection of blood from the left ventricle is rapid at first. As the rate of pressure change decreases, the rounded maximum of the curve is obtained. The peak aortic pressure during systole is a function of left ventricular stroke volume, the peak rate of ejection, and the distensibility of the walls of the aorta. In a diseased heart, ventricular contractability and rigid atherosclerotic arteries produce unwanted rises in blood pressure.

When the systolic period is completed, the aortic valve is closed by

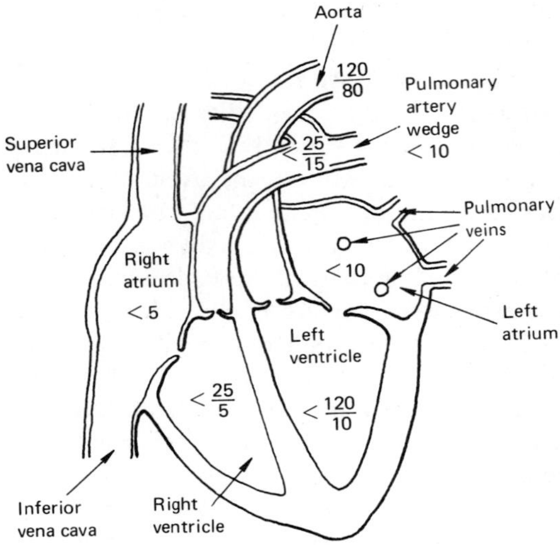

Fig. 8–1 Schematic representation of typical normal blood pressures.

the back pressure of blood (against the valve). This effect can be seen on the pressure pulse waveform as the *dicrotic notch.* When the valve is closed completely, the arterial pressure gradually decreases as blood pours into the countless peripheral vascular networks. The rate at which the pressure falls is determined by the pressure achieved during the systolic interval, the rate of outflow through the peripheral resistances, and the diastolic interval.

The form of the arterial pressure pulse changes as it passes through the arteries. The walls of the arteries cause damping and reflections; and as the arteries branch out into smaller arteries with smaller cross-sectional areas, the pressures and volumes change and hence the rate of flow also changes. The peak systolic pressure gets a little higher and the diastolic pressure flatter. The mean pressure in some arteries (e.g., the brachial artery) can be as much as 20 mm Hg higher than that in the aorta.

As the blood flows into the smaller arteries and arterioles, the pressure decreases and loses its pulsatile character. Pressure in the arterioles can vary from about 60 mm Hg down to 30 mm Hg. As the blood enters the venous system after flowing through the capillaries, the pressure is down to about 15 mm Hg.

In the venous system, the pressure in the venules decreases to approximately 8 mm Hg, and in the veins to about 5 mm Hg. In the vena cava, the pressure is only about 2 mm Hg. Because of these differences in pres-

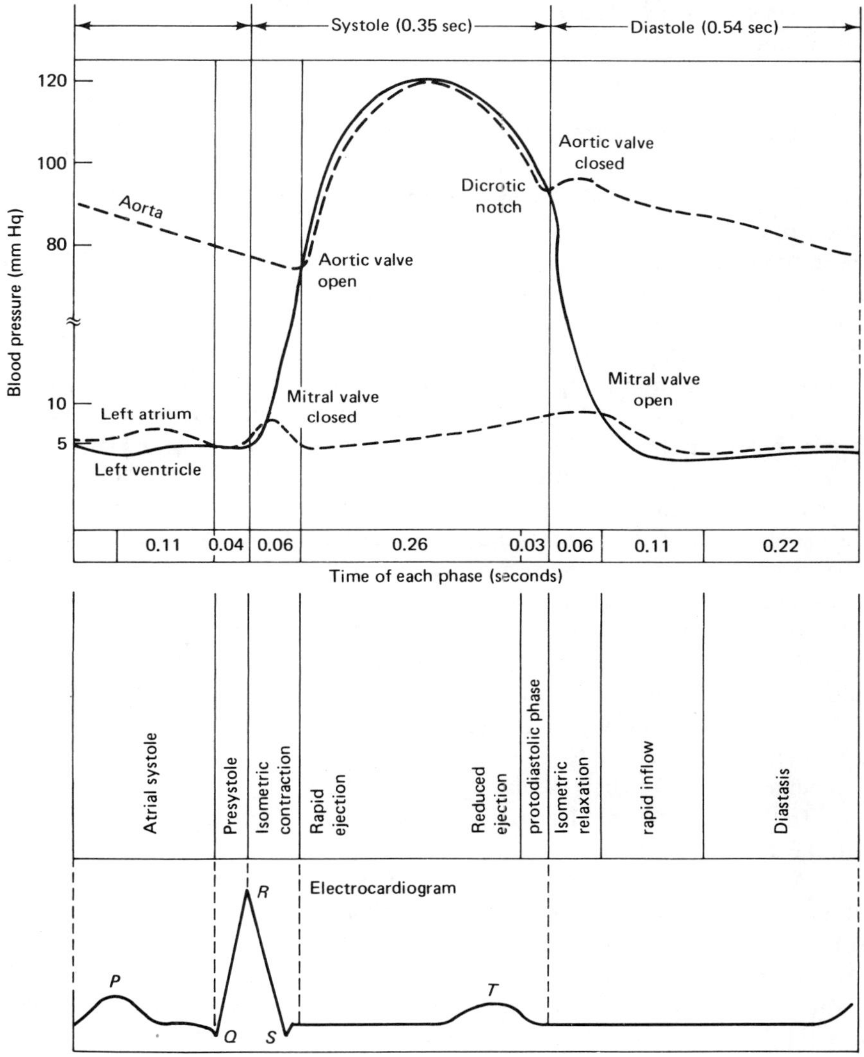

Fig. 8–2 Blood pressure variations as a function of time.

sure, measurement of arterial blood pressure is quite different from that of venous pressure. For example, a 2-mm Hg error in systolic pressure is only on the order of 1.5%. In a vein, however, this would be a 100% error. Also, because of these pressure differences, the arteries have thick walls, while the veins have thin walls. Moreover, the veins have larger internal diameters. Since about 75 to 80% of the blood volume is contained in the venous system, the veins tend to serve as a reservoir for the body's blood supply.

8.2 Indirect Measurement of Blood Pressure

As one of the physiological variables that can be quite readily measured, blood pressure is considered a good indicator of the status of the cardiovascular system. A history of blood pressure measurements has saved many an individual from an untimely death by providing warnings of dangerously high blood pressure (*hypertension*) in time to provide treatment.

In routine clinical tests, blood pressure is usually measured by means of an indirect method using a *sphygmomanometer* (from the Greek *sphygmos,* meaning pulse). This method is easy to use and can be automated. It has, however, certain disadvantages in that it does not provide a continuous recording of pressure variations and its practical repetition rate is limited. Furthermore, only systolic and diastolic arterial pressure readings can be obtained, with no indication of the details of the pressure waveform. The indirect method is also somewhat subjective and often fails when the blood pressure is very low (as would be the case when a patient is in shock).

Methods for direct blood pressure measurement, on the other hand, do provide a continuous readout or recording of the blood pressure waveform and are considerably more accurate than the indirect method. They require, however, that a blood vessel be punctured in order to introduce the sensor. This fact limits their use to those cases in which the condition of the patient warrants invasion of the vascular system.

In this chapter only the indirect methods are discussed. Direct methods are the subject of the next chapter.

As stated earlier, the familiar indirect method of measuring blood pressure involves the use of a sphygmomanometer and a stethoscope. The sphygmomanometer consists of an inflatable pressure cuff and a mercury or aneroid manometer to measure the pressure in the cuff. The cuff consists of a rubber bladder inside an inelastic fabric covering that can be wrapped around the upper arm and fastened with either hooks or a Velcro® fastener. The cuff is normally inflated manually with a rubber bulb and deflated slowly through a needle valve. A wall-mounted sphygmomanometer is shown in Figure 8-3. These devices are also manufactured as portable units.

The sphygmomanometer works on the principle that when the cuff is placed on the upper arm and inflated, arterial blood can flow past the cuff only when the arterial pressure exceeds the pressure in the cuff. Furthermore, when the cuff is inflated to a pressure that only partially occludes the brachial artery, turbulence is generated in the blood as it spurts through the tiny arterial opening during each systole. The sounds generated by

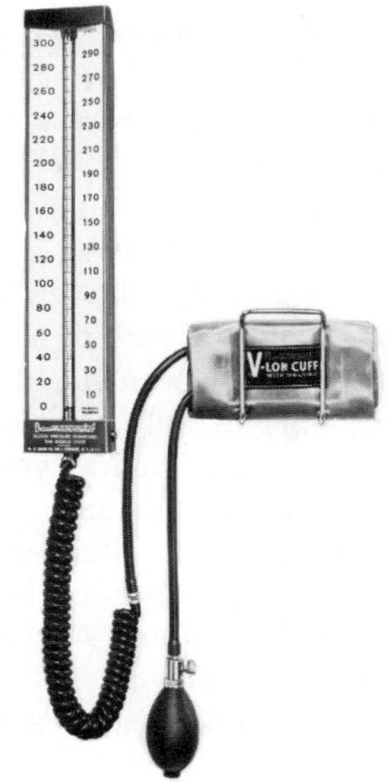

Fig. 8–3 Wall-mounted sphygmomanometer. *(Courtesy of W. A. Baum, Inc., Copiague, New York.)*

this turbulence, called *Korotkoff* sounds, can be heard through a stethoscope placed over the artery downstream from the cuff.

In order to obtain a blood pressure measurement with a sphygmomanometer and a stethoscope, the pressure cuff on the upper arm is first inflated to a pressure well above systolic pressure. At this point no sounds can be heard through the stethoscope, which is placed over the brachial artery, for that artery has been collapsed by the pressure of the cuff. The pressure in the cuff is then gradually reduced. As soon as cuff pressure falls below systolic pressure, small amounts of blood spurt past the cuff and Korotkoff sounds begin to be heard through the stethoscope. The pressure of the cuff that is indicated on the manometer when the first Korotkoff sound is heard is recorded as the systolic blood pressure.

As the pressure in the cuff continues to drop, the Korotkoff sounds continue until the cuff pressure is no longer sufficient to occlude the vessel during any part of the cycle. Below this pressure, the Korotkoff sounds disappear, marking the value of the diastolic pressure.

This familiar method of locating the systolic and diastolic pressure values by listening to the Korotkoff sounds is called the *auscultatory method* of sphygmomanometry. An alternate method, called the *palpatory method,* is similar except that the flow of blood is identified in the artery by palpating the pulse of the patient downstream from the cuff instead of listening for Korotkoff sounds. Although systolic pressure can easily be measured by the palpatory method, diastolic pressure is much more difficult to identify. For this reason, the auscultatory method is more commonly used. Figure 8-4 shows a blood pressure measurement, using the auscultatory method.

Because of the trauma imposed by direct measurement of blood pressure (described in Chapter 9) and the lack of a more suitable method for indirect measurement, attempts have been made to automate the manual procedure. As a result, a number of automatic or semiautomatic systems have been developed. Most devices are of a type that utilizes a pressure transducer connected to the sphygmomanometer cuff, a microphone placed beneath the cuff (over the artery), and a standard physiological recording system on which cuff pressure and the Korotkoff sounds are recorded. The basic procedure parallels the manual method. The pressure cuff is automatically inflated to about 220 mm Hg and allowed to deflate slowly. The microphone picks up the Korotkoff sounds from the artery near the surface, just below the compression cuff. The instrument either superimposes the signal of the Korotkoff sounds on the voltage recording that

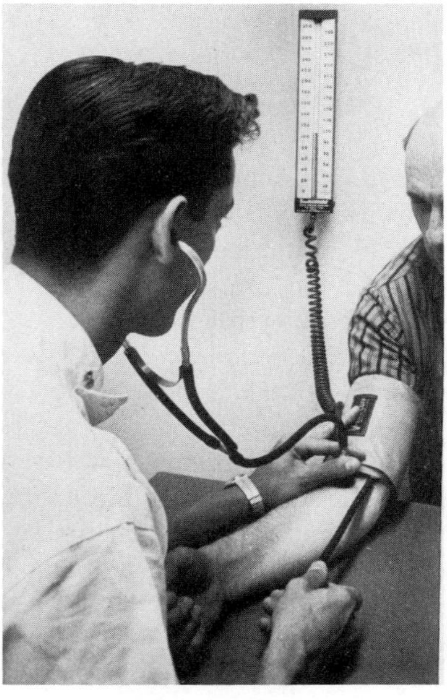

Fig. 8–4 Measurement of blood pressure using a sphygmomanometer. *(Courtesy of W. A. Baum, Inc., Copiague, New York.)*

represents the falling cuff pressure or records the two separately. The pressure reading at the time of the first sound represents the systolic pressure; the diastolic pressure is the point on the falling pressure curve where the signal representing the last sound is seen. This instrument is actually only semiautomatic, for the recording thus obtained must still be interpreted by the observer. False indications—caused, for instance, by motion artifacts—can often be observed on the recording. Fully automated devices use some type of signal-detecting circuit to determine the occurrence of the first and last Korotkoff sounds and to retain and display the cuff pressure readings for these points, either electronically or with mercury manometers that are cut off by solenoid valves. These devices, by necessity, are more susceptible to false indications caused by artifacts. Methods other than those utilizing the Korotkoff sounds have been tried in detecting the blood pulse distal to the occlusion cuff. Among them is impedance plethysmography (see Chapter 12), which indicates directly the pulsating blood flow in the artery, and ultrasonic Doppler methods, which measure the motions of the arterial walls.

Many of the commercially available automatic blood pressure meters work well when demonstrated on a quiet, healthy subject but fail when used to measure blood pressure during activity or when used on patients in circulatory shock.

In recent years a new approach that utilizes ultrasound to measure the pulsatile motion of the brachial artery wall has been developed. The principle is similar to sonar. High-frequency sound energy is transmitted into the patient's arm and is reflected back from the arterial walls. By means of the Doppler effect (see explanation in Chapter 12), the movement of the arterial walls can be detected as they snap open and closed with each pulsation of blood.

An advantage of this type of instrument is that results closer to direct measurements (discussed in Chapter 9) are obtained. Also, it can be used for patients under shock and in intensive care units, when direct measurement would not be suitable for the patient. Because vessel-wall movement is sensed, blood flow is not a requirement for measurement.

One such instrument is the Arteriosonde®, manufactured by Hoffman-La Roche, Inc., Nutley, New Jersey. It has a cloth cuff and air bag with an electric air pump to supply the pressure; the pump can be regulated by a front-panel control. The cuff is placed on the arm in the same fashion as the sphygmomanometer except that there is a transducer array under the cuff. These transducers are arranged as alternate transmitters and receivers. The motion of the artery produces a so-called Doppler shift, which identifies the instant the artery is opened and closed with each beat between systolic and diastolic pressure. It is analogous to the Korotkoff sound.

The first signal is used to stop the mercury fall in the first of two manometers to indicate systolic pressure. The second manometer is stopped at the point of disappearance of the pulses to indicate diastolic pressure. Hence both readings can be noted simultaneously.

8.3 Care and Techniques of Measurements

At best the sphygmomanometer is only as accurate as the person taking the measurement. Unfortunately, there is a small discrepancy from one person to another. The authors have conducted experiments of different people taking blood pressure measurements on the same subject and found that these variations exist. Also, the same person taking measurements on different days might get different results.

In the indirect method, extreme accuracy is not too important, since a "normal" blood pressure is not usually defined as an exact value. Instead a range of "normal" values is specified. In considering the condition of a patient, it is the change in blood pressure that is important rather than the actual level. Some hypertensive people have spent their entire lives with blood pressure of 180/140 mm Hg. A physician or nurse who is unfamiliar with the patient could, on taking a reading and being unaware of this condition, assume that problems exist that actually do not.

Three items of equipment are normally used: the stethoscope, the bag and cuff, and the manometer. The stethoscope is a very robust instrument. However, its condition should be watched, particularly for a cracked diaphragm or for deteriorated condition of the rubber tubing. The biggest problem with the stethoscope is not the instrument itself but the interface of the instrument with the ear of the observer. If the Korotkoff sounds are not absolutely clear, duplicate readings should always be taken. The medical condition of the observer can affect readings—slight deafness after a cold, for example. Normally the bell provides the most sensitive determination of the relatively low-frequency Korotkoff sounds.

The cuff surrounds an inflatable bag. One problem that exists, but not too frequently, is inadequate cuff width. Most sets have a standard cuff, but a smaller-width type is available for children or people with small arms. Wide cuffs for obese people or for thigh measurements are also available.

If the cuff is too narrow, the blood pressure reading will be high; whereas if it is too wide, there is a possibility of a low reading. A rule of thumb is to use the standard cuff, usually 12 to 14 cm wide, unless it is obvious that the limb is too small or too large. In that case, use a small cuff (available down to about 2.5 cm) or large ones (available up to 20 cm wide).

Although the bag is elastic, the cuff should not be of stretch-type material, since it is necessary to apply even pressure. The cloth-bandage type used for many years should encircle the arm several times. However, the newer cuffs have Velcro® fasteners in which the surfaces of the mating fabrics interlock. The bag and its inflating system should also be watched for leaks. Erratic inflation or deflation usually means a leak.

In hospitals and doctors' offices, most manometers are of the mercury column type, although, for portability, an aneroid manometer can also be used. The latter is not as accurate as the mercury type and should be calibrated over its entire range reasonably frequently. With the mercury column type, care should be taken that no mercury is lost. In addition, the columns should be completely vertical.

In taking readings, it is important that the nurse become proficient in recognizing the Korotkoff sounds; also, in the case of the mercury column manometer, the reading of mercury level should be taken with the eye opposite the meniscus of the column.

In general, the patient should be placed in a chair or on a bed with the forearm either horizontal on a table or on the bed at approximately the level of the heart. There are postural effects on blood pressure. With wall manometers, the patient's bed should be in a high position. However, a consistent technique is the most important variable, and satisfactory documentation of blood pressure can be obtained as long as all staff have patients at the same level. The main point is to be consistent in the way measurements are taken. The patient should sit quietly, without distractions, in a comfortable position for 5 to 10 minutes prior to the reading. Factors that can affect blood pressure readings include eating, smoking, alcohol, temperature, anxiety, and pain—or a pretty nurse. Those that cannot be avoided should be written on the patient's chart so that they may be taken into account for later analysis (with the possible exception of the last).

The way in which the stethoscope is used is important. It should be placed firmly on the antecubital space over the brachial artery. Too much pressure might distort the sounds, whereas too little can result in a space between the stethoscope and the arm, thus making some soft sounds inaudible. The cuff, with the bag on the inside of the arm, should have the lower edge 2 to 3 cm above the spot where the stethoscope will be placed.

On inflating the bag, with stethoscope in position, the pressure should be watched carefully as it is raised. About 30 to 40 mm Hg above expected results is the highest level to which it should be raised. More accurately, the radial pulse can be palpated on a preliminary run, and about 30 mm Hg above the point in which it disappears can be used. Patients sometimes become apprehensive if the cuff becomes too tight. Pressure should be released at a rate of about 2 mm Hg/second.

The Korotkoff sound becomes audible in the stethoscope as the pressure falls, and four definite phases can be detected. The first phase is the period at which the sounds appear as a faint tapping that gradually increases in intensity. This phase is followed by a period of "swishing" sounds. The systolic pressure is the point at which the tapping is heard for at least two consecutive beats. During the third phase, the sounds are crisper and still increasing; then there is an abrupt muffling of the sound, which becomes softer and of a blowing quality. This phase is the best index of diastolic pressure. The final stage is when the sound becomes inaudible. The precise moment is hard to ascertain. Although most blood pressure readings indicate only systolic/diastolic, it has been recommended that the fourth and fifth phase pressures should both be noted. For example, 122/82/76 would be noted. If the fourth and fifth phase are identical, such as 122/82/82, only the two levels are used.

Many people take the blood pressure reading for both arms. If one happens to give higher readings than the other, that arm should be used, to be on the safe side. The right arm will have the higher arterial pressure in most people.

8.3.2 Clinical Problems in Indirect Measurements

Several special problems should be noted. Before discussing them, it is important to mention again that since all blood pressure measurements are relative, it is important to establish a base or reference reading for a given patient. *Basal blood pressure* is obtained when a patient is under conditions as ideal as possible—for example, at home or after a few days of rest in the hospital. It should be taken with the patient free of all mental, emotional, or physical stimuli. The person taking the blood pressure measurements should try to avoid talking or doing anything with the patient that might influence the reading.

As mentioned, a different-sized cuff is important for obese or small persons and for children. In the latter case, additional factors must be considered, such as providing some diversion for the child so that he or she is not distressed; a bottle may be necessary for infants. If a child cries, the blood pressure can rise considerably. It is sometimes preferable in hospital cases to leave the cuff on until the patient is asleep.

In children, the muffling sound mentioned as phase four is better than the complete cessation of sound for the diastolic pressure reading. In very young infants, the sounds may be too faint and special techniques are often necessary. It is important to continue to run the cuff pressure down slowly following cessation of Korotkoff sounds. In hypertension, an "auscultatory gap" may occur in which the Korotkoff sounds reappear following initial cessation.

Ocasionally there is a problem in obtaining blood pressure in the arms, such as with upper-extremity amputees; and the thigh may be used instead.

A cuff about 6 mm wider than the arm cuff is used, depending on the diameter of the thigh. The patient must lie face down on the abdomen; then the cuff is wrapped around the thigh a few centimeters higher than the artery in the popliteal fossa where the stethoscope is placed. The bag is on the posterior side of the thigh. The large cuffs usually record systolic pressure in the thigh as higher than that in the arms, whereas the diastolic tends to be lower.

In the presence of frequent premature ventricular contractions, atrial fibrillation, and certain other cardiac arrhythmias causing beat-to-beat variations of cardiac output, the arterial blood pressure may be significantly lower. Serial determinations should be made for accurate documentation.

If a patient is in shock, the Korotkoff sounds will be diminished or completely absent; consequently, blood pressure readings cannot be taken by this method. Since the blood pressure can be a critical parameter for determining the conditions that resulted in shock, a percutaneous method of direct measurements via a major artery (Chapter 9) is indicated. If this method is too traumatic, the ultrasonic method can also be used.

9

Direct Measurement of Blood Pressure

In 1728 Hales inserted a glass tube into an artery of a horse and crudely obtained the first direct measurement of arterial blood pressure. Poiseuille substituted a mercury manometer for the long glass tube of Hales; later, Ludwig added a float and devised the kymograph, which allowed continuous recording of blood pressure. It is only recently that strain gage transducers and complex electronic systems have replaced the manometer and kymograph. Sophisticated and safe invasive techniques of vessel catheterization have become common in both diagnostic and patient care areas.

A discussion of direct blood pressure measurements in the clinical setting must necessarily be concerned with specifics if it is to be of any use to the practitioner. This chapter describes blood pressure measurement instrumentation, plus the specific patient-care concerns inherent in direct monitoring of central venous and pulmonary artery and wedge pressures, as well as left atrial and central arterial pressures.

9.1 Direct Measurement Technology

Direct measurement of blood pressure requires the use of *invasive* methods. That is, a transducer or a catheter leading to a transducer must be introduced into the cardiovascular system with the sensing tip at the point of measurement (the location from which the measurement is to be made). A *catheter* is a thin, flexible tube designed for entry into the blood stream.

Any one of three methods can be used to gain access to the point of measurement:

1. Percutaneous insertion of a short catheter or small bore needle into a vessel is a method used where the point of measurement is near the point of penetration. The catheter or needle is connected to a pressure transducer external to the body.
2. A catheterization technique which involves guiding a long catheter through the artery or vein to the point of measurement, which may be in one of the major vessels or in the heart itself. Again, the pressure transducer is external to the body.
3. Location of the transducer itself at the point of measurement where the transducer is installed at the tip of the catheter and is called a *catheter tip transducer*.

The first two methods employ a fluid column to transmit the pressure encountered at the tip of the catheter or needle to the transducer. In the third method, the transducer encounters the pressure inside the vessel directly.

Percutaneous insertion and catheterization usually involve minor surgical techniques. Figures 9-1 and 9-7 give a general idea of both methods.

Typically, for percutaneous insertion, a local anesthetic is injected near the site of invasion. The vessel is occluded and a needle inserted at a slight angle toward the vessel. When the needle is in place, a catheter is fed through the needle, usually by means of a flexible guide. When the catheter is securely in place in the vessel, the needle and guide are withdrawn. For some measurements, the needle is attached to a tube, so that the needle can be left in the vessel and the transducer or manometer connected to the tube.

Catheterization of blood vessels was first developed in the late 1940s and has become a major technique for obtaining information about the functioning of the heart and other parts of the cardiovascular system. The technique requires that the vessel to be cannulated be made visible by venous or arterial cutdown methods. Apart from obtaining blood pressures

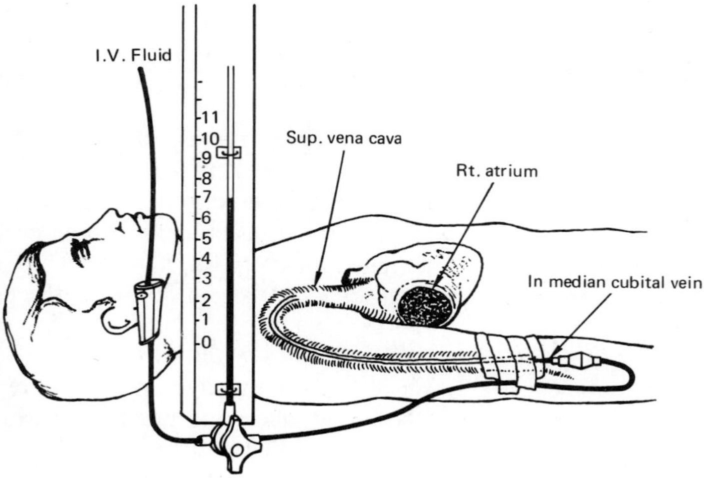

Fig. 9–1 Catheterization of the right atrium for central venous pressure determinations via the median cubital vein.

in the heart chambers and great vessels, this technique is also used to obtain blood samples from the heart in order to measure its oxygen content or to detect the location of abnormal blood flow pathways or shunts. Also, catheters are used to inject radiopaque dyes for X-ray studies, substances for indicator dilution studies, and the administration of vasoactive drugs directly into the heart and certain vessels.

When the pressure transducer is external to the body (extracorporeal), a sterile solution, such as 5% dextrose in water or normal saline is introduced into the catheter so that the fluid pressure can be transmitted to the transducer.

In both fluid-column measurements and measurements obtained with a transducer at the point of measurement, a complete pressure system includes provisions for balancing the transducer-amplifier system and for adjusting the gain or sensitivity. Balancing is achieved by adjusting the system to indicate zero pressure when the actual pressure is zero. The sensitivity or gain setting adjusts the system to indicate a given pressure when that pressure is applied to the transducer.

9.1.1 Transducers

As introduced in Chapter 2, a *transducer* is a device that converts a physiological variable, such as blood pressure, into an electrical signal. In direct blood pressure measurements, the transducer is used to convert the blood pressure variations into voltage variations that can be displayed as the pressure waveform or converted into a numeric display of blood pressure values.

Blood pressure transducers can be categorized as resistive, inductive or capacitive, depending on the type of electrical element used.

The fluid that applies pressure to the transducer is in contact with a thin flexible diaphragm which bends in proportion to the pressure. In a *resistive* transducer, more commonly called a *strain-gage transducer,* the bending of the diaphragm stretches some fine wires, increasing their resistance in proportion to the applied pressure. At the same time the stretching of some other wires is decreased, lowering the resistance of those wires. The wires in the transducer are connected to form a bridge circuit as shown in Figure 9-2. The operation of a bridge circuit is described in Section 3.9.1.

When the transducer is connected to a blood-pressure amplifier or monitor, an excitation voltage (either ac or dc) is applied to the bridge. When the bridge is properly balanced and calibrated, a voltage proportional to the pressure applied to the transducer will appear between terminals A and B. The balancing and calibration of the transducer bridge are described in Section 9.1.3.

Not all blood pressure transducers are of the strain-gage type. Inductive and capacitive transducers are also available. One type of inductive transducer frequently used in patient care utilizes a *linear variable differential transformer (LVDT).* Although they may look very much like their strain-gage counterparts, LVDT transducers are based on an entirely different operating principle. These devices utilize a special type of transformer (see Section 3.7.4) which produces an output voltage proportional to the applied pressure. Because a transformer is involved, ac excitation is required. Thus, the signal conditioning equipment used with a strain-gage transducer may not be usable with an LVDT transducer. Although it is used in a manner quite similar to that of the strain-gage unit, the LVDT transducer produces a greater output voltage for a given excitation voltage.

In a typical capacitive transducer, the diaphragm moved by the pressure variations is connected to a movable plate of a variable capacitor.

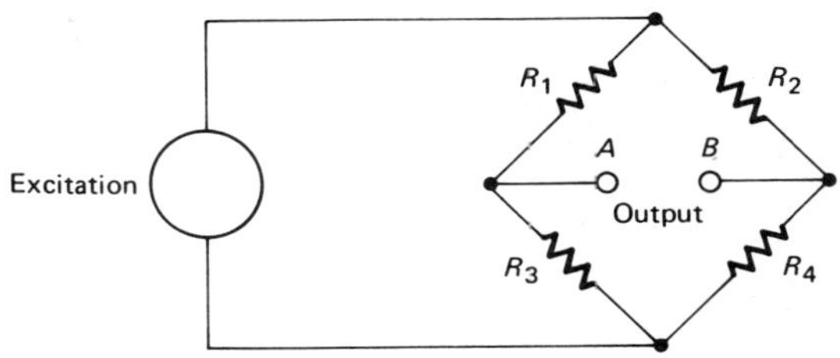

Fig. 9–2 Resistance strain-gage bridge.

When this plate is moved with respect to a fixed plate, the resulting changes in capacitance reflect variations in the measured blood pressure. These capacitance changes are converted to voltage changes by circuitry contained within the transducer itself. In this case, the control for zero (baseline) adjustment is also located on the transducer.

Blood Pressure Measurements Employing a Fluid Column. Figures 9-3 and 9-4 show two typical transducers that use a fluid column in order to measure pressure. Figure 9-3 illustrates a standard-size Statham Model P23ID transducer, while Figure 9-4 shows a miniature model.

The electrical connection to the strain-gage bridge inside the transducer is made via a cable at the bottom of the transducer. Pressure connections to the catheter are made at the top through *Luer fittings* in the transparent dome, which also provide a means of flushing the transducer. The dome is transparent so that air bubbles can be detected and eliminated. The transducer itself is of the strain-gage type.

Strain-gage blood pressure transducers are available in many types.

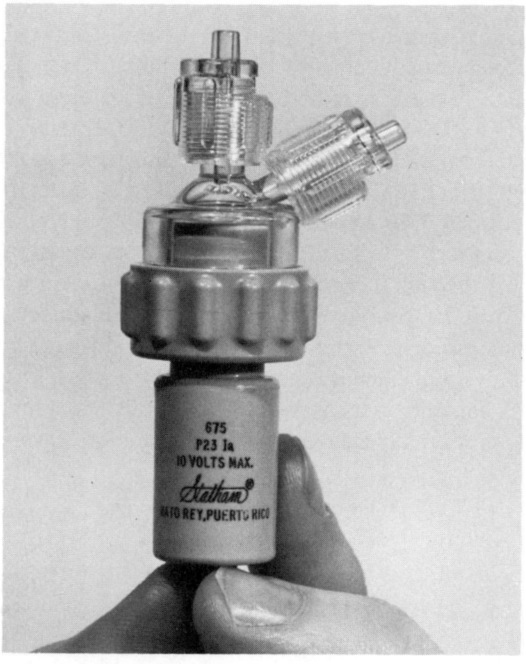

Fig. 9–3 Fluid-column blood pressure transducer, Statham Model P23ID. *(Courtesy of Gould, Inc., Statham Instruments Division, Oxnard, California.)*

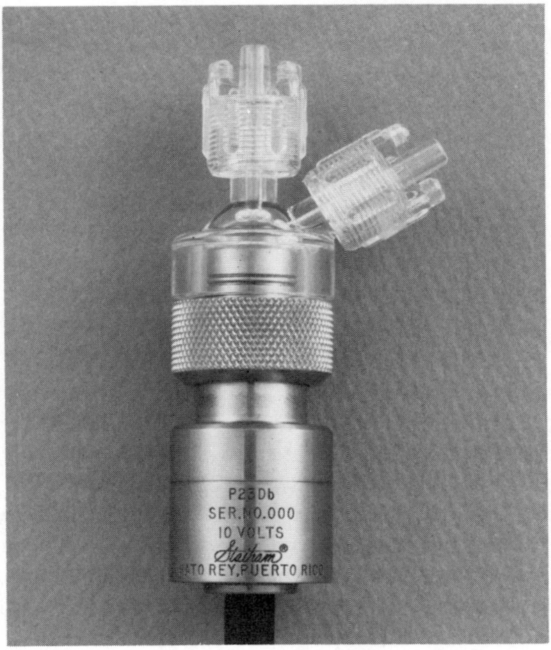

Fig. 9–4 Fluid-column blood pressure transducer, Statham Model P23Db. *(Courtesy of Gould, Inc., Statham Instruments Division, Oxnard, California.)*

There are general-purpose models for arterial pressure (0 to 330 mm Hg) and venous pressure (0 to 50 mm Hg), and special models with differing sensitivities, volume displacement characteristics, and mechanical arrangements.

These transducers can be flushed to remove air bubbles and to prevent blood from clotting at the end of the catheter. These procedures will be discussed in more detail in the next section.

The fluid column used with a transducer of this type has a natural frequency or resonance of its own that can affect the frequency response of the system. Care must be taken in selecting a transducer and catheter to be used together so that the frequency response of the complete system will be adequate.

Pressure transducers are normally mounted on a suitable manifold (see Section 9.1.2) near the patient's bed. It is important to keep the transducer at the same height as the point at which the measurements are to be made in order to avoid errors due to hydrostatic pressure differences. If a *differential pressure* is desired, two transducers of this type may be used at two different points, and the difference in pressure may be obtained as the difference of their output signals. Figure 9-5 shows a typical infusion manifold incorporating transducers, a flushing system, and syringes for blood specimen withdrawal.

The signal-conditioning and display devices for these transducers are available in a variety of forms. However, each must provide a method of excitation for the strain-gage bridge or the LVDT, a means of zeroing or balancing the bridge, necessary amplification of the output signal, and a display device, such as a monitor scope, a recorder, panel meter, or digital readout device. Most modern systems permit many possible combinations. Figure 9-6 depicts a typical readout system for direct pressure monitoring.

Blood Pressure Measurement At The Site. In order to avoid the frequency-response problem often inherent in measuring blood pressure through a fluid column, a "catheter-tip" transducer can be positioned at the site at which the blood pressure is to be measured. One such transducer makes use of a variable inductance principle. The tip of the transducer is placed directly in the bloodstream so that the blood presses on a membrane surrounded by a protective cap. The membrane is connected to a magnetic core that is free to move within a coil assembly, thereby changing the inductance of the coil as a function of the pressure on the membrane. The inductance changes are converted into voltage changes which are proportional to the changes in blood pressure.

Another type of transducer has a strain-gage sensor built into the tip of a cardiac catheter. Pressure variations at the site itself produce resistance changes in the strain gage. Measurements at the site are usually performed for diagnostic purposes.

Percutaneous Measurements. An example of a percutaneous blood pressure measuring system is shown in Figures 9-7 and 9-8. Figure 9-7 shows the transducer applied, while Figure 9-8 provides an exploded view showing the dome and stopcocks. The plastic dome with the three-way stopcock permits flushing of the needle, withdrawal of blood samples, and, in certain circumstances, the administration of drugs. This transducer is usually employed to measure arterial pressures (e.g., radial artery) but may also be used to measure venous pressures or the pressures of other physiological fluids by direct attachment to a needle at the point of measurement. It can be used with a continuously self-flushing system without appreciable degradation of the signal. The transparent plastic dome permits observation of air bubble formation and facilitates their removal. Another advantage of this transducer is the fact that it can be connected to a standard intravenous infusion system.

Another type of blood pressure transducer is shown in Figure 9-9. This device has a strain-gage sensor built into the tip of a No. 6 French catheter.

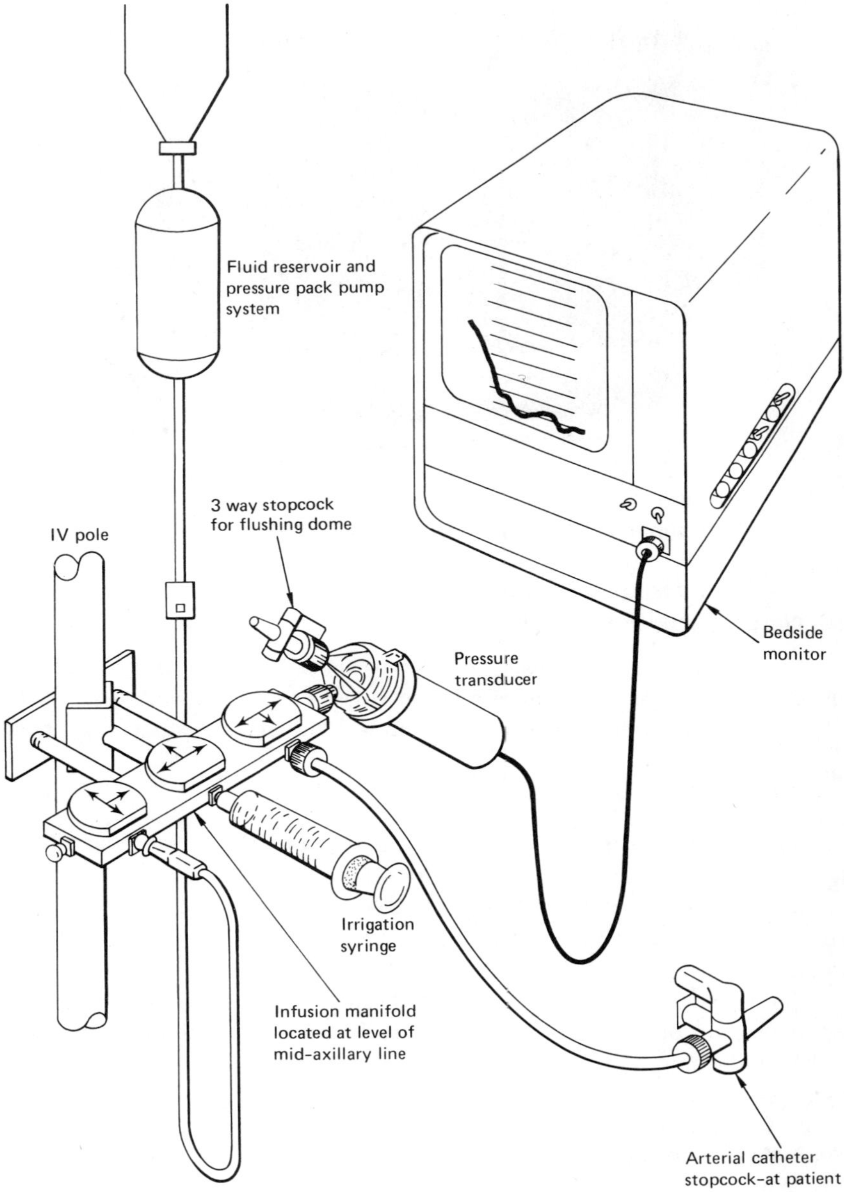

Fig. 9–5 Infusion manifold with transducer, flushing system and syringe. *(Courtesy of Michael Tomeo, UCLA Medical Center.)*

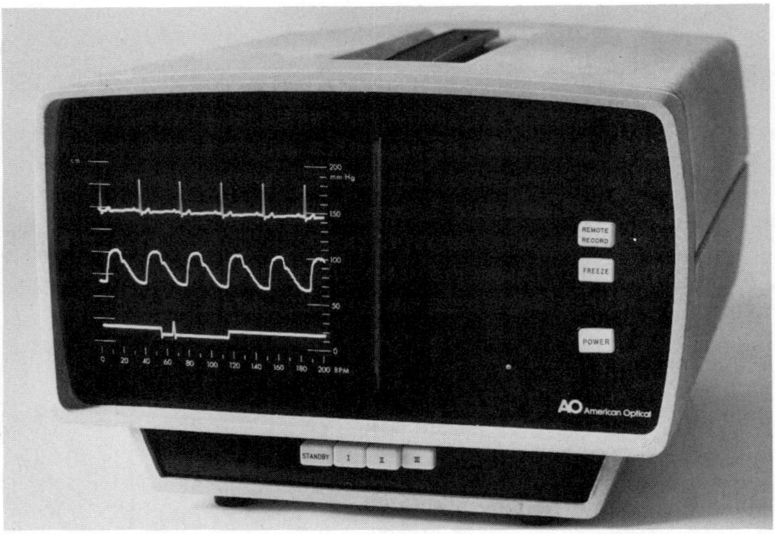

Fig. 9–6 Blood pressure amplifier and display. *(Courtesy of American Optical Corporation, Medical Division, Newport Beach, California.)*

The frequency response of this transducer is sufficiently high to measure both pressure and heart sounds.

Implantable Transducers. Figure 9-10 shows a type of transducer that can be implanted into the wall of a blood vessel or into the wall of the heart itself. This transducer, however, is limited to long-term research in animals.

9.1.2 The Infusion Manifold

The knowledgeable use of both transducers and the measurement techniques employed constitutes a very important factor in accurate pressure monitoring. Central to the use of transducers are an intact, safe, and conveniently organized infusion manifold and an accurately balanced and calibrated transducer.

To prevent system blockages and ensure patency of the system, heparinized normal saline or 5% dextrose in water is commonly employed as the fluid column. *Patency* is the absence of clots or obstructions that might prevent or limit flow. The concentration of heparin may vary, but 500 units per 250 cc of solution is an effective anticoagulant concentration. In addition, a flushing system utilizing one or more three-way stopcocks and syringes in series with the fluid reservoir and the patient provides a means by which blood specimens can be withdrawn, ensures patency, and allows periodic calibration of the transducer. The manifold must be at the level of the patient's right atrium if fluid column measurement of *central*

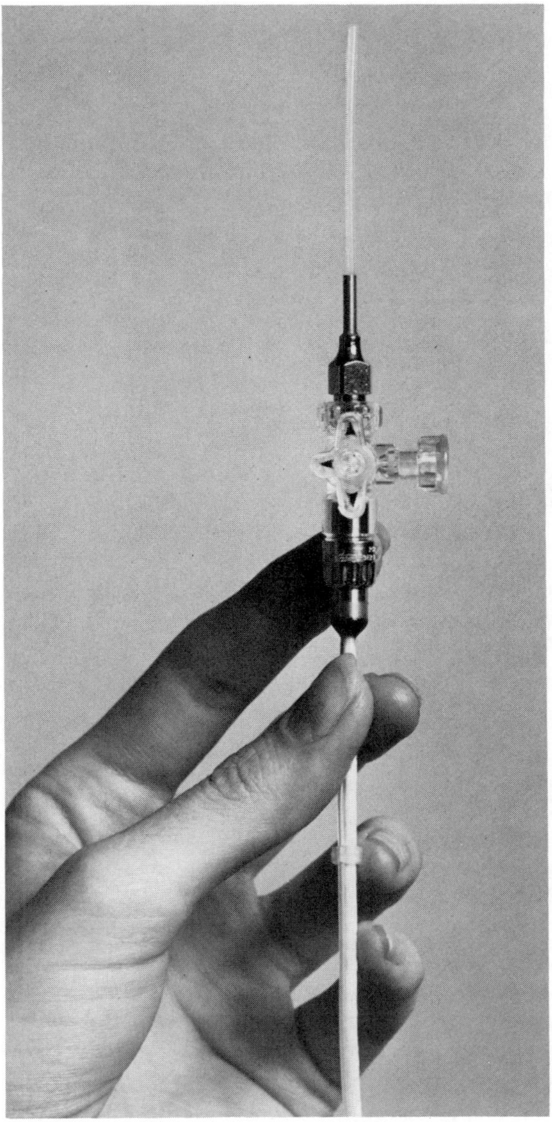

Fig. 9–7 Percutaneous blood pressure transducer. *(Courtesy of Gould, Inc., Statham Instruments Division, Oxnard, California.)*

venous pressure (CVP) is to be accomplished; positioning the manifold in this way reduces the error due to differences in hydrostatic pressure. In addition, the manifold must be sturdy and vibration resistant. Transducers

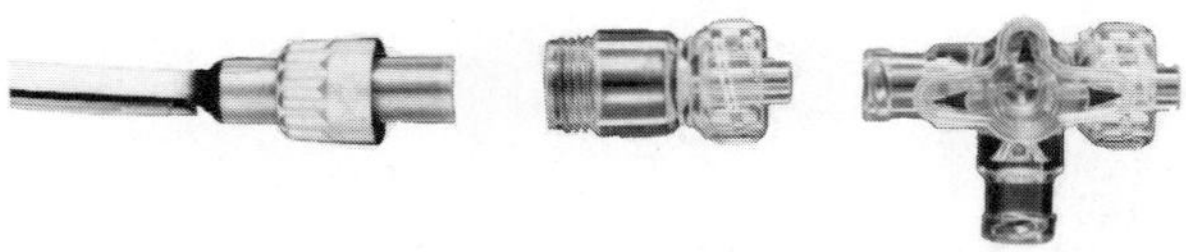

Fig. 9–8 Exploded view of blood pressure transducer. *(Courtesy of Gould, Inc., Statham Instruments Division, Oxnard, California.)*

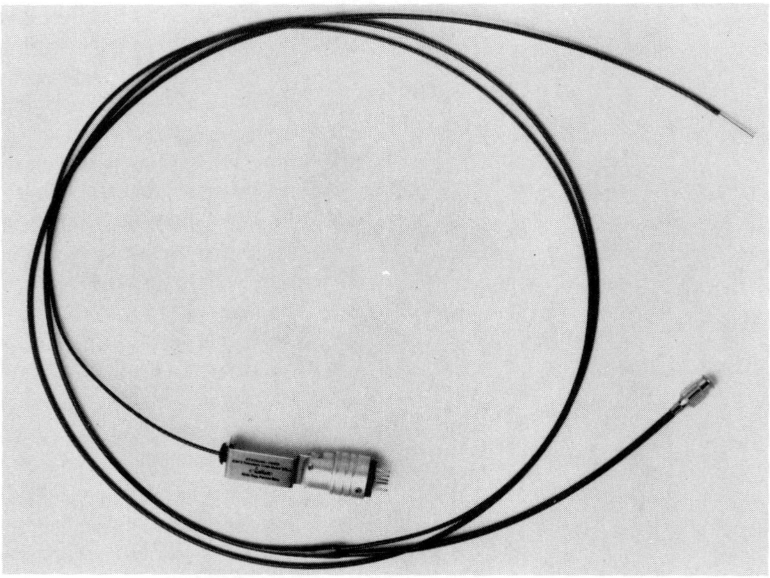

Fig. 9–9 SF-1 blood pressure sensor. *(Courtesy of Gould, Inc., Statham Instruments Division, Oxnard, California.)*

may be mounted horizontally or vertically in such a way that they are not readily bumped by personnel or equipment and so that air bubbles may be easily removed. All equipment that comes in contact with the fluid reservoir, and hence with the patient, must be sterile, including the transducer. Rigid tubing connects the transducer to the vessel to be monitored. Rigidity is necessary to prevent measurement errors.

In addition, a system for continuous slow infusion of heparinized

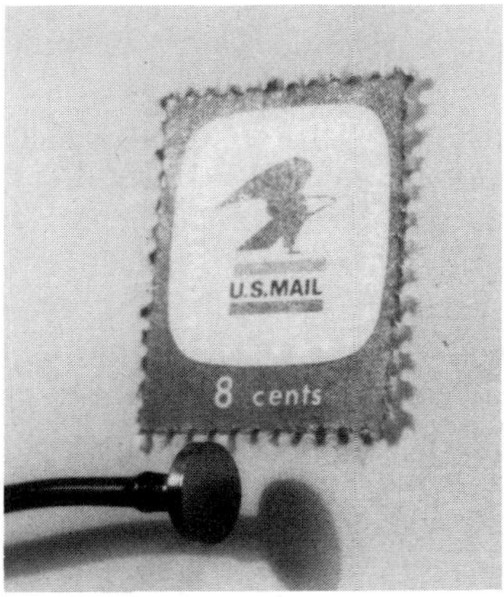

Fig. 9–10 Implantable pressure transducer. *(Courtesy of Konigsberg Instruments, Pasadena, California.)*

solution into monitoring lines may be employed. This system may be automatic or manual, in the form of an infusion pump or pressurized transfer pack for high-pressure vessels. Although patency is further ensured by using such equipment, it should be realized that the use of any additional line-powered electrical equipment in conjunction with the fluid column in the catheter increases the risk of exposing a patient to electric shock. The subject of electrical safety is covered in Chapter 18.

Figure 9-4 shows a typical infusion manifold with transducers, flushing equipment and a pressurized pack rèservoir.

9.1.3 Balancing and Calibration of Transducers

As discussed earlier, most blood pressure transducers used in critical care are of the strain-gage type in which pressure variations are converted into changes in the resistance of wires inside the transducer. The wires are interconnected to form a bridge circuit. Although the resistances in the bridge are matched as perfectly as possible at the time of manufacture, it is still necessary to compensate for slight differences that still exist. Further, when ac excitation is used, differences in capacitance must also be balanced out. For these reasons, the amplifier or monitor may include one or more controls to permit *balancing* of the bridge. In the balancing procedure, the controls are adjusted so that a zero pressure reading is obtained when the pressure being sensed is zero.

Calibration refers to adjustment of the gain or sensitivity of the amplifier so that the indicated pressure value will agree with the pressure actually sensed. In some systems, it is possible to obtain a numerical *calibration factor* for each transducer used. Then when a given transducer is to be used, its calibration factor is simply dialed into the appropriate control on the panel of the instrument to ensure that the equipment is properly calibrated.

Balancing and calibration should be performed before a patient is connected to the system and periodically during monitoring to ensure accurate readings. The methods by which these procedures are accomplished will vary, depending on the type of transducers and signal conditioning equipment used. In fact, some patient monitors provide automatic balancing so that manual balancing is not required. A typical balancing and calibration procedure is outlined in Appendix B. However, for specific information the reader is referred to the manufacturers' instruction manuals.

When more than one pressure transducer is used on a patient, it is useful to label each waveform on the monitor. This practice will help prevent mistaking the central venous pressure (CVP) or pulmonary artery pressure for a central arterial reading. For the most part, personnel should record the values shown on the readout rather than from the monitor scope, since the latter may be subject to baseline drift and artifacts due to patient movement. A possible exception to this practice might be the documenting of end diastolic pressure contours, which would not be shown on the meter.

9.2 Clinical Application of Direct Measurement Technology

9.2.1 *Monitoring Central Venous Pressure*

Central venous pressure (CVP) is the pressure exerted by blood in a central vein, usually the right atrium, superior vena cava, or subclavian. Depending on catheter placement, the normal range of values is from 0 to 5 cm H_20 in the right atrium and from 6 to 12 cm H_20 in the superior vena cava or subclavian. More important than the actual value itself, however, is the trend or movement indicated by a series of pressure values. For example, an upward or downward trend of 6 cm H_20 over a few hours may be significant, even though the values themselves remain within normal limits. Water manometric measurement will give a mean or average value, whereas a transducer measurement provides the actual fluctuations due to undulating changes in right heart and intrathoracic pressure.

Central venous pressure contributes information about circulating blood volume, vascular tone, and the effectiveness of the right heart as a pump. This technique is widely utilized in acute care settings because of the ease of catheter placement and monitoring. Probably the most useful aspect of this method is the continuous evaluation of fluid replacement therapy in situations involving *extracardiac* disease, such as acute hypovolemic, vasogenic, or neurogenic shock. For example, fluid replacement in a severely burned patient during the first critical 48 hours is guided primarily by urinary output and CVP. When vasopressors or volume expanders are utilized in other clinical situations, CVP can document efficacy of treatment, since cardiac output and, ultimately, tissue perfusion are an outcome of optimal blood volume returning to the heart.

It must be remembered that the cardiac competency reflected in the CVP applies only to the right heart; indeed, failure of the left ventricle may precede failure of the right by several hours. For this reason, CVP values must be utilized in conjunction with other assessment parameters, such as arterial blood pressure, direct measurement of pulmonary artery wedge or left atrial pressures, apical pulse (especially third heart sounds and tachycardia), and breath sounds (assessing basilar rales and tachypnea). It should be noted that the use of CVP is especially limited in the patient with a decompensating heart due to cardiac disease. Consequently, the acutely ill patient with *myocardial infarction* (MI) should be monitored through pulmonary artery techniques, which more accurately reflect left ventricular status. This method is discussed later.

Either a percutaneous or venous cutdown technique may be used to insert a radiopaque polyethelene catheter into a central vein. The physician may use a subclavian approach, or he may choose to use a large vein in the arm, such as the basilic or median cubital. Occasionally the jugular vein is used. The catheter is threaded into the desired location and connected to the transducer (or water manometer). Fluctuations with heartbeat or ventricular ectopics may indicate that the catheter has traversed the tricuspid valve and entered the right ventricle. In this case, withdrawing the catheter a few centimeters will produce the desired placement. A chest X-ray will usually be done after a subclavian procedure so as to determine the presence of a pneumothorax, a frequent complication of this approach.

Figure 9-11 represents a typical system for measurement of CVP by means of a water manometer. Basically, three elements are involved: (a) a fluid reservoir to ensure patency, (b) a three-way stopcock to divert fluid into the water manometer and then isolate the fluid column from the reservoir so that it becomes continuous with the tip of the catheter, and (c) the secured CVP catheter with a sterile dressing placed over the point of entry.

CVP is usually monitored with the patient in a flat position, although positional modifications may be incorporated as long as specific notations are made on the flow sheet or nursing notes and consistency is maintained.

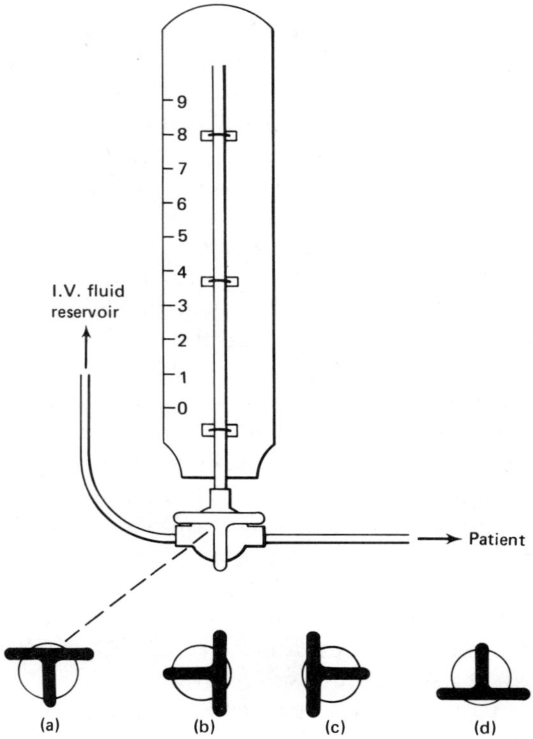

Fig. 9–11 Typical manometric system for measuring central venous pressure demonstrating positioning of the stopcock to (a) maintain patency only; (b) fill the manometer with reservoir fluid; (c) obtain isolated readings; and (d) to obtain continuous readings while maintaining patency.

As mentioned earlier, the transducer is to be located at the level of the right atrium, which is usually 5 cm below the sternum or at the midaxillary line. Marking this point with a pen on the skin of patients is also helpful.

The technique for monitoring CVP is relatively straightforward. With a few simple considerations, safe and accurate readings can be ensured. Any amount of air in the manometer (or transducer dome) or in the fluid column connected to the patient will affect the measurements. Air embolization, even in small amounts, can be dangerous and may be lethal to the patient with a right-to-left circulatory shunt. When the manometer is connected to the patient, fluctuations of 0.5 to 2 cm H_20 should be apparent with respiration. The fluid will rise with changes in interpulmonic pressure. Such fluctuations should be indicated on the flow sheet. Poor fluctuation of the fluid level, as well as slow equilibration, generally indicates lack of patency and requires flushing of the line with reservoir fluid. Excessive force should never be used in flushing the line because of the danger of embolization. If the patient is receiving assistance in respiration, his CVP will be higher than if he were not. However, most patients may be removed from the ventilator for a few seconds while the reading is taken. Straining and coughing will also increase the reading.

Because of the placement of the catheter tip, care and judgment must be used both in infusion of medications and in maintaining sterility. Drugs like potassium chloride, isoproterenol, and aminophylline can produce cardiac irritability and potentially dangerous arrhythmias when given through central venous lines. On the other hand, drugs such as cephalothin may be especially desirable to infuse via the central line for patients with subacute or acute bacterial endocarditis. The practitioner should always determine what medications are to go through the CVP line. Any medications (especially antibiotics) may effectively shorten the life of the line and distort readings as well. For the same reason, it is not wise to use a CVP line to withdraw blood specimens. Although it may be convenient, especially with the patient who has poor peripheral veins, this practice results in clotted lines and inaccurate measurements.

In order to maintain sterile conditions, meticulous care is necessary in all efforts relating to the CVP. This is especially true in the preparation of IV additives and care of the infusion site, in order to prevent endocardial disease. Some centers routinely change CVP and other infusion catheter site dressings daily, painting the area with an antibacterial solution and ointment. Dressings should be occlusive but not constrictive and should hold the catheter in a stable position. In spite of the best technique, however, the chance of central contamination is always present, particularly in high-risk patients with prosthetic valves and suture lines in the endocardial area. Thus nonfluctuating CVP lines through which fluid may still be infused should be quickly removed unless fluid repletion is still critical and dependable peripheral venous access is not possible.

9.2.2 *Monitoring Pulmonary Artery and Pulmonary Capillary Wedge Pressures*

The bedside monitoring of *pulmonary artery pressure* (PAP) and *pulmonary capillary wedge pressure* (PCWP) is increasing in use. This technique measures the pressure exerted by blood volume in a small pulmonary artery and the pulmonary capillary bed, respectively. The PCWP measurement is a direct indicator of left ventricular filling pressure. Thus, it provides a more accurate index of left ventricular competency. Normal values of pulmonary artery pressure are less than 25 mm Hg at systole and less than 15 mm Hg at diastole. The mean pressure is less than 18 mm Hg. The pulmonary capillary pressure usually has a mean value of less than 15 to 18 mm Hg. As was the case with CVP determinations, changes over time provide important information regarding changes in cardiac status. Water manometric methods may be used to obtain mean pressure values. However, since the clinician is still more frequently concerned with systolic and diastolic waveforms and values as well as mean values, a transducer/amplifier/display system is usually employed.

Like CVP monitoring, the monitoring of pulmonary artery pressures (PAP) and pulmonary capillary wedge pressures (PCWP) contributes important information on circulating blood volume and vascular tone; in addition, it provides accurate data about the competency of the left ventricle. During diastole, when the mitral valve is open, there is a continuous pool of blood or *lacuna* from the left ventricle to the pulmonary vein (where there are no valves), to the pulmonary capillary bed, and thus to the pulmonary artery. In Figure 9-12, it can be seen that small, undesirable increases in left ventricular filling pressure will be readily indicated by increases in the wedge pressure.

Like CVP measurements, the PA and PCW pressures are considered in combination with other parameters, such as arterial blood pressure, apical rate, breath sounds, and heart sounds. The practitioner who bases his

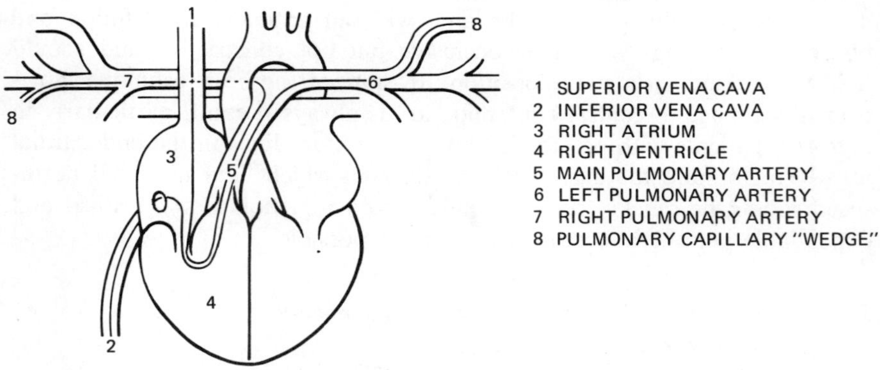

Fig. 9–12 Right heart catheterization. The chambers and vessels which may be catheterized during a right heart catheterization, including positioning of catheters in the pulmonary capillary wedge position, and their course when passed from the arm (superior vena cava) and leg (inferior vena cava). *(Courtesy from Hoechst-Roussel Pharmaceuticals, Inc., Somerville, New Jersey.* "Directions in Cardiovascular Medicine—Part 4. Cardiac Catheterization" Fig. 18, p. 25.)

assessment on only one type of measurement is unlikely to diagnose patient problems accurately.

Placement and Monitoring Technique. The construction of specialized, multiple-lumen "floatation" catheters has made insertion and continuous monitoring of pulmonary artery pressures feasible in most clinical settings. This type of catheter was designed by Drs. Swan and Ganz of the Cedars-Sinai Medical Center in Los Angeles and bears their names. Although specialized models are available, the basic catheter is approximately 110 cm in length and consists of a double-lumen tube with an inflatable balloon tip (see Figure 9-13).

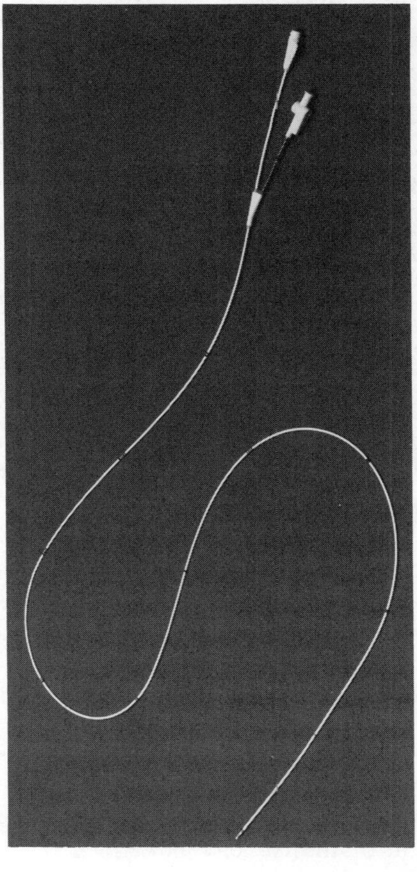

Fig. 9–13 Swan-Ganz monitoring catheter for measurement of pulmonary artery and pulmonary capillary wedge pressures: (a) full view; (b) balloon. *(Manufactured by Edwards Laboratories, Santa Ana, California.)*

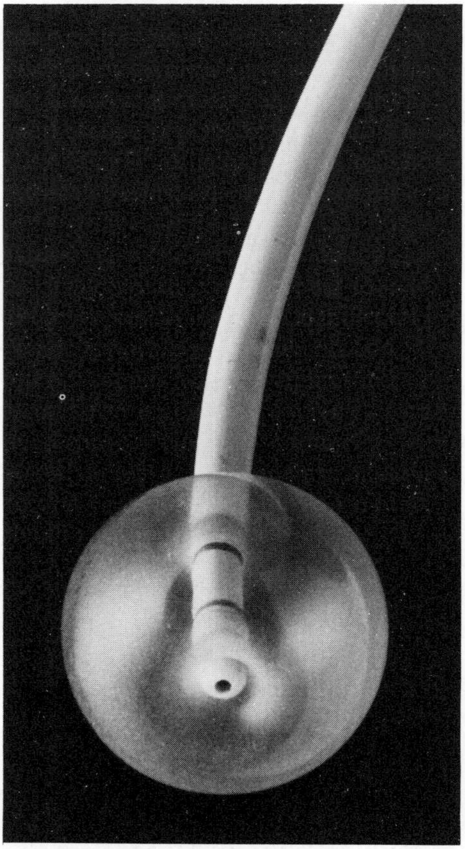

Fig. 9–13 (Continued.)

The catheter may be inserted percutaneously or via a venous cutdown in the antecubital area. By using continuous pressure and electrocardiographic (ECG) monitoring, the catheter is threaded into the subclavian vein with the balloon deflated. At this point, the balloon is partially inflated to half capacity (0.4 to 0.6 cc of CO_2 or air) and carried downstream to the right atrium by the flow of blood. The balloon is then fully inflated (0.8 cc) and advanced again so that the blood flow propels it through the tricuspid valve into the right ventricle. From there it is carried through the pulmonary valve into the pulmonary artery where the balloon wedges in a distal artery branch. The position of the catheter is verified by the pressure tracing, which shifts from a pulmonary artery pressure indicator to the "wedged" pressure waveform position. Under ideal circumstances it should take the physician no more than one minute to float the catheter from full balloon inflation in the right atrium to the wedge position. During insertion, the fully inflated balloon covers the hard tip of the catheter, distributing pressure forces evenly across a broad area of the endocardium. In this manner, the catheter's construction precludes the occurrence of premature ventricular contractions (PVCs) which are often encountered with stimulation of the right ventricular endocardium and tricuspid regions. Once the catheter has wedged, PCWP is recorded and the balloon is deflated. A continuous display of the PAP waveform should then be evident. The catheter is usually sutured to the skin in the area of insertion, and a secure dressing that includes antibiotic ointment is applied.

Essentially the same considerations apply for monitoring PA and PCW pressures as were described earlier for CVP. A constant, slow flow of heparinized 5% dextrose in water or saline ensures patency. Location of the transducer at the midaxillary line ensures consistency of measurements. The infusion of solution in the line (automatically or manually) is accomplished under pressure in order to overcome the higher pressures encountered in the pulmonary artery. The transducer, infusion reservoir, and PA line may then be secured to the infusion manifold discussed earlier. Accurate labeling of lines is vital, especially on the infusion manifold itself, in order to prevent errors involving the administration of medication or sampling of blood.

Limitations of PA and PCW Pressure Monitoring. Much has been said about the relevance of PA and PCW pressures in the accurate measurement of left ventricular capability. There are, however, some significant limitations of the method that must be noted. In obstructive conditions such as mitral stenosis, accuracy may be impaired in measuring this parameter. In addition, catheter placement is hampered in patients with severe cardiogenic shock or low right-heart flow rates. In cases of pulmonary artery hypertension (e.g., acute or chronic cor pulmonale) associated with a dilated right ventricle and pulmonary artery, insertion of the catheter is more difficult. Perforation of the pulmonary artery during floatation catheter insertion has been reported in patients with severe pulmonary artery hypertension. This occurrence was attributed to a rupture of the pulmonary artery and alveoli during wedging due to the direct effect of high pressure in the vascular system. Aneurysmal dilatation of the pulmonary artery itself due to chronic increased pressure might be another contributing factor.

Complications and Related Care. *Perforation of the pulmonary artery* is quite unusual with the Swan-Ganz® floatation catheter. This problem is largely confined to clinical situations involving pulmonary hypertension or deviations from the prescribed technique. For example, if the catheter should be floated into the pulmonary artery without the balloon being fully inflated, the catheter tip may be propelled through the vessel wall, thus producing serious hemorrhage. No deaths specifically attributable to this cause have been reported in the literature, but personnel on duty should be aware of some cardinal signs relating pulmonary artery perforation and concomitant alveolar rupture. These signs include hemoptysis, auscultation of bubbly rales over the area, shortness of breath, and diminished blood pressure. In one situation, the patient first complained of bubbling "windpipe" sensations and a sweet taste in her mouth. It should be obvious from this discussion that situations causing an increase of pressure in the area of this small pulmonary artery set the stage for rupture of the vessel.

Pulmonary infarction is another important complication. Again, the problem is frequently related to an improper technique or to unintentional wedging of the catheter tip. If air is used in the balloon, nursing personnel must be sure to deflate the balloon following notation of the wedge pressure. Otherwise, after approximately 3 minutes, blood flow will be reduced to the affected area of lung to the extent that ischemia and infarction will result. The likelihood of this problem can be diminished by using CO_2 as the medium in the balloon instead of air. Because CO_2 is more diffusable than air, it will diffuse through the balloon wall at a rate that reduces the balloon diameter at a rate of approximately 0.5 mm/min.

An early indication of inadvertent wedging of the catheter tip is a loss of systolic/diastolic fluctuation when the catheter is in the pulmonary artery location. When this happens the physician must withdraw the catheter a few centimeters until this fluctuation is again evident. In addition to the continuous wedge reading, symptoms of pulmonary infarction are similar (although possibly less severe) to those attributable to pulmonary embolization. These symptoms include acute pain, dry cough, which might be productive of pink sputum, and shortness of breath.

Balloon rupture and air embolization may be a dangerous occurrence in patients who have right-to-left circulatory shunting, which is possible in an atrial or ventricular septal defect. Because of its diffusibility, carbon dioxide should be used as the balloon medium in clinical situations where the possibility of right-to-left shunting exists. Because of the small size of the balloon, care should be taken to avoid inadvertent rupture during routine inflation. Only that amount of air necessary to obtain a wedge pressure display on the monitor should be inserted. Under no circumstances should the inflation volume printed on the catheter be exceeded. To check whether air is present in the balloon, always empty the balloon completely before injecting air. Interestingly, even though balloon rupture may occur, the pulmonary arterial pressure data may still be relevant. Prerupture data can be used to compare the earlier wedge determinations with the PA diastolic pressure. If they correlate well, the latter figure may be used to give a less direct but fairly accurate picture of left ventricular function.

Microembolization and in situ thrombosis are important complications that must be considered, especially when the catheter has been in place for more than 72 hours. Anticoagulation is usually required if the catheter is to remain in place for such extended periods of time. Signs and symptoms would primarily relate to resulting pulmonary infarction, discussed earlier. In clinical situations involving right-to-left circulatory shunting, embolization of air or blood clots may cause coronary artery occlusion and systemic arterial occlusive damage—for example, cerebral or renal infarction—any of which will produce disastrous results.

Other complicating hazards include local or systemic infection and looping or kinking of the catheter tubing. In general, the latter problem occurs during placement and may be confirmed by use of fluoroscopy. Such an occurrence may be due to the insertion of an excessive length of catheter, or use of a catheter that might have undergone crushing during storage. Consequently, each catheter should be carefully examined prior to insertion. Pulmonary artery lines are not to be used for the injection of medications. Diagnostic dyes for cardiac output determinations, however, may be injected.

Pitfalls of PA and PCW Pressure Monitoring. Previously, a number of problems that can contribute to errors in the measurement of blood pressure or that might affect patient safety were discussed. Some additional difficulties involving *pressure damping* and certain *pressure artifacts* can also result in inaccurate readings.

Pressure damping is defined as a reduction of the higher frequency components of the pressure waveform. It generally results in a distorted waveform and often produces pressure values that are much lower than the pressures actually encountered by the transducer. Certain features, such as the dicrotic notch and the sharp systolic peak, may be lost. Figure 9-14 shows the effect of damping during pressure monitoring of the pulmonary artery.

Pressure damping is almost always due to increased hydraulic resistance in the fluid column between the transducer and the catheter tip. This resistance may be due to a blood clot within the catheter itself or at the distal orifice, or an occlusion of the catheter orifice as it rests against a vessel wall. In addition, bubbles or kinks anywhere in the system can generate resistance. It must be realized that a low PA pressure reading might be due to a pathological condition, such as a sudden blood loss, as well as to a damped fluid column. It is therefore important that other pressure readings be checked along with any other factors that might indicate the pathology before attributing the difficulty to a damped line.

In the absence of a pathological problem, the following remedies might be initiated. First, having secured a syringe containing 10 cc of flushing solution from the heparinized fluid reservoir on the infusion manifold (refer to Figure 9-4), clear the line by withdrawing fluid from it. Never simply

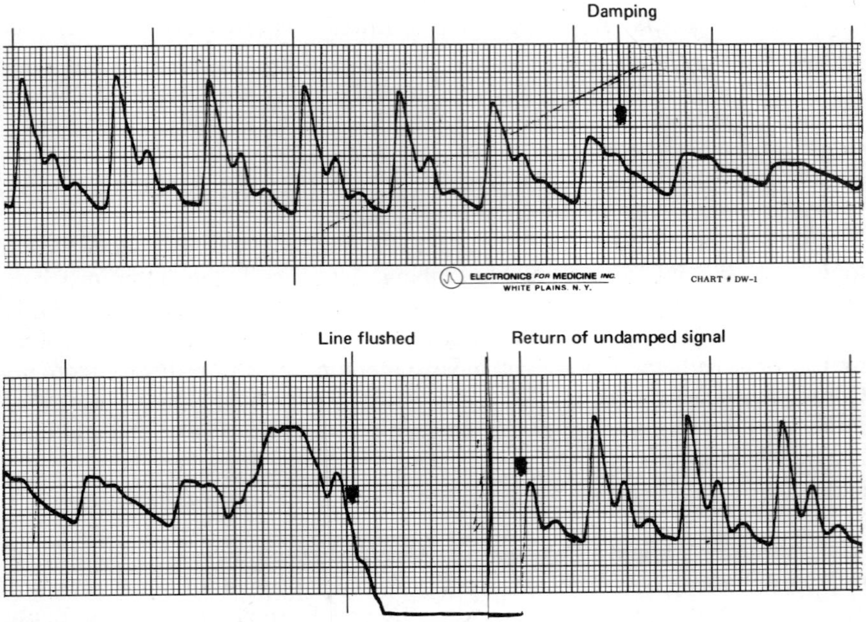

Fig. 9–14 Typical waveforms encountered with damping phenomenon including the flush artifact and the undamped tracing. *(Courtesy of Cedars-Sinai Medical Center, Los Angeles, California.)*

push the solution against the resistance, since to do so increases the possibility of embolization or PA rupture. With fluid return evident on withdrawal, flush the system with approximately 10 cc. The amount of flushing solution may vary, depending on the fluid status of the patient. If the line is still not clear and if resistance is encountered during flushing, reposition the patient to remove the catheter tip from its proximity to a vessel wall. At the same time the physician may withdraw the line slightly. If the system can be flushed adequately but damping is still evident, check for bubbles or kinks. Should some improvement be noted after flushing, repeat this procedure. When all efforts to this point fail, repositioning the patient and/or catheter tip may produce the desired result (if this has not already been attempted). If all efforts are fruitless, and if no use can be made of the distorted patient data, the line must be removed. As a last resort, such factors as blood viscosity or the injudicious use of distensible or large-bore connecting tubing might also be considered. See Figure 9-15 for a schematic representation of the troubleshooting procedure when damping is encountered.

Pressure artifacts: Critical care personnel should be familiar with two kinds of artifacts commonly encountered in all transducer-mediated direct pressure monitoring. The first is the so-called *whip* phenomenon, which is

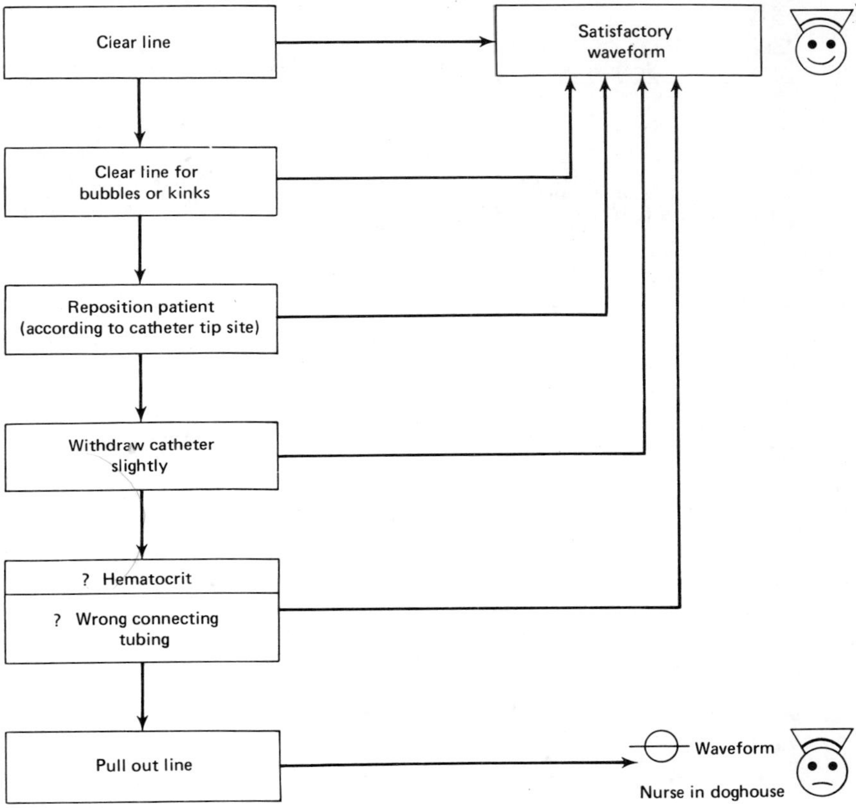

Fig. 9–15 Trouble-shooting schema for a damped line.

caused by movement of the catheter tip within the blood vessel being monitored. Because of the wide excursions or "spiking" that occur in this situation, it is especially difficult to obtain accurate diastolic readings. Depending on the severity of spiking, the physician may be able to interpret the diastolic values by adding a few mm Hg to the distorted whip values. If he should feel uncomfortable with such an estimate, he may elect to pull the catheter back a bit, which may bring some improvement.

A second important artifact is attributable to movement of the tubing between the patient and the transducer. Within the limits of patient comfort and safety, such artifacts can be prevented by proper positioning of the tubing itself. Figure 9-16 illustrates these commonly encountered artifacts.

9.2.3 *Monitoring Left Atrial Pressure*

With increased use of pulmonary capillary wedge pressure monitoring in critical care settings, it can be anticipated that the direct assessment of

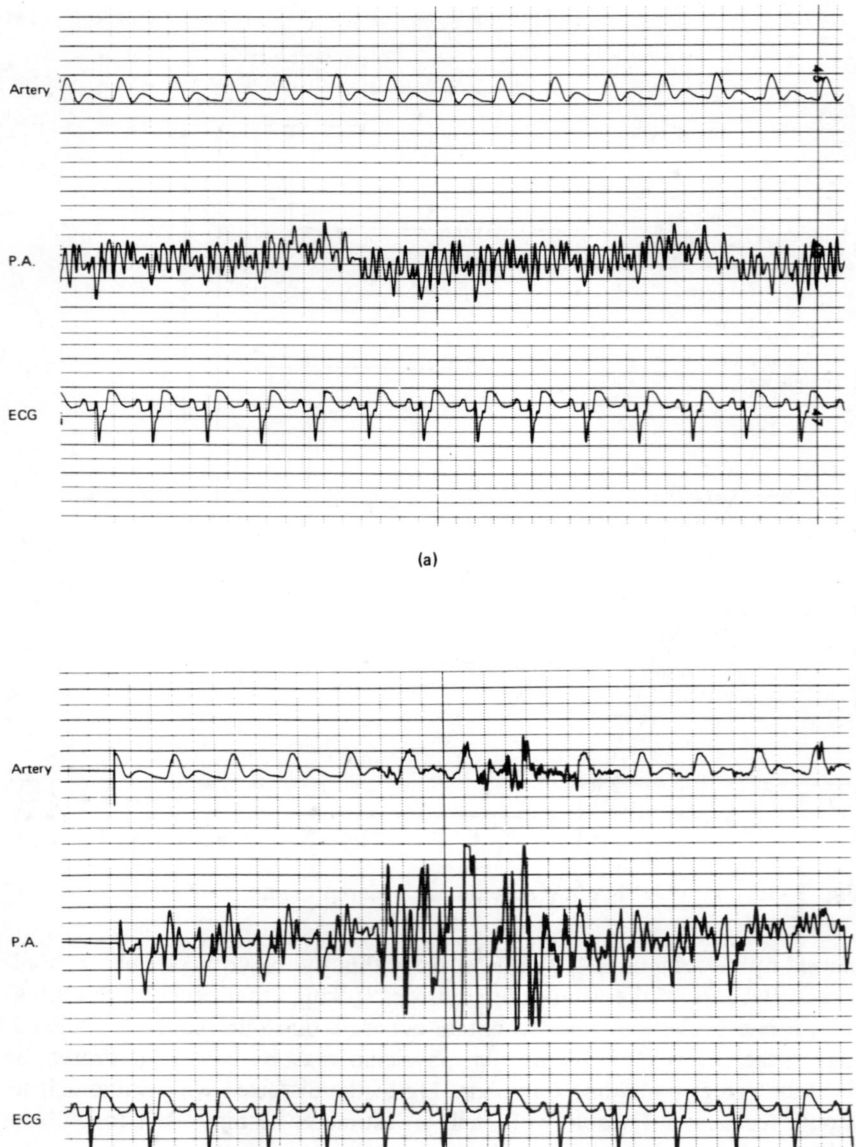

Fig. 9–16 a. A pulmonary artery tracing (middle) demonstrating the "whip" phenomenon as well as pressure changes due to respirations. b. A pulmonary artery tracing (middle) demonstrating artifact consistent with tubing movement, or of someone bumping into the infusion manifold. *(Courtesy of Cedars-Sinai Medical Center, Los Angeles, California.)*

left atrial pressure may suffer a concomitant decline. Both methods provide essentially the same patient information (left ventricular end-diastolic or filling pressure). Like PCWP, left atrial pressure reflects the competency of the left ventricle to handle a volume load in order to provide optimal cardiac output to the systemic circulation. Because the left atrium is a continuation of the pulmonary capillary bed and no valves exist in the pulmonary veins, the PCWP and left atrial pressure are about the same; similarly, a series of readings is more relevant than isolated measurements. In short, the same physiological parameters may be monitored, although the technique of left atrial cannulation limits its use to selected patient situations.

Placement and Monitoring Techniques. The monitoring of left atrial pressure usually involves the insertion of a small catheter directly into the left atrium. This technique is largely confined to thoracic surgery patients in which the catheter can be brought out through the incision and sutured securely to the skin. In these situations, a very small catheter must be used, since it will ultimately be removed from the left atrium without further surgery. Consequently, the surgeon can receive this vital patient data only after the operative procedure has begun. With the earlier insertion of a floatation catheter into the pulmonary artery, the surgical team can be provided with essentially the same information during the period of anesthesia induction, which is an especially vulnerable time for patients with already poor hemodynamic status. During cardiac catheterization for diagnostic purposes, the left atrium may be entered in a transseptal maneuver from the right atrium. This procedure is called the *Brockenbrough technique*. Also, retrograde catheter passage may be accomplished through the left ventricular wall and mitral valve or via retrograde passage from a point distal to the ascending aorta. Needless to say, such techniques are generally not indicated for long-term monitoring because of the inherent risk of ventricular irritability and lethal embolization.

As in the other methods discussed earlier, the left atrial line must have rigid tubing from the transducer to the catheter; similarly, a slow drip of heparinized dextrose and water or saline solution should also be used to ensure patency. Figure 9-12(b) shows the usual placement of the left atrial catheter. Salient physiological data may be evaluated more readily by critical care personnel when central arterial and left atrial pressures or PCWP are displayed together.

Problems and Related Care. The threat of *air embolization,* even in amounts of less than 0.5 cc, can be lethal because of the relative proximity of the catheter tip to the sinus of Valsalva in the ascending aorta from which the coronary arteries originate. *For this reason, any attempt to clear the left atrial line must be performed with extreme caution.* The specific technique for clearing the line is the same as that described for pulmonary artery lines; however, the critical care practitioner must continuously be alert to the danger of embolization of blood clots to the coronary and renal arteries or to other parts of the systemic circulation. Again, if gentle aspiration of the line does not result in a return of blood flow, no force should be used to flush it. The physician would be notified so that he can manipulate the line or else totally withdraw it.

Premature clotting of left atrial lines is probably the most widely encountered difficulty inherent in their use. This fact is not surprising when the size of the catheter lumen is considered. If possible, an automatic slow infusion of heparinized solution should be used to prolong the life of the line.

Another potential problem stems from the technique necessitated by this method. The catheter affords a direct pathway for endocardial contamination from the mediastinum and the body surface. In addition to meticulous technique in infusing solution to ensure patency, meticulous sterile techniques must be practiced during such procedures as dressing changes and catheter or chest tube manipulation. In these situations patients should always be given prophylactic antibiotic coverage.

During removal of the line, the critical care staff should be particularly alert to potential problems of bleeding and cardiac tamponade, as well as breakage or embolization of the catheter tip. In addition, thrombi adherent to the catheter might be dislodged at this time, producing systemic or coronary arterial occlusion.

As in pulmonary artery pressure monitoring, left atrial pressures that are transducer-mediated may suffer the same electrical artifacts and pitfalls already discussed. Intervention is not unlike the methods previously mentioned. Similarly, medications other than heparin are never given through the line, and accurate, clear labeling is mandatory to preclude this possibility.

9.2.4 Monitoring Arterial Pressure

As already noted, the use of arterial pressure measurements is appropriate when an auscultated blood pressure measurement is impossible to obtain or might be misleading in its value. Either condition may exist during circulatory shock, which is characterized by low cardiac output, hypotension, or both. According to findings by Drs. Weil and Shubin of the University of Southern California Shock Research Unit, the loudness of the Korotkoff sounds are markedly altered during shock states. Under such conditions blood flow through the partially occluded vessel causes distortion in both diastolic and systolic values. Such is not the case in patients with normal or hypertensive blood pressures. Therapy with vasopressors, as well as inherent physiological compensatory mechanisms that cause peripheral vasoconstriction, may contribute to the inaccuracies associated with auscultated pressure readings. For these reasons, direct arterial blood pressure determinations are utilized in critical care situations where circulatory shock is an everpresent threat.

The reader should refer to Figure 8-2, which shows the pressure/time relationships in a central arterial system. In monitoring the patient in shock the mean pressure is more important than the systolic and diastolic values. This pressure can be calculated when only the systolic and diastolic pressure values are known by adding one-third of the pulse pressure to the diastolic pressure. The mean pressure falls closer to the diastolic value because systole is shorter than diastole.

Another important reason for monitoring arterial pressure is a by-product of the first. Displaying the arterial pressure waveform permits the observation of the predicrotic and dicrotic notches, which represent the behavior of the aortic valve. It is not uncommon, following aortic valve replacement, for the surgeon to keep a close watch on these features to note early changes that might be indicative of possible thrombus formation or malfunction of the valve itself.

Placement and Monitoring Techniques. Arterial pressure monitoring is generally instituted by the insertion of a small, short catheter into a peripheral artery (usually the radial). For more central arterial readings, the femoral artery may be used. One major factor in the placement of these catheters is the danger to arterial circulation distal to the point of entry. Serious complications can result from blood clot embolization from an arterial catheter tip. The higher the placement of the catheter, especially on the arm, the more extensive would be the results, should thrombus formation at the site or embolization distal to the site occur.

As in the other transducer-mediated methods previously described, the arterial line must be secured to the transducer and infusion manifold system. Again the transducer should be at the same height as the point of measurement. Water column methods are never used for ongoing direct monitoring of arterial blood pressure, because the fluid level can't respond to the wide fluctuations between systolic and diastolic pressures. Rigid tubing is used to connect the catheter to the transducer. The dressing that covers the arterial puncture site is secured in order to provide both sterility and protection and to avoid premature removal of the line. Usually the arterial catheter is sutured to the skin and the rigid connecting tubing is looped and again secured, so as to avoid direct pull on the point of entry. Care must be taken not to impede patency of the line with such looping; otherwise damping of the pressure curve and clotting in the catheter will result.

The transducer is connected to the amplifier-display system, and normally both numerical and waveform data are provided. The numerical readout provides accurate systolic, diastolic, and mean pressure values at the flip of a switch. The undamped pressure waveform can be observed on the monitor screen. Waveforms must be accurately labeled on the appropriate channel, as well as the individual lines coming from the patient. Figure 9-17 shows some typical arterial pressure waveforms and a numerical readout system.

Problems and Related Care. In addition to earlier comments regarding accuracy and safety, some precautions related to the withdrawal of blood for blood gas measurements and other purposes through arterial pressure monitoring lines must be discussed. In order to obtain a good specimen that is not diluted with heparinized infusion fluid, the "dead space" in the tubing between the syringe and the patient's artery must be aspirated first. This "dead space" blood must be withdrawn with a different syringe from that used for the specimen. Following the collection of the specimen, the flushing syringe on the infusion manifold is filled and the arterial line is quickly cleared of blood to prevent clotting. To minimize the chance of blood clot embolization and contamination, it is not advisable to reinject the dead space fluid first. In fact, some centers require a written order from a doctor to do so. It should be reiterated that the amount of fluid that is infused in order to restore and/or maintain patency of arterial and other lines must be minimized. In patients with very limited cardiac reserve, the difference between restoration to health and death may be determined by this factor. Accurate records of the patient's fluid status are also extremely important.

Staff personnel must be aware of the arterial pressure waveforms, just as they are of cardiac arrhythmias. In addition to recognizing damping and artifact, they should be able to assess changes associated with respirations (especially if the patient is on a ventilator), premature ventricular contractions, cardiac tamponade, atrial fibrillation, aortic valve incompetency, and diminished stroke volume.

Patients who have arterial lines in place should not be left alone for any period of time, particularly if they are restless or unable to summon assistance. Should the arterial line become disconnected or the catheter become dislodged, the patient may suffer blood loss. The degree of bleeding may be severe if the patient has been anticoagulated or is markedly hypovolemic to begin with. At the very least, such an event will interrupt pressure monitoring for a time, during which no accurate determination of cardiac status may be made. In addition to maintaining the competency of the line, the staff should assess the status of the extremity distal to the point of insertion. Such observation should be done at least hourly and should include palpation of pulses, assessment of color, blanching of nail beds, warmth, and the presence of edema. Edema would probably result from an

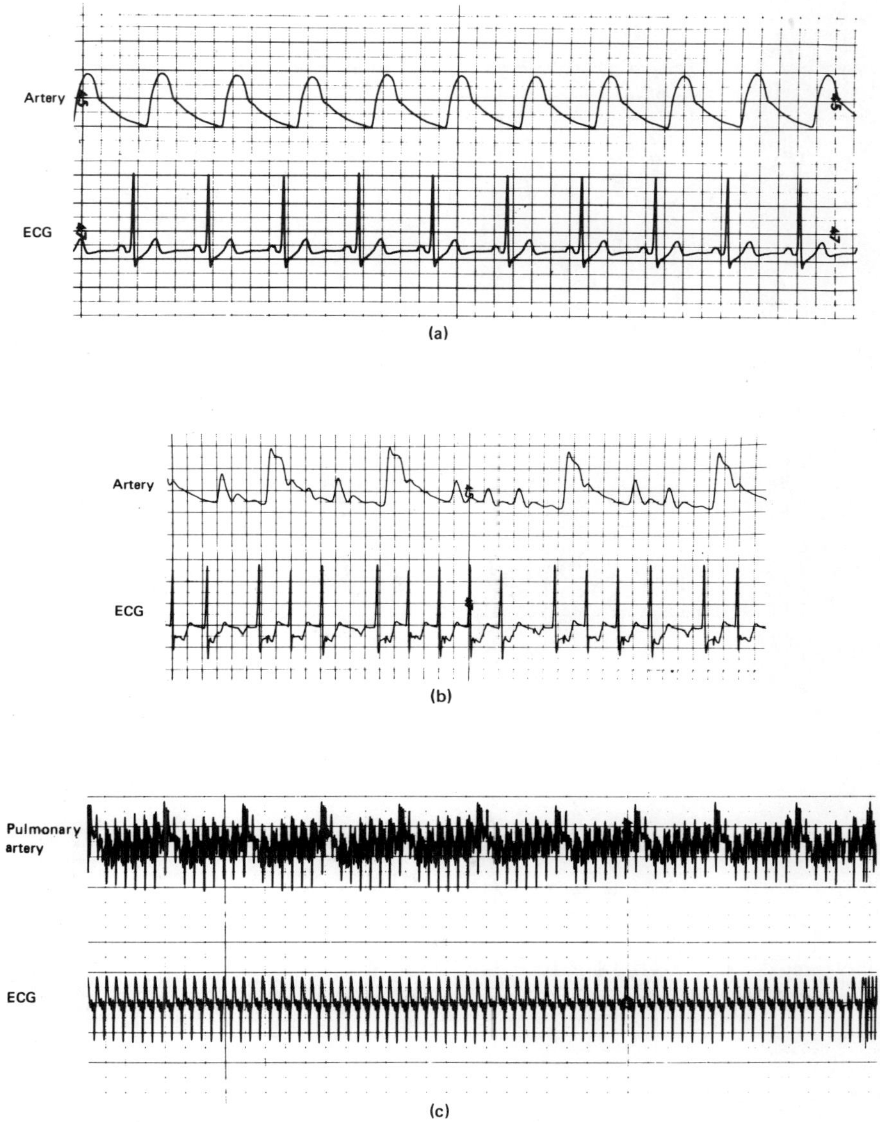

Fig. 9–17 Pressure waveforms commonly encountered in critical care settings: (a) Normal arterial tracing and EKG; (b) intermittent pacemaker capture with resulting changes in cardiac output; (c) changes in pulmonary artery pressure due to respirations recorded at a slow speed; (e) effect of premature ventricular contractions (PVCs) upon cardiac output; (f) frequent PVCs progressing to ventricular tachycardia, then fibrillation with profound drop in cardiac output. Note: all tracings have been reduced in size and were taken at a paper speed of 25mm/sec. unless otherwise indicated. *(Courtesy of Cedars-Sinai Medical Center, Los Angeles, California.)*

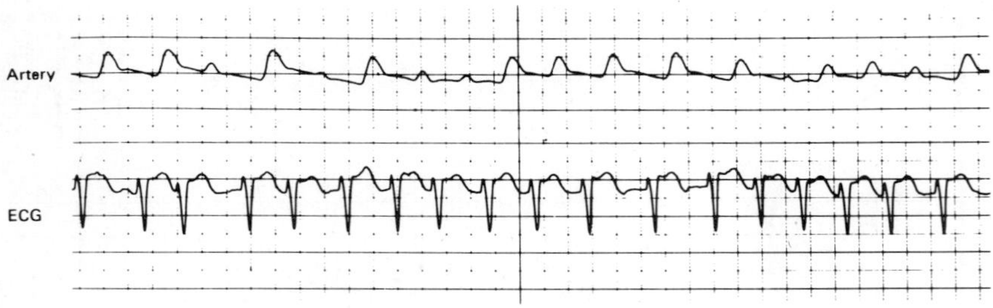

(d)

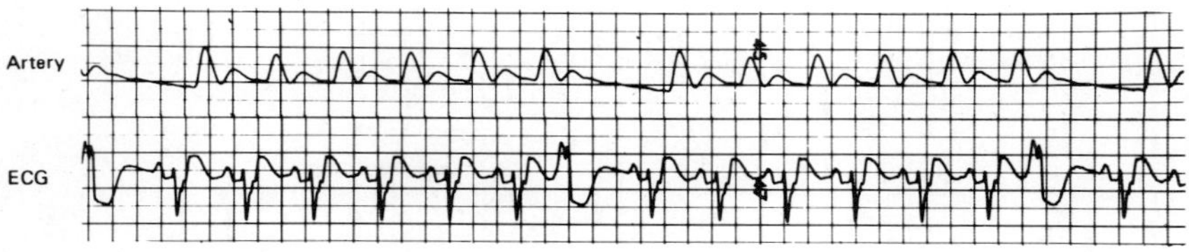

(e)

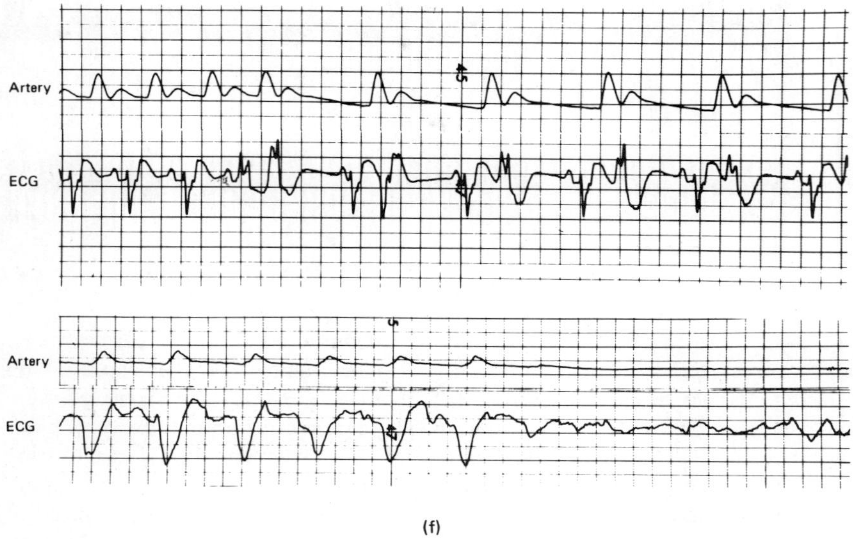

(f)

Fig. 9–17 (Continued.)

overly constrictive dressing rather than local thrombus formation or embolization. The staff should be particularly alert to such conditions as absence of pulses, complaints of pain, pallor, and slow blood return with blanching. If any of these signs should occur, the physician should be notified immediately. At times arterial spasm can occur. This painful condition is as dangerous to the patient as clot formation. In this case, the physician may inject an alpha adrenergic blocking agent, such as Regitine,® to relax the spasm and improve blood flow. *This is the only situation in which a medication other than heparin should be injected into the arterial line.*

The arterial line may be removed by either the physician or the nursing staff, depending on hospital policy. Care must be taken to avoid extravasation of blood into surrounding tissues, a process that may promote thrombus formation by pressure and diminished flow within the artery. When the catheter is removed, thrombi adhering to its walls may be knocked loose, possibly to occlude distal or local arterial vessels. Firm pressure must be applied to the area for 15 minutes following intentional or unplanned catheter withdrawal. A pressure dressing should then be applied. The staff should continue to check distal pulses and look for signs of arterial inadequacy of the extremity.

A number of parameters dealing with direct pressure monitoring have been discussed in this chapter. They provide salient data regarding physiological adaptations and responses to therapy. Critical care flow sheets that incorporate pressure variables are used in most units and provide a clear documentation of the patient's hemodynamic status at any point in time.

10

Cardiac Pacemaker Systems and Defibrillators: Mobile Emergency Care

More than a half million people fall victim to heart attacks in the United States every year and thousands more are critically injured in accidents. Taking care of these patients in special care units of hospitals involves the use of several types of specialized equipment, among which are cardiac pacemakers and defibrillators. Defibrillators and cardiopulmonary resuscitation equipment are also required away from the hospital, in an ambulance or at the scene of an emergency.

In the past few years electronic pacemaker systems have become extremely important in saving and sustaining the lives of cardiac patients whose normal pacing functions have become impaired. Depending on the exact nature of a cardiac dysfunction, a patient may require temporary artificial pacing during the course of treatment or permanent pacing in order to lead an active, productive life after treatment.

The need to manage critically ill persons can occur anywhere and at any time. In fact, about half the fatal heart attacks occur away from the hospital, where emergency care and equipment are not present. It is estimated that if proper emergency care were given these victims within 20 minutes of the onset of their affliction, most would survive. Public service departments of many communities have now established mobile special care units to meet such emergencies. Manned by specially trained personnel, these units contain equipment similar to that found in special care units of hospitals. Thus personnel are able to render on-site diagnoses, resuscitation, and preliminary treatment of victims of heart attacks and accidents.

This chapter deals with the various types of cardiac pacemakers, defibrillators, and mobile emergency care equipment. In addition to describing each device, the chapter also discusses its basic purpose, the physiological conditions under which it is required, and the ways in which it is used.

10.1 Cardiac Pacing and Irregularities

The heart's electrical activity is described in Chapter 5, but a brief review at this point will be helpful in understanding the need for artificial cardiac pacing. The rhythmic action of the heart is initiated by regularly recurring action potentials (electrochemical impulses) originating at the natural cardiac pacemaker, located at the sinoatrial (SA) node. Each pacing impulse is propagated throughout the myocardium, spreading over the surface of the atria to the atrioventricular (AV) junctional tissue—which is located within the septum, adjacent to the atrioventricular valves—and depolarizing the atria. After a brief delay at the AV junction, the impulse is rapidly conducted to the ventricles to depolarize the ventricular musculature.

A normal sinus rhythm (NSR) depends on the continuous, periodic performance of the pacemaker and the integrity of the neuronal conducting pathways. Any change in the NSR is called an *arrhythmia* (abnormal rhythm). Should the SA node temporarily or permanently fail because of disease (SA node disease) or a congenital defect, the pacing function may be taken over by pacemakerlike cells located near the AV junction, producing what is called a *junctional rhythm.* However, under certain conditions, cells in the conduction system (an *idioventricular focus*) may pace the ventricles instead. Similarly, an area in the excitable ventricular musculature may try to control the heartbeat. Unfortunately, the junctional focus and the idioventricular foci pace at a much slower rate than normal, ranging between 30 and 50 beats per minute (BPM). The result is a condition called *bradycardia* (slow heart) in which the heart cannot provide sufficient blood circulation to meet the body's physical demands. During the transition period from an NSR to a slow rhythm, dizziness and loss of consciousness (syncope) may occur because of diminished cardiac output.

Heart block occurs whenever the conduction system fails to transmit the pacing impulses from the atria to the ventricles properly. In *first-degree block* an excessive impulse delay at the AV junction occurs that causes the P-R interval to exceed 0.2 s for normal adults. *Second-degree block* results in the complete but intermittent inhibition of the pacing impulse, which may also occur at the AV node. Total and continuous impulse blockage is called *third-degree block*. It may occur either at the AV node or elsewhere in the conduction system. In this case, the ventricles usually continue to contract but at a sharply reduced rate (40 BPM) because of the establishment of an idioventricular escape rhythm or because of impulses that only periodically originate from the atria. In all these conditions, an artificial method of pacing is generally required in order to ensure that the heart beats at a rate that is sufficient to maintain proper circulation.

10.2 Pacemaker Systems

A device capable of generating artificial pacing impulses and delivering them to the heart is known as a *pacemaker system* (commonly called a *pacemaker*) and consists of a *pulse generator* and appropriate *electrodes*. Pacemakers are available in a variety of forms. *Internal pacemakers* may be permanently implanted in patients whose SA nodes have failed to function properly or who suffer from permanent heart block because of a heart attack. An internal pacemaker is defined as one in which the entire system is inside the body. In contrast, an *external pacemaker* usually consists of an externally worn pulse generator connected to electrodes located on or within the myocardium.

External pacemakers are used on patients with temporary heart irregularities, such as those encountered in the coronary patient, including heart blocks. They are also used for temporary management of certain arrhythmias that may occur in patients during critical postoperative periods and in patients during cardiac surgery, especially if the surgery involves the valves or septum.

Internal pacemaker systems are implanted with the pulse generator placed in a surgically formed pocket below the right or left clavicle, in the left subcostal area, or, in women, beneath the left or right major pectoralis muscle. Internal leads connect to electrodes that directly contact the inside of the right ventricle or the surface of the myocardium. The exact location of the pulse generator depends primarily on the type of electrode used, the nature of the cardiac dysfunction, and the method (mode) of pacing that may be prescribed. Pacing electrodes and modes are described later in this chapter. Since there are no external connections for applying power, the pulse generator must be completely self contained, with a power source capable of continuously operating the unit for a period of years. A typical internal pulse generator is shown in Figure 10-1 with six self-contained

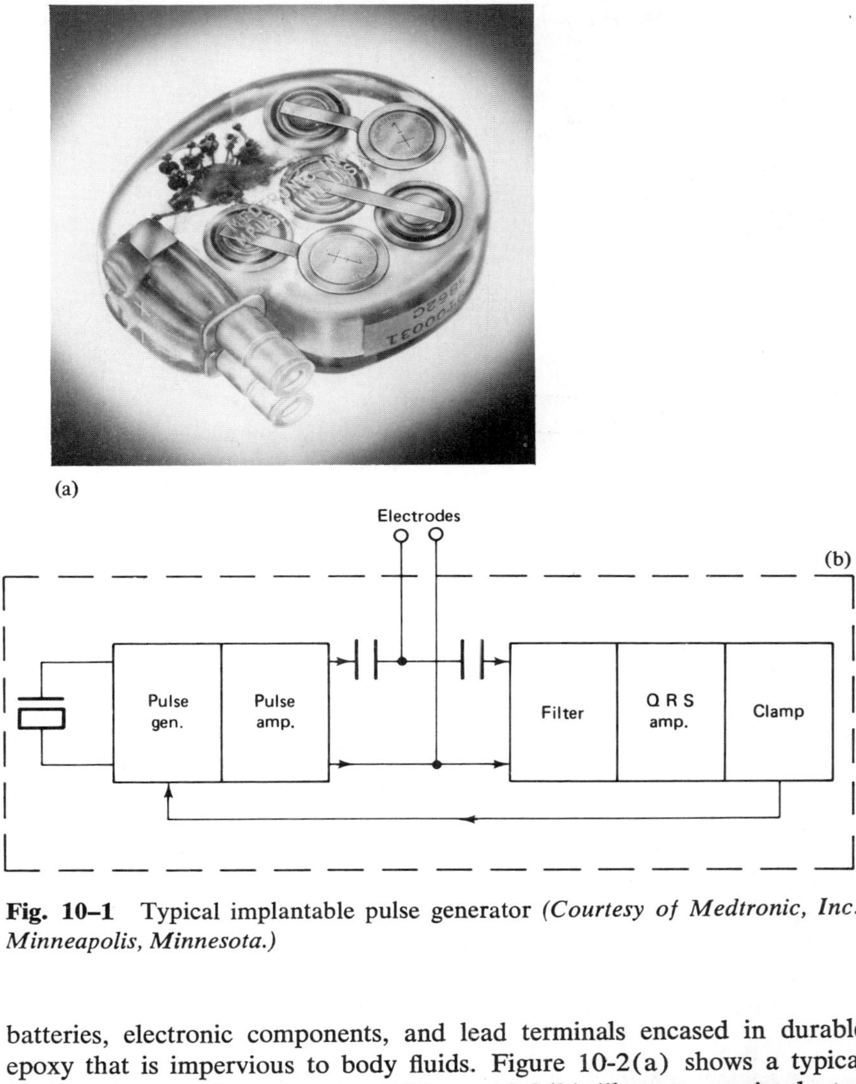

Fig. 10–1 Typical implantable pulse generator *(Courtesy of Medtronic, Inc., Minneapolis, Minnesota.)*

batteries, electronic components, and lead terminals encased in durable epoxy that is impervious to body fluids. Figure 10-2(a) shows a typical implanted pacemaker system, and Figure 10-2(b) illustrates an implanted pulse generator with its transvenous electrode lodged in the right ventricle.

External pacemakers, which include all types of pulse generators located outside the body, are normally connected through wires introduced into the right ventricle via a cardiac catheter, as shown in Figure 10-2. The pulse generator may be strapped to the lower arm of a patient who is confined to bed, or worn at the midsection of an ambulatory patient, as shown in Figure 10-3. A detailed view of the external pulse generator appears in Figure 10-4.

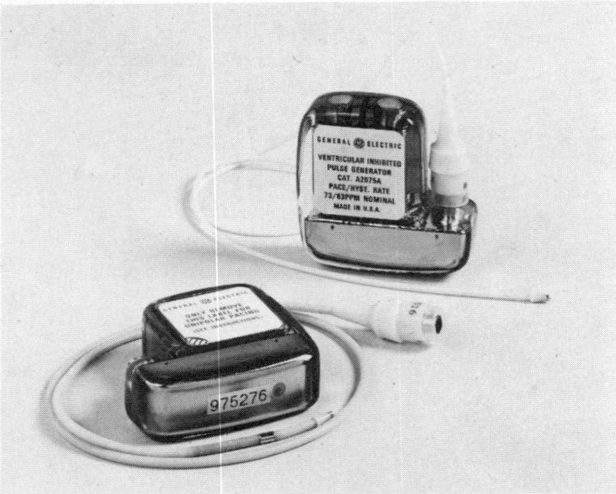

(a)

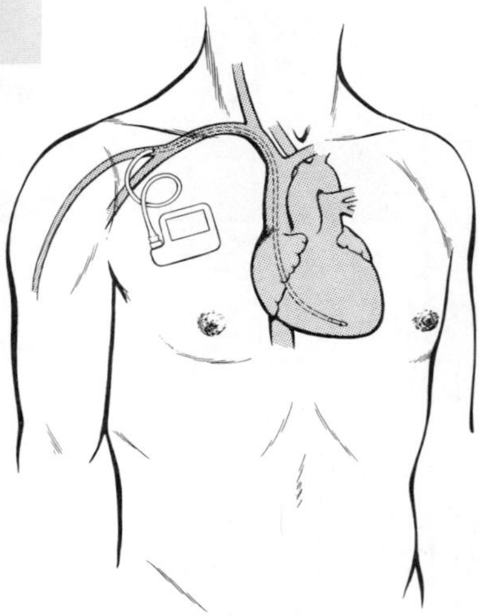

(b)

Fig. 10–2 (a) Pacemaker system with catheter electrode; (b) implanted pulse generator with catheter electrodes inserted through the right cephalic vein. *(Courtesy of General Electric Company, Medical Systems Department, Milwaukee, Wisconsin.)*

10.3 Pacing Modes and Pulse Generators

Several pacing techniques are possible with both internal and external pacemakers. Of these techniques, the two basic modes shown in Figure 10-5 are most frequently used today. They are the *competitive* and *noncompetitive* pacing modes. The noncompetitive method, which uses pulse generators that are either *ventricular programmed* or programmed by the atria, is more popular. Ventricular-programmed pacemakers are designed to operate either in a *demand* (R-wave inhibited) or *standby* (R-wave triggered) mode, whereas atrial-programmed pacers are always synchronized with the P wave of the ECG.

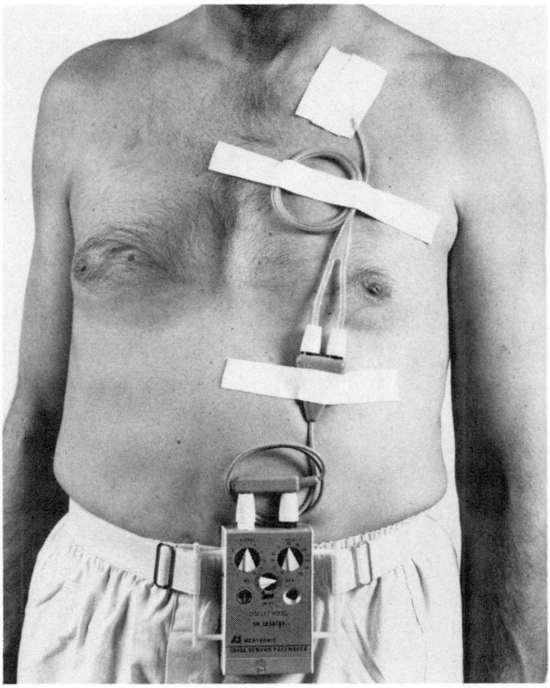

Fig. 10–3 Portable external pacemaker. Patient is being temporarily paced with an external pulse generator and intravenous pacing catheter. *(Courtesy of Medtronic, Inc., Minneapolis, Minnesota.)*

The first (and simplest) pulse generators were *fixed-rate* or *asynchronous* (not synchronized) devices that produced pulses at a fixed rate (set by the physician or nurse) and were independent of any natural cardiac activity. The pacemaker shown in Figure 10-2 is of this type. Asynchronous pacing is called *competitive* pacing because the fixed-rate impulses may occur along with natural pacing impulses generated by the heart and would therefore be in competition with them in controlling the heartbeat. This competition is largely eliminated through use of ventricular- or atrial-programmed pulse generators.

Fixed-rate pacers are sometimes installed in elderly patients whose SA nodes cannot provide proper stimuli. They are also used temporarily to determine the amplitude of impulses needed to pace or *capture* the heartbeat of a patient prior to or during the implantation of a more permanent unit. The amplitude at which capture occurs is referred to as the pacing *threshold.* While the implantable fixed-rate units tend to fail less frequently than the more sophisticated demand or standby pacers, their battery life (if the

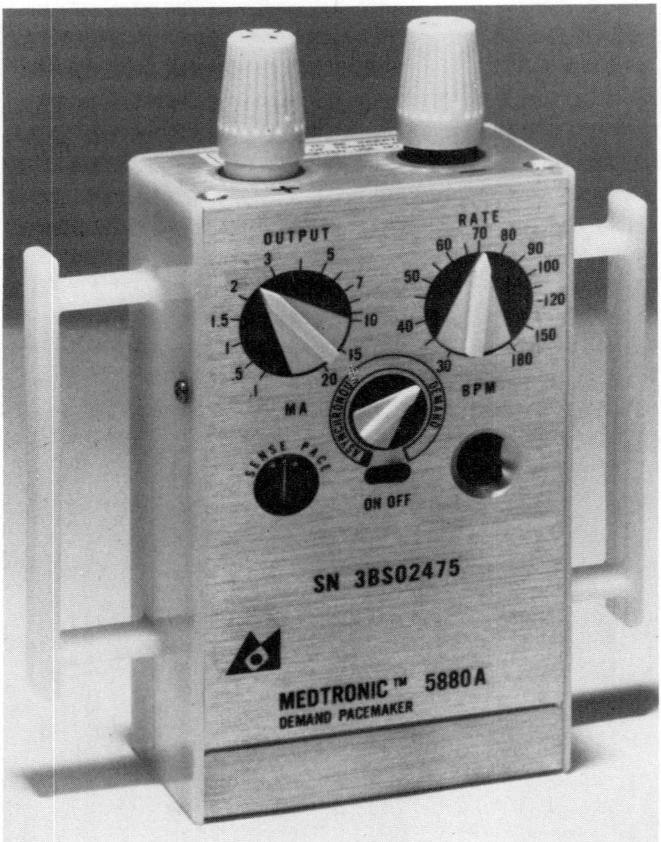

Fig. 10–4 Detail view of external demand pacemaker showing adjustment controls and output terminals. *(Courtesy of Medtronic, Inc., Minneapolis, Minnesota.)*

batteries are not rechargeable) is generally shorter because they are in constant operation.

The problems of shorter battery life and competition for control of the heart led, in part, to the development of ventricular-programmed (demand or standby) pulse generators. The external pacemaker shown in Figure 10-4 is of the *demand* type. Either type of ventricular-programmed pulse generator, when connected to the ventricles via electrodes, is able to sense the presence (or absence) of a naturally occurring R wave. The output of an R-wave inhibited (demand) unit is suppressed (no output pulses are produced) as long as natural (intrinsic) R waves are present. Thus its output is held back or inhibited when the heart is able to pace itself. How-

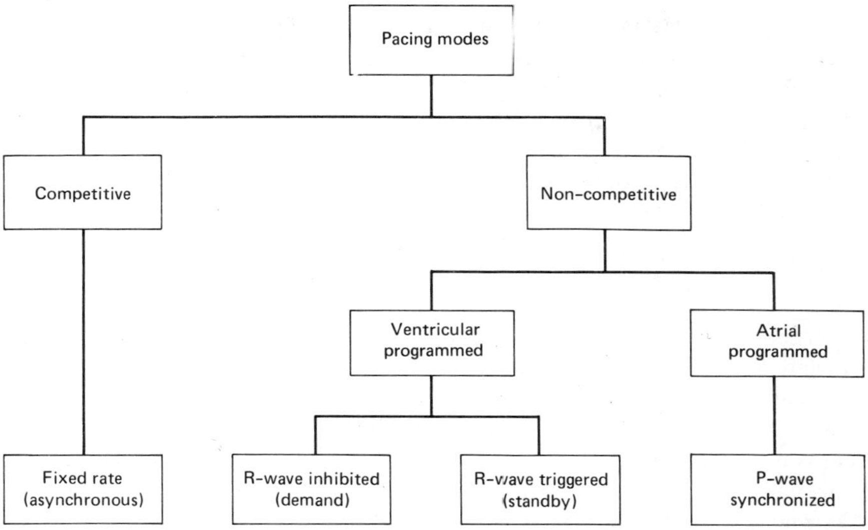

Fig. 10–5 Types of pacing modes.

ever, should standstill occur, or should the intrinsic rate fall below the preset rate of the pacer (around 70 BPM), the unit will automatically provide an output to pace the heart after an escape interval at the designated rate. In this way, ventricular-inhibited pacers are able to pace on demand. Some external demand-mode pacers may be adjusted to operate in a fixed-rate mode by means of an accessible mode control of the type shown on the unit in Figure 10-4. Other controls allow the setting of the pacer's rate between 30 and 180 BPM, as well as the amplitude of output pacing pulses between 0.1 and 20 mA. Some external demand pacers have a sense-pace indicator that deflects for each detected R wave or pacer-initiated impulse. The ON-OFF switch of some external pacers is provided with an interlock mechanism to prevent the unit from being accidentally turned off.

A demand pacer, in the absence of R waves, automatically reverts to a fixed-rate mode of operation. For testing purposes at the time of implantation and for evaluation later, implanted demand pacers are purposely placed in a fixed-rate mode, usually by means of a magnet provided by the manufacturer. When placed over the skin layer covering the pacer, the magnet activates a magnetically operated switch that prevents the pacer from sensing R wave activity. This process causes the pacer to operate in a fixed-rate mode at a slightly higher rate (about 10 BPM higher than the demand-mode pacing rate that had been preset). For a patient with a normal sinus rhythm, this procedure is used to ensure that an implanted demand pacer whose output is normally inhibited is capable of providing pacing pulses when needed. Evidence of the presence of pacing impulses is obtained from the electrocardiogram. Pacing impulses appear as *pacing artifacts* or *spikes*. Occasionally they may seriously distort the recorded QRS complex.

When required, the basic pacing rate of some of the earlier implanted pacers (both fixed-rate and demand types) may be changed with the use of a needlelike screwdriver (a Keith surgical skin needle) that is inserted transcutaneously in order to turn a rate control in the pulse generator. The amplitude of the impulses may also be adjusted in some earlier pacers by using the same type of needle in the appropriate control. In a newer type of pacer, these adjustments are accomplished by means of coded impulses that are magnetically coupled to the implanted pulse generator from the skin surface, thus eliminating the need to puncture the skin. To adjust this pacemaker, a special programming device with an attached coil is placed over the implanted pulse generator. Appropriate controls on the programmer allow the unit to transmit coded signals that cause the pacer to change its basic rate and vary the amplitude of its impulses. The basic rate and impulse amplitude of other recent implantable pulse generators are fixed by the manufacturer and cannot be changed, however.

As explained earlier, R-wave triggered pulse generators, like the R-wave inhibited units, also sense each intrinsic R wave. However, this pacer emits an impulse with the occurrence of each sensed R wave. Thus the unit is triggered rather than inhibited by each R wave. The pacing impulses are transmitted to the myocardium during its absolute refractory period, however, so that they will have no effect on normal heart activity. Should the intrinsic heart rate fall below the preset rate of the pacer, the pacer will automatically operate asynchronously at its preset rate to pace the heart. Thus this pacemaker stands by to pace when needed. Ventricular-triggered pacing is used less frequently than inhibited-mode pacing. Evidence of pacing impulses from this type of pacer is present on the patient's ECG, although some monitoring modes that utilize greater filtering may distort and even block the pacer artifact. In this case, one should document the ventricular complex following a pacer spike and compare it to the complex in question.

In cases of complete heart block where the atria are able to depolarize but the impulse fails to depolarize the ventricles, atrial synchronous pacing may be used. Here the pulse generator is connected through wires and electrodes to both the atria and the ventricles. The atrial electrode couples atrial impulses to the pulse generator, which then emits impulses to stimulate the ventricles via the ventricular electrode. In this way, the heart is paced at the same rate as the natural pacemaker. When the SA node rate changes because of vagus or sympathetic neuronal control, the ventricle will change its rate accordingly but not above some maximum rate (about 125 per minute).

Pulses applied directly to the heart are usually rectangular in shape with a duration of from 0.15 to 3 ms, depending on the type of pulse generator used and the needs of the patient. Depending on the value of impulse current required to capture, pulse amplitudes may range from 5 to 15 mA for adults, while infants and children require less. If, in an emergency, pacing must be done through the intact chest wall, amplitudes ten times as great are required. These higher values of current are often painful and may cause burns and contractions of the chest muscles and diaphragm. The amplitude of impulse required to capture the heartbeat of a patient is affected by the duration of the pulse. For example, an impulse of 2-ms duration may capture when its amplitude is only 3 mA. On the other hand, a 0.8-ms pulse may reach 6 mA before capture occurs.

The ability to capture and hence the threshold value of a pacer impulse that has a given amplitude and duration also depend on the electrical quality of the contact between the electrode and the heart. Capture will occur at a higher threshold value for a poor contact than for a good electrical contact at the electrode-heart muscle interface.

The quality of the electrode-heart muscle contact also affects a demand pacer's inhibition capability or *sensitivity*. A good contact will permit the pacer's output to remain inhibited for smaller values of sensed R waves.

The performance of pulse generators can be checked with the use of a special tester. In one type of tester, pacing impulses are indicated by a lamp that blinks at the pacing rate. In another type, the pacer's pulse rate, amplitude, width, and interval are displayed in digital form. This type of tester is also able to generate impulses used to check the inhibition capability of a demand pacer.

10.4 Pacing Electrodes

Implanted or external pulse generators make contact with the heart either through *endocardial* or *myocardial (epicardial)* electrodes. However, during certain surgical procedures, both types may be used. An endocardial electrode, also called a *catheter electrode* or *pacing electrode,* is placed transvenously inside the heart, as shown for the implanted pulse generator in Figure 10-2. In general, when properly placed, its tip lies wedged into trabeculations at the apex of the right ventricle. For temporary pacing, the catheter may be inserted into the basilic vein, then guided through the subclavian vein, into the right ventricle. An alternate route may be taken through the external jugular vein.

Myocardial electrodes are attached directly to the anterior surface of the heart, as shown in Figure 10-6. This process requires thoracotomy to allow the electrodes to be sutured directly to the left ventricle. Epicardial electrodes are always required for use with implanted atrial synchronous

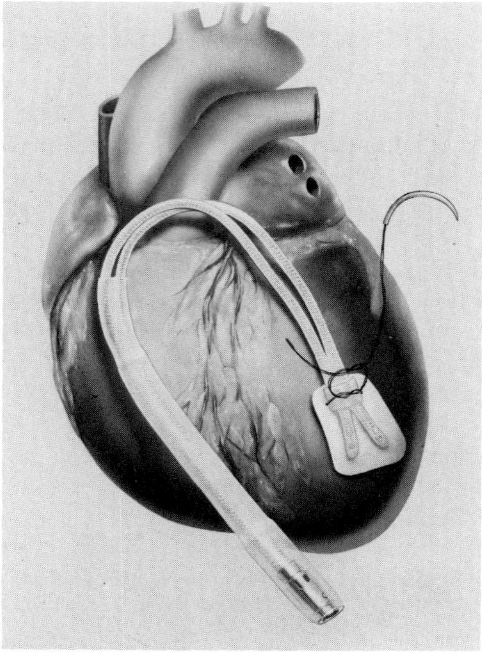

(a)

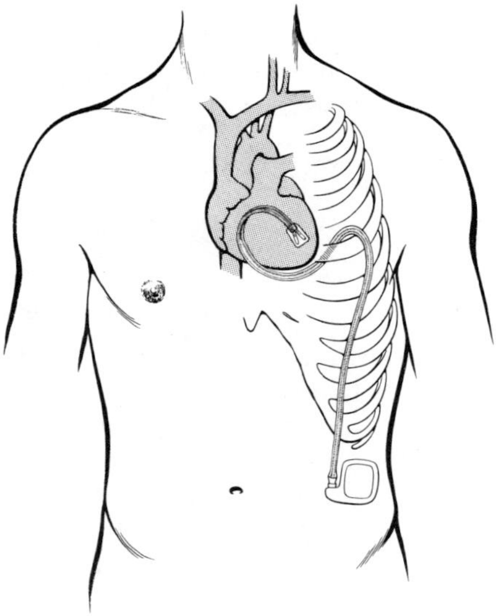

(b)

Fig. 10–6 (a) Myocardial electrodes attached to the ventricles; (b) electrodes with pulse generator implanted in abdomen. *(Courtesy of General Electric Company, Medical Systems Department, Milwaukee, Wisconsin.)*

pulse generators because endocardial electrodes for atrial sensing have not proven reliable.

Both *unipolar electrodes,* in which one electrode is placed on or in the heart and the other (reference) electrode is located somewhere away from the heart, and *bipolar electrodes,* in which both electrodes are on or in the heart, are used for pacing. For some types of implantable pulse generators, the reference electrode is a stainless steel plate that forms one side of the case. Since the pacing pulses from pulse generators are short bursts of direct current, the output terminals of some external pulse generators are polarized and identified with plus and minus signs. When connecting the end wires of the catheter electrodes to the pacer, care must be taken that the electrode wire at the tip is connected to the negative terminal. Reversal of these connections may lead to an undesirable electrochemical action at the distal electrode that will affect the ability of the device to pace or sense properly. To ensure that the electrode lead connections cannot be reversed accidentally, most implanted pacers utilize keyed connectors that fit together in only one way. The electrodes of R-wave programmed pacers both sense and pace but at different times.

It should be remembered that, when connected to an indwelling pacing catheter, the terminals that connect to an external pacemaker provide a direct electrical path to the heart. In order to prevent undesirable stray currents from accidentally reaching the heart, these terminals should be covered with a surgical glove that may be held in place by a rubber band. Also, rubber gloves should be worn when the need arises to handle the pacer or the pacing wires.

10.5 Power Sources and Electromagnetic Interference

The type of power source used for a pulse generator depends on whether the unit is an external or an implantable type. Today most of the manufactured external pulse generators are battery powered, although earlier units that receive power from the ac power line are still in use. Because of the need to electrically isolate patients with direct wire connections to their hearts from any possible source of power-line leakage current (see Chapters 3 and 18), and for portability, battery-powered units are preferred. Implantable pulse generators commonly use mercury batteries whose life span ranges between 2 and 3 years, after which a new pulse generator must be installed. Recognizing the need to develop longer-lasting batteries for pacing use, the industry has developed the lithium-iodide battery, which has an estimated life expectancy of 5 years. A pulse generator with rechargeable batteries whose life span is estimated at 10 years is now available.

A rechargeable pacemaker system and its recharging unit are shown in Figure 10-7. For a short period of time once each week, the patient dons a

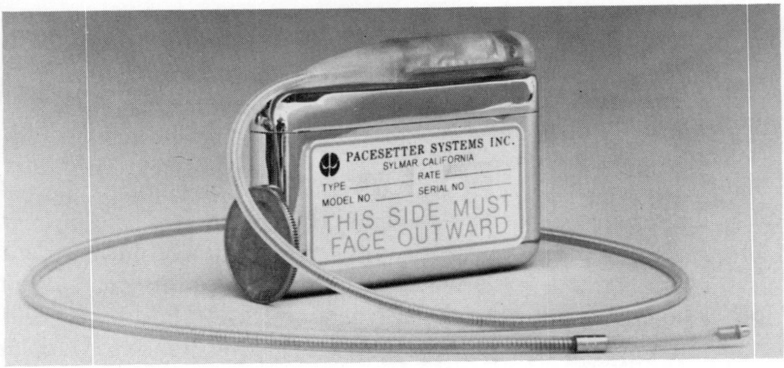

(a)

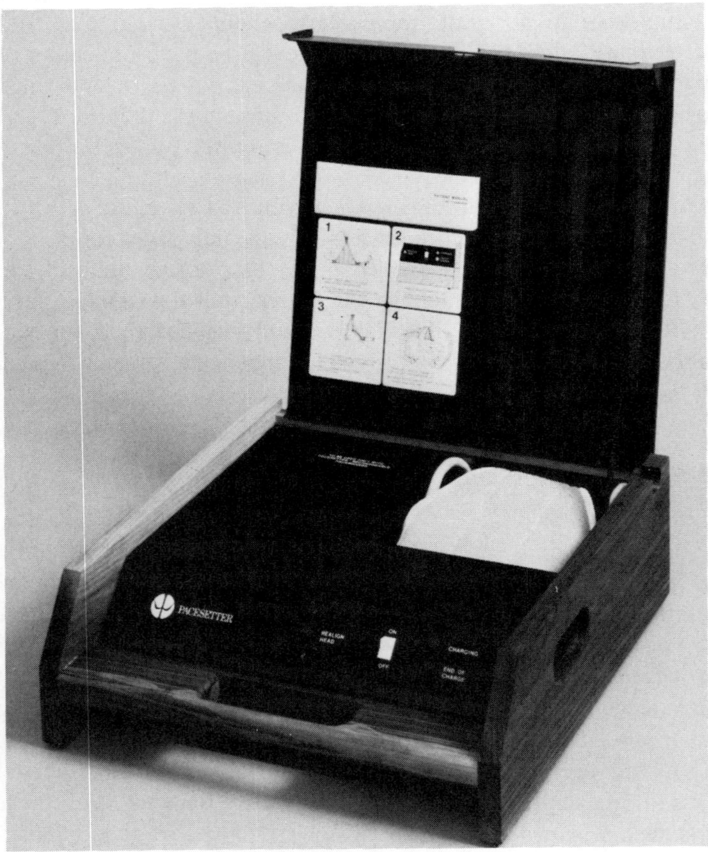

Fig. 10–7 (a) Rechargeable implantable pacemaker system; (b) charging unit. *(Courtesy of Pacesetter Systems, Inc., Sylmar, California.)*

(b)

vest, thus ensuring the correct positioning of a charging head over the implanted pulse generator. Through magnetic coupling between the charging head and the pacer, the pacer's batteries can be recharged. Afterward the pacer signals the charging unit that the process is completed. The weekly charge provides a pacing safety margin of approximately 6 weeks.

Another technological advance in implantable power sources has been the introduction of nuclear-powered pulse generators. In these devices, heat generated by the decay of radioactive plutonium is converted into direct current that is used to power the pacemaker. These units have an estimated useful life of at least 10 years, with negligible radiation danger to the patient.

Sources of electromagnetic energy, such as microwave ovens, diathermy, electrosurgical units, and auto ignition systems, may affect the operating mode of implanted or external pacemakers. Under certain circumstances such electrical noise signals may be strong enough to mimic the R wave in demand-mode pacers, thus inhibiting their outputs. Some implantable units are shielded in order to minimize the effects of extraneous noise. Nevertheless, patients with demand pacers should be warned about approaching microwave ovens or other obvious sources of electrical interference.

10.6 Defibrillators

As discussed earlier in this chapter, the heart is able to perform its important pumping function only through precisely synchronized action of the heart muscle fibers. The rapid spread of action potentials over the surface of the atria causes these two chambers of the heart to contract together and pump blood through the two atrioventricular valves into the ventricles. After a critical time delay, the powerful ventricular muscles are synchronously activated to pump blood through the pulmonary and systemic circulatory systems. A condition in which this necessary synchronism is lost is known as *fibrillation.* During fibrillation the normal rhythmic contractions of either the atria or the ventricles are replaced by rapid irregular twitching of the muscular wall. Fibrillation of atrial muscles is called *atrial fibrillation;* fibrillation of the ventricles is known as *ventricular fibrillation.*

Under conditions of atrial fibrillation, the ventricles can still function normally, but they respond with an irregular rhythm to the nonsynchronized bombardment of electrical stimulation from the fibrillating atria. Since most of the blood flow into the ventricles occurs before atrial contraction, there is still blood for the ventricles to pump. Thus even with atrial fibrillation circulation is still maintained, although not as efficiently. The sensation produced, however, by the fibrillating atria and irregular ventricular action can be quite traumatic for the patient.

Ventricular fibrillation is far more dangerous, for under this condition the ventricles are unable to pump blood; and if the fibrillation is not corrected, death will usually occur within a few minutes. Unfortunately, fibrillation, once begun, is not self-correcting. Hence a patient susceptible to ventricular fibrillation must be watched continuously so that the medical staff can respond immediately if an emergency occurs. This is one of the reasons for cardiac monitoring, which is discussed in Chapter 11.

Although mechanical methods (heart massage) for defibrillating patients have been tried over the years, the most successful method of defibrillation is the application of an electric shock to the area of the heart. If sufficient current to stimulate all musculature of the heart simultaneously is applied for a brief period and then released, all the heart muscle fibers enter their refractory periods together, after which normal heart action may resume. The discovery of this phenomenon led to the rather widespread use of defibrillation by applying a brief (0.25 to 1 s) burst of 60-Hz ac at an intensity of around 6 A to the chest of the patient through appropriate electrodes. This application of an electrical shock to resynchronize the heart is sometimes called *countershock*. If the patient does not respond, the burst is repeated until defibrillation occurs. This method of countershock was known as *ac defibrillation*.

There are a number of disadvantages in using ac defibrillation, however. Successive attempts to correct ventricular fibrillation are often required. Moreover, ac defibrillation cannot be successfully used to correct atrial defibrillation. In fact, attempts to correct atrial fibrillation by this method often result in the more serious ventricular fibrillation. Thus ac defibrillation is no longer used.

About 1960, a number of experimenters began working with direct-current defibrillation. Various schemes and waveforms were tried until, in late 1962, Dr. Bernard Lown of the Harvard School of Public Health and Peter Bent Brigham Hospital developed a new method of *dc defibrillation* that has found common use today. In this method, a capacitor is charged to a high dc voltage and then rapidly discharged through electrodes across the chest of the patient (see Chapter 3).

It was found that dc defibrillation is not only more successful than the ac method in correcting ventricular fibrillation, but it can also be used successfully for correcting atrial fibrillation and other types of arrhythmias. The dc method requires fewer repetitions and is less likely to harm the patient. A typical dc defibrillator is shown in Figure 10-8.

Depending on the defibrillator energy setting, the amount of electrical energy discharged by the capacitor may range between 100 and 400 watt-seconds or joules. The duration of the effective portion of the discharge is approximately 5 ms. The energy delivered is represented by the typical

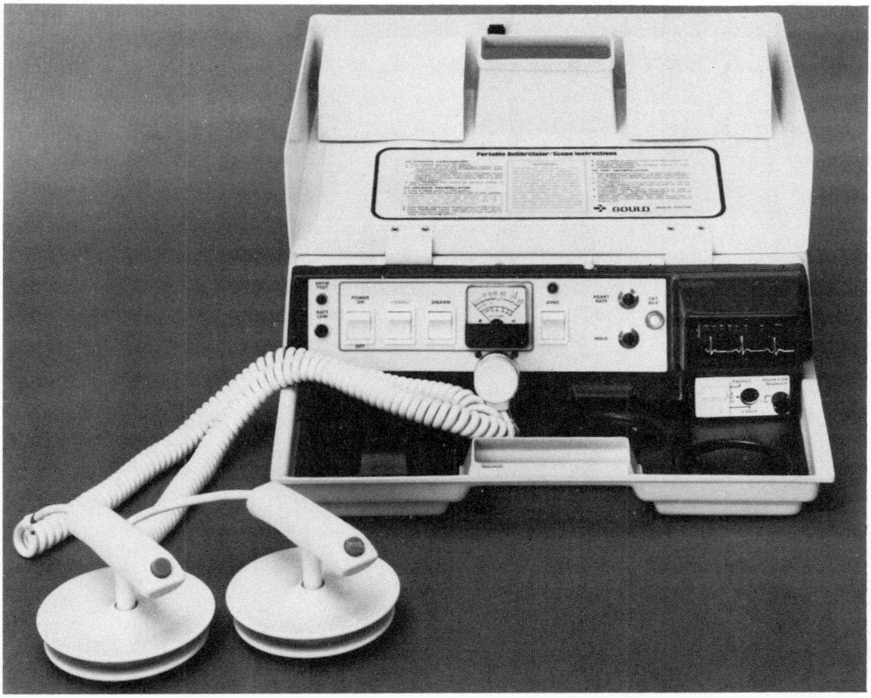

Fig. 10–8 DC defibrillator with paddles. This portable unit incorporates a defibrillator, electrocardioscope and pacemaker. *(Courtesy of Gould Medical Systems, Sunnyvale, California.)*

waveform shown in Figure 10-9 as a time plot of the current forced to flow through the thoracic cavity. The area under the curve is proportional to the energy delivered. It can be seen that the peak value of current is nearly 20 A and that the wave is essentially *monophasic*, since most of its excursion is above baseline. An inductor in the defibrillator is used to shape the wave in order to eliminate a sharp, undesirable current spike that would otherwise occur at the beginning of the discharge.

Even with dc defibrillation there is danger of damage to the myocardium and the chest walls because peak voltages as high as 6000 V may be used. To reduce this risk, some defibrillators produce dual-peak waveforms of longer duration (approximately 10 ms) at a much lower voltage. When this type of waveform is used, effective defibrillation can be achieved in adults, with lower levels of delivered energy (between 50 and 200 watt-seconds). A typical dual-peak waveform is shown in Figure 10-10.

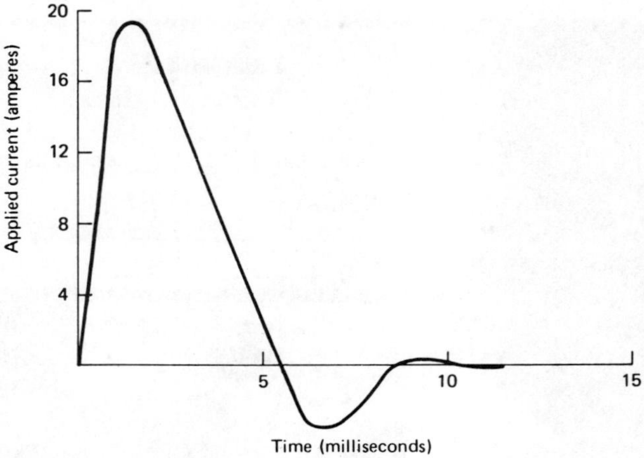

Fig. 10–9 DC defibrillator discharge waveform (Lown).

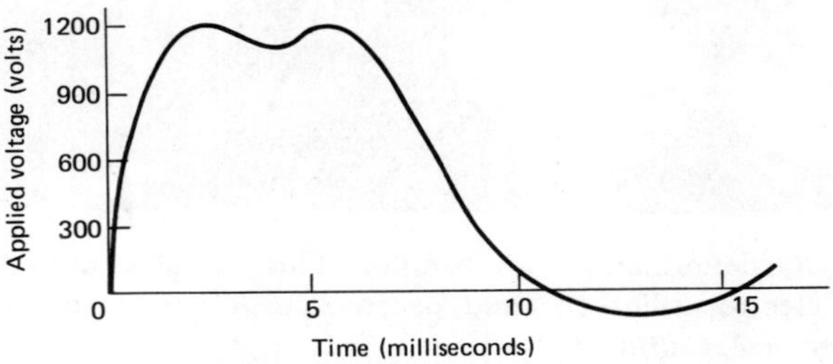

Fig. 10–10 Dual-peak monophasic defibrillator discharge waveform.

Effective defibrillation at the desirable lower-voltage levels is also possible with the *truncated* waveform shown in Figure 10-11. The amplitude of this waveform is relatively constant, but its duration may be varied in order to obtain the amount of energy required.

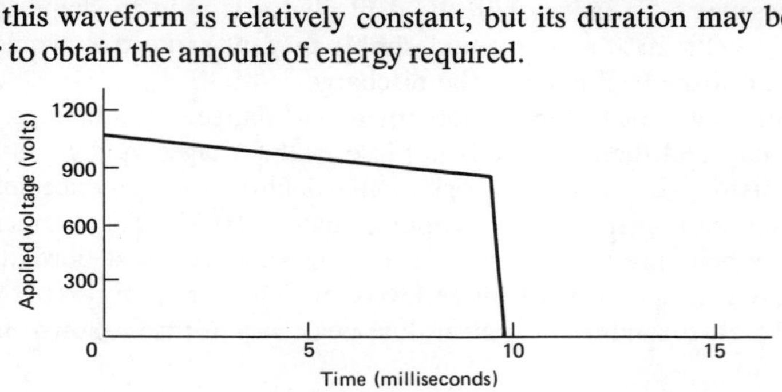

Fig. 10–11 Truncated defibrillator discharge waveform.

In order to deliver the large current discharge applied through the skin properly, large electrodes are used. These electrodes, called *paddles,* have metal disks that usually measure from 8 to 10 cm (3 to 4 in.) in diameter for external (transthoracic) use. For internal use (direct contact with the heart) or for use on infants, smaller paddles are applied. In external use, a pair of electrodes is firmly pressed against the patient's chest. Conductive jelly or a saline-soaked gauze pad (the latter is preferred) is applied between each paddle surface and the skin to prevent burning. However, if conductive jelly is applied to the paddles prior to electrode placement, care must be taken that, when the paddles are applied, the jelly does not accidentally form a conductive bridge between the paddles. If it does, the defibrillation attempt may not be successful. With either of the preceding conductive materials, care must be taken that they will not dry out with repeated discharges.

To protect the person applying the electrodes from accidental electric shock, special insulated handles are provided. A thumb switch, located in one (or both) of the handles, is generally used to discharge the defibrillator when the paddles are properly positioned. This device prevents the patient, or someone else, from receiving shock prematurely. In earlier equipment, a foot switch was used instead. The possibility of someone accidentally stepping on the foot switch in the excitement of an emergency, before the paddles are in place, makes the thumb switches in the handles preferable.

The method by which defibrillators are programmed to become charged (or recharged after use) varies widely. For example, in some defibrillators the charging process is accomplished by means of a charge switch (or push button) located on the front panel of the unit. A newer model, however, has the charge switch located in the handle of one of its paddles. In a few defibrillators the charging process begins automatically (and immediately) after discharge. Whatever the method, it is important that the person using the defibrillator follow the manufacturer's instructions in order to operate the unit safely. Additionally, to ensure the safety of the medical team that is immediately caring for the patient, the user should verbally indicate that the defibrillator is about to be discharged.

The two defibrillator electrodes applied to the thoracic walls are called either *anterior-anterior* or *anterior-posterior* paddles. With anterior-anterior paddles, both paddles are applied to the chest. Anterior-posterior paddles are applied to both the patient's chest wall and back so that the energy is delivered through the heart. This method of paddle application offers better control over arrhythmias that occur as a result of atrial activity. A pair of anterior-posterior paddles consists of the anterior paddle already described and a flat posterior paddle that has a larger electrode diameter than the anterior paddle. Internal paddles, as mentioned above, may be applied directly to the myocardium (during open-chest surgery), or they may be applied to the chest of an infant. Such paddles are flat and are usually available in several sizes, with diameters ranging from 5 to 10 cm. In these applications, the energy levels required for defibrillation may range from 10 to 50 watt-seconds. Special *pediatric paddles* are available with diameters ranging from 2 to 6 cm. Internal paddles can be either gas sterilized or autoclaved.

Most defibrillators include watt-second (or joule) meters to indicate the amount of energy stored in the capacitor prior to discharge. For some defibrillators, however, this indication is not assurance that the amount of energy to which the unit is set by the user will, in fact, be delivered to a patient. Some of the energy indicated on the meter is lost or dissipated as heat in components (mainly inductors) inside the unit and, to a lesser extent, at the electrode-skin interface. As a result, the patient always receives less energy than the amount indicated on the meter. For example, a user may set a defibrillator to deliver 300 watt-seconds of energy to a patient (as shown by the meter). The actual amount of energy delivered, however, may be only 240 watt-seconds, which represents a 20% loss of energy. In some defibrillators, the loss may reach 40% or more. This inherent drawback of some defibrillators makes it difficult to determine accurately the amount of energy needed for various countershock procedures. For this type of defibrillator, a calibration chart can be prepared (by an engineer or a biomedical equipment technician) as an aid in setting them to accurate levels of delivered energy.

Within the last few years defibrillators whose delivered energy levels essentially equal their preset levels have bcome available. Their output waveforms are of types shown in Figures 10-10 and 10-11.

Because of the large amount of energy released into the body, an implanted pacemaker pulse generator located immediately beneath a defibrillator paddle could be damaged during a discharge. Furthermore, the lump beneath the skin may reduce the effective skin contact area of the paddle and increase the danger of burns. Thus care should be taken to avoid placement of a paddle over or near the pulse generator.

Electrocardiographic evidence of a heart in ventricular fibrillation is characterized by an irregular pattern of low amplitude in which P waves, QRS complexes, and T waves are not present. As explained earlier, if defibrillation does not take place within a very few minutes after the onset of fibrillation, severe brain damage or death will occur. Thus the defibrillator charge must be delivered to the patient as quickly as practicable. Since no normal ECG pattern is present in ventricular fibrillation, no attempt is made to synchronize the defibrillator discharge with the patient's ECG.

Defibrillators are also used to convert other potentially dangerous arrhythmias to an NSR or to one that is easily managed. This process is referred to as *cardioversion*. For this procedure, anterior-posterior paddles are generally used. For example, a defibrillator discharge may be used to convert a *tachycardia* (fast heart) arrhythmia to a normal rhythm. Unlike the ECG for a heart in ventricular fibrillation, the electrocardiogram for a fast heart contains QRS complexes. To avoid the possibility of ventricular fibrillation resulting from the application of the dc pulse in cardioversion, the discharge must be synchronized with the electrocardiogram. The optimum time for discharge is during or immediately after the downward slope of the R wave when the heart is in its absolute refractory period (see Chapter 5). This synchronization will ensure that the countershock is not delivered during the middle of the T wave, which is called the heart's *vulnerable period.* During this time, since it is partially refractory, the heart is susceptible to ventricular fibrillation by the introduction of artificial stimuli.

Most modern defibrillators include a provision for synchronizing the discharge pulse with the patient's ECG. The ECG signal is fed to an amplifier from either a patient monitor or an electrocardiograph. In some cases, the patient's ECG electrodes are connected directly to the amplifier. When properly programmed, the defibrillator will discharge only at the desired portion of the ECG waveform. The closing of the thumb switches on the paddles applied to the patient allows the defibrillator to discharge at the next occurrence of the R wave.

10.7 Mobile Emergency Care

The need to provide immediate around-the-clock medical care to heart attack and accident victims in the community has resulted in the use of *mobile emergency care* units. Manned by personnel trained to administer first aid as well as emergency cardiopulmonary resuscitation techniques, these vehicles are equipped with instruments and medication similar to that used in the special care units of hospitals. Because these units are in constant radio contact with community organizations (police and fire departments) and with hospitals, they are able to reach an accident scene or the location of a stricken citizen in a short period of time. Typically, on arrival, a portable electrocardiograph (often with an oscilloscope display) is quickly applied to obtain an evaluation of the patient's ECG and heart rate. An indication of cardiac standstill or pulmonary failure will initiate emergency cardiopulmonary resuscitation procedures. After airway clearance and assisted breathing are ensured, defibrillation or cardioversion may be required by a portable defibrillator. The victim's heart may then be temporarily paced by a portable pacer. Some instruments, such as the defibrillator shown in Figure 10-8, are capable of performing the three functions—monitoring of ECG display, defibrillation (or cardioversion), and pacing. The condition of the patient may then be radioed to personnel in the special care unit of a nearby hospital while his ECG is simultaneously transmitted to the unit's display and recording equipment via telemetry (see Section 13.3.3). In a short time, after a detailed diagnosis is made, instructions returned by radio may prescribe specific medication or additional resuscitation techniques. If the patient is in standstill and cannot breathe, adequate blood circulation can be maintained by means of a mechanical cardiopulmonary resuscitation unit. When the patient is able to be transported to a hospital, his vital signs are monitored by appropriate equipment inside the vehicle. In this way, a seriously stricken individual is able to receive timely special care away from the hospital.

11

Instrumentation in Critical Care Units

The need for intensive care and patient monitoring has been recognized for centuries. The 24-hour nurse for the critically ill patient has become a familiar part of the hospital scene over the years. But only in the last few years has equipment been designed and manufactured that is reliable enough and sufficiently accurate to be used extensively for patient monitoring. The nurse is still there, but her role has changed somewhat. She now has powerful tools at her disposal for acquiring and assimilating information about the patients under her care. Thus she is able to render better service to a larger number of patients, as well as to react promptly to an emergency. With the capability of providing an immediate alarm in the event of certain abnormalities in the behavior of a patient's heart, monitoring equipment makes it possible to summon a physician or nurse in time to administer emergency aid, often before permanent damage can occur. With prompt warning and by providing such information as the electrocardiogram prior to, during, and after the onset of cardiac difficulty, the monitoring system enables the physician to give the patient the correct drug rapidly. In some cases, even this process is automated.

Physicians do not always agree among themselves as to which physiological parameters should be monitored. The number of parameters monitored must be carefully weighed against desired care, personnel, cost, complexity, and reliability of the equipment. There are, however, certain parameters that provide vital information and that can be reliably measured at relatively low cost. For example, all cardiac-monitoring units continuously measure the electrocardiogram from which the heart rate is easily derived. The electrocardiogram waveform is usually displayed on a cathode-ray tube and may be recorded on paper.

As noted in Chapter 1, the concept of intensive coronary care had little practicality until the development of electronic equipment that was capable of reliably measuring and displaying the electrical activity of the heart on a continuous basis. With such cardiac monitors, instant detection of potentially fatal arrhythmias finally became feasible. Combined with stimulatory equipment to reactivate the heart in the event of an arrhythmia, a full system of equipment to prevent sudden death in such cases is now available. Today coronary care, intensive respiratory care, medical and surgical intensive care units, cardiac catheterization laboratories, to name but a few, fall under the heading of what is conventionally known as critical care. These areas as well as certain other diagnostic or care units, such as the stress-testing laboratory and postcoronary care unit, all have two features in common: they are heavily instrumented with electronic equipment and they are staffed with personnel familiar with its use.

In these critical care areas, monitoring equipment is installed beside the bed of each patient to measure and display the electrocardiogram, heart rate, and other parameters being monitored from the patient. In addition, information from several bedside stations is usually displayed on a central console at the nurses' station.

Blood pressure measurements are frequently monitored, displayed, and recorded along with the electrocardiogram. Other physiological parameters, such as temperature, respiration, and cardiac output, are also monitored by electrical instrumentation. Generally it is desirable that such instrumentation should

1. Operate accurately across a wide range of both normal and abnormal physiological states; for example, provide systolic blood pressure data in a range of 0 to 300 mm Hg.
2. Be simple and sturdy in design so as to facilitate its use by nontechnical personnel.
3. Possess capabilities for monitoring more than one parameter simultaneously, such as ECG, blood pressure, and temperature, or be compatible with other monitoring equipment in use.
4. Possess appropriate safety alarms that are adjustable for individual patient needs.

5. Be economical in terms of both cost and space requirements.

This chapter describes the various elements that compose a critical care monitoring system, as well as some of the problems often encountered with this type of equipment. It should be noted that there is some repetition of material already covered in Chapters 7, 9, and 10, but this repetition is intentional, since these discussions are in the context of the critical care unit.

11.1 The ECG Monitor

Whenever the patient is monitored in the critical care area, in nearly all cases the first and most central parameter to be monitored is the electrocardiogram, frequently abbreviated ECG (or sometimes EKG). In addition to monitoring the ECG waveform, most instruments provide the patient's heart rate as well, which is easily derived from the electrical signal. The ECG waveform is usually displayed on a cathode-ray tube (CRT) for visual observation by the staff. Normally there are provisions for permanently recording the waveform on paper. Figure 11-1 shows the front view of a typical ECG monitor.

The ECG monitor can perform several useful and necessary functions for proper patient care. In order to perform these functions, the monitor

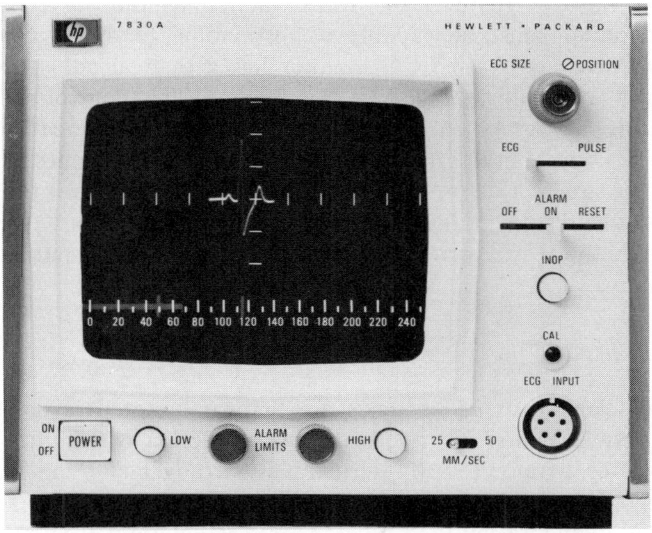

Fig. 11–1 ECG monitor. *(Courtesy of Hewlett-Packard Company.)*

must contain the necessary controls and adjustments so that it can be equally useful across a wide spectrum of cardiac arrhythmias as well as normal rhythms. The basic functions that the ECG monitor must provide are described below.

11.1.1 ECG Display

The fundamental requirement of the patient monitor is its ability to display the patient's ECG waveform accurately, without artifact and with sufficient size to be viewed from a distance. The two most common methods of display are the *bouncing ball* and the *nonfade* display. The nonfade display has numerous advantages over the bouncing ball display, although it is also more expensive. The major advantages of the bouncing ball instrument are its simplicity, small size, and lower cost.

It is important that the display be sufficiently bright and that the viewing surface be nonglare and nonreflective to permit clear observation of the tracing even in well-illuminated areas.

11.1.2 Magnitude of the ECG

Typically, the magnitude of the ECG at the surface of the body is about 1 mV; however, this value varies greatly from one patient to another. The ECG of a critically ill patient may be as low as 0.1 mV or as high as 3 mV. Even higher values of the ECG may be obtained from within the heart. Whatever the source and magnitude of the ECG, the patient monitor must be capable of responding to and accepting these values. Consequently, an ECG monitor has a manual adjustment for the purpose of controlling the size of the display. This control is located on the front of the instrument. Different manufacturers may call this control by various names, but the function is the same. Typical names for the ECG size control are ECG *size, gain,* and *sensitivity.* In addition to controlling the size of the display, this control also ties in with the heart rate computer so that only the R waves are detected and counted for the purpose of heart rate display.

11.1.3 Lead Selector

The selection of which leads are being monitored is determined by medical requirements. Therefore the lead selection capabilities may vary from monitor to monitor. In the simplest arrangement, the monitor will have only three wires to be connected to the patient. The selection of which lead configuration is to be monitored is determined by the choice of location of the electrodes (see Chapter 7 for further details). Thus if the two active electrodes are placed on the left and right arms and the reference electrode is placed on the right leg, the monitor will display the lead I ECG. Similarly, if the active electrodes are placed on the right arm and left leg, the display will be lead II. In order to eliminate the need for removing and reapplying electrodes, some monitors incorporate a switch to select the required lead configuration that must be monitored. Thus by placing five electrodes on the patient, and with the aid of the lead selector switch, it becomes possible to view any required lead at any time.

As shown in Figure 11-2, the lead selector switch is usually located on the front of the instrument, where it is accessible. However, on some instruments, the lead selector switch is not located on the instrument but is mounted at a remote location nearer the patient. Also, the lead selector switch may have only a limited lead selection, such as leads I, II, and III.

11.1.4 Heart Rate Computer and Alarms

Most ECG monitors also provide the patient's heart rate. Normally, for every heartbeat, there is one QRS complex. Thus by counting the number of QRS complexes it is possible to obtain the patient's heart rate. Most heart rate computers (*cardiotachometers*) are almost automatic in their operation and do not require any adjustments. Once the proper ECG size is displayed on the monitor screen, the heart rate computer is able to count the QRS complexes and display the patient's heart rate. The heart

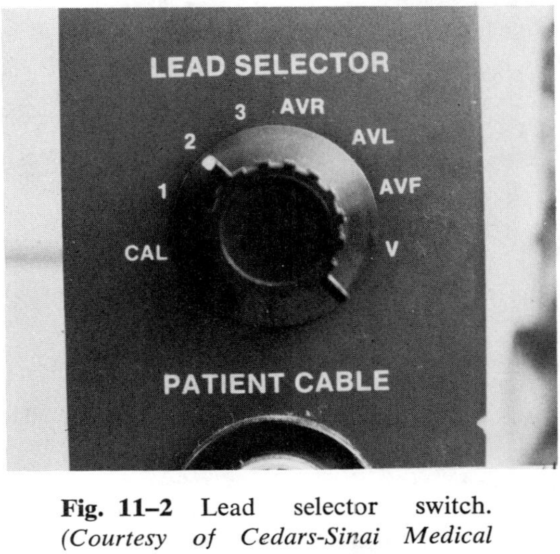

Fig. 11–2 Lead selector switch. *(Courtesy of Cedars-Sinai Medical Center, Los Angeles, California.)*

rate can be displayed on a digital display, as shown in Figure 11-3(a), or it can be displayed on a conventional meter [Figure 11-3(b)].

The advantages of the digital heart rate indicator are its greater accuracy and ease in viewing, both from nearby as well as from a distance.

In addition to heart rate, the heart rate computer permits certain alarm criteria to be established based on the patient's heart rate. Since the indication of heart rate is in beats per minute (BPM), it becomes a

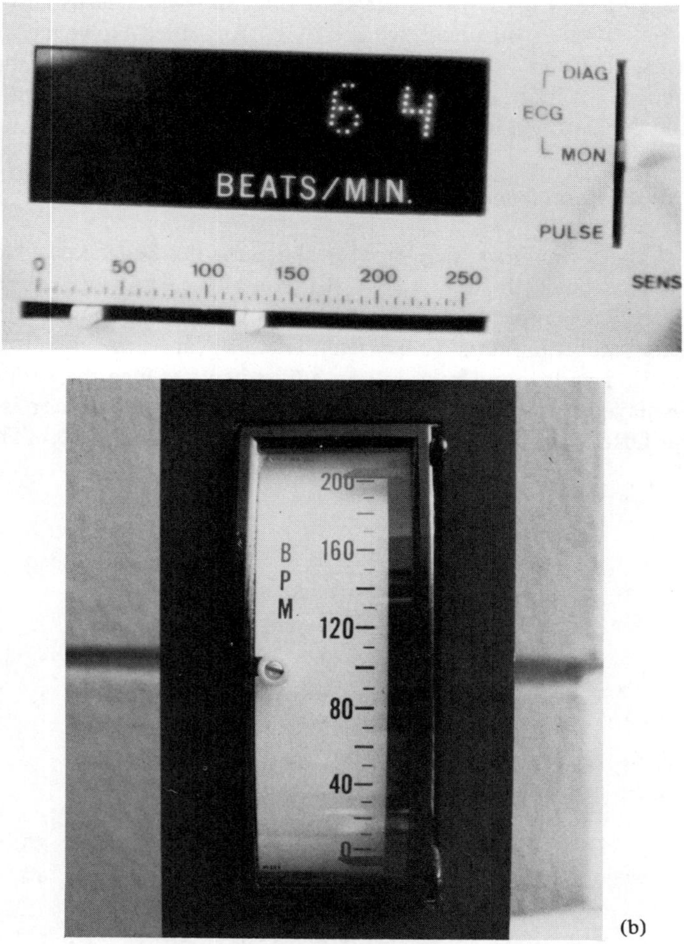

(a)

(b)

Fig. 11–3 (a) Digital heart rate indicator; (b) conventional heart rate monitor. *(Courtesy of Cedars-Sinai Medical Center, Los Angeles, California.)*

relatively easy matter to establish some upper and lower rate limits. Then if the limits are exceeded, an automatic alarm is activated to alert the staff. The upper and lower limits are always adjustable so as to provide individualized patient criteria for an alarm condition. For example, if a patient's normal heart rate is 64, the upper limit might be set at 80 and the lower limit at 50. Under no circumstances should the rate alarms be set too far in either direction. This action would make the alarm useless should the patient suddenly show a ventricular tachycardia or heart block, for example. For most hearts that are behaving normally, an alarm setting of 50 and 100 should provide the desired safety effect with minimal false alarms.

Of cardinal importance to the effectiveness of any critical care unit is proper activation of alarms, whether ECG, spirometer alarms, and so on. Under the usual clinical conditions, when an alarm is turned off, vital information becomes relatively inaccessible to the staff. Just as every nursing student is admonished to place the nurse call button within easy reach of the patient, so the critical care nurse must maintain the calling capability of the patient's alarms.

11.1.5 Diagnostic and Monitor Modes of Display

The bedside patient monitor can be used in two basic operating modes. The first is the *monitoring mode,* used where a gross observation of the electrical activity of the patient's heart is necessary, with little analysis or detail. In the monitoring mode, the frequency response of the monitoring instrument is somewhat limited in order to reduce the undesirable effects of two common artifacts:

1. *Motion artifact,* which can be observed as rapid and random spikes on the displayed ECG waveform. This type of artifact, if allowed to persist and be picked up by the monitor, may activate the heart rate computer, causing a false high rate and inappropriately activating the alarms.
2. *Baseline variation artifact* results from variations in the electrode potentials between the electrodes and the body surface. Baseline artifact is observed as a slow up and down movement (called *wandering*) of the displayed baseline. Although this artifact will not activate the alarms, it makes observation of the waveform difficult. One of the problems associated with baseline artifact is the difficulty in recording the waveform on paper. When the baseline wanders, the recording stylus in the paper recorder will also wander, reaching the edges of the paper and producing poor tracings.

In the *diagnostic mode,* the monitor must display an accurate presentation of the electrical activity of the patient's heart. In this mode, the frequency response of the monitor is wider, thus allowing a truer presentation of all the necessary details in the ECG waveform. Figure 11-4 shows the difference of a simulated ECG waveform when recorded in the diagnostic and monitoring modes of display.

When a detailed analysis of the patient's ECG is necessary, the diagnostic mode of monitoring must be used. For instance, in order to observe S-T segment elevation or depression or to document pacemaker function accurately, it is absolutely necessary to use the instrument in the diagnostic mode. Failure to do so will result in inaccurate information.

For most continuous monitoring, the instrument should be set to the monitoring mode. This setting will reduce the number of false alarms resulting from artifacts.

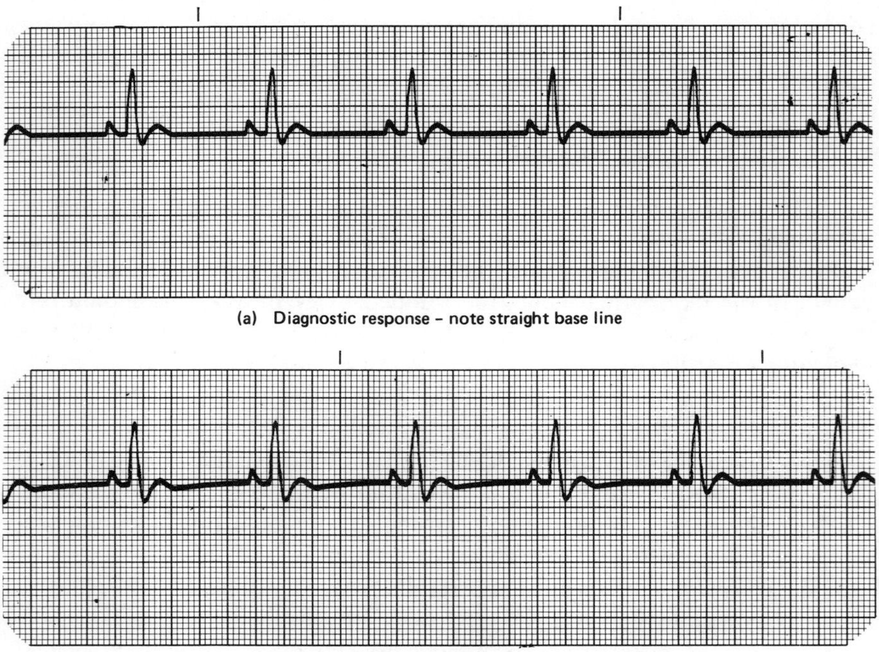

(a) Diagnostic response - note straight base line

(b) Monitor response - note slanted base line

THE EFFECT OF DIAGNOSTIC AND MONITOR
FREQUENCY RESPONSE ON AN ECG COMPLEX

Fig. 11–4 (a) ECG waveform—diagnostic; (b) ECG waveform—monitoring. *(Courtesy of Cedars-Sinai Medical Center, Los Angeles, California.)*

11.1.6 1 mV Cal

One of the most useful but most infrequently used controls on a patient monitor is the 1 mV cal (Calibration) button or switch. As stated previously, the patient's ECG may vary in magnitude as well as waveform. In order to obtain a meaningful pattern, the size of the display must be adequate. But what if the display is not large enough and cannot be increased further with the aid of the ECG size control? Is the instrument defective? Are the leads applied improperly? Or is a low-amplitude ECG signal coming from the patient? The 1 mV cal can be used to answer most of these questions. By depressing the calibration button, a reference voltage of 1 mV is applied to the input of the patient monitor. If this reference signal can be adjusted to its proper size on the monitor screen, then the user knows that the monitor is functioning properly and that it has the necessary gain in order to display the ECG at an acceptable size. It is then probable that the problem is associated with lead placement and/or that a low-amplitude ECG signal is coming from the patient. Based on these criteria, the staff can take the necessary steps to correct the situation.

In addition to these "go, no-go" checks that can be performed with the calibration button, more sophisticated tests can also be performed in order to determine the frequency response of the monitoring system. The details for such tests are not covered in this book.

11.1.7 Leads-Off Indicator/Alarm

Some bedside monitors utilize a relatively new device, the *leads-off indicator*. Problems involving the interface of the electrodes with the patient and the integrity of the patient leads are often encountered in patient monitoring. The function of the leads-off indicator is to verify the quality of the patient-equipment interface and indicate whether this interface is poor or marginal. Thus, in case of difficulty, the nursing staff can rapidly determine the nature of an improper ECG display. It also serves as a useful reminder to the nursing staff when patients have been temporarily removed from their monitor to walk or to change the electrodes. Under such circumstances the alarm indicator will indicate a problem with the leads. Care must be taken to reactivate the alarm setting, which is usually turned off during the electrode change; a separate indicator also shows whether or not the alarm is set in such equipment, thus reminding the staff to correct the situation.

11.2 Defibrillator/Cardioverter

An extremely important lifesaving instrument in the critical care area is the defibrillator. Although this device was discussed in Chapter 10, certain concepts are mentioned here in the context of the critical care area. Unlike the instrumentation mentioned thus far, the prime purpose of the defibrillator is to intervene during ventricular fibrillation. This condition is lethal unless quickly corrected, since the heart muscle literally quivers in a haphazard manner due to widespread electrical discharging of the muscle cells.

Most defibrillators in common use in critical care have a synchronizer component and appropriate ECG-monitoring attachments to make them useful for *cardioversion,* another technique commonly utilized in critical care. Unlike defibrillation, which is an emergency technique, cardioversion is usually attempted on patients on an elective basis for such problems as atrial fibrillation. Because these patients have normally synchronized ventricular activity, it is imperative that the discharge of electrical current applied across the chest be *synchronized* with the patient's QRS complexes. Failure to do so might result in ventricular fibrillation should the current traverse the heart during its vulnerable period. A synchronizer on the defibrillator/cardioverter automatically times the discharge to occur at the time of the R wave rather than during or near the T wave.

The staff must be sure that their defibrillator/cardioverter synchronizer switch is normally in the OFF position; otherwise no discharge will occur when defibrillating under emergency circumstances. This instrument should be checked at low watt-second levels at least daily to ensure its effectiveness when needed. Normal safety considerations apply here and will be elaborated on in Chapter 18.

11.3 The Central Nurses' Station

In addition to the bedside ECG monitor and the defibrillator, the next most important group of instruments is found at the central nurses' station. In practice, the central station is an extension of the bedside equipment and provides information from all patients at one location. By observing the central monitor, all patient activities can be observed at a glance. In addition, a paper recorder at the central station can be activated, manually or automatically, in order to record patient information permanently. Typical equipment at the central station consists of the following devices:

1. Large multitrace central monitor
2. Paper recorder

3. Patient selector for the paper recorder
4. Frequently, heart rate indicators.

11.3.1 The Central Monitor

The central monitor is usually a large multitrace instrument capable of displaying several traces at the same time. Generally this monitor is a slave to the bedside equipment and has very few controls. As a rule, it will have only a power ON-OFF switch, brightness control, and position controls for each of the traces. Since it is a slave-type instrument, the necessary calibrations are performed at bedside and should not be altered at the central station. This monitor is of extreme importance, since it permits the nurse or arrhythmia technician to view any patient as required and without having to move from the station. Should an abnormality be observed, the patient can be attended immediately.

11.3.2 The Paper Recorder and Patient Selector

Perhaps the most valuable central station instrument is the strip chart recorder. It permits the nurse to record permanently, on paper, the patient's physiological data. Besides being useful for immediate observation and analysis, these records become part of the patient's permanent medical records. In critical care areas it is common practice to obtain the patient's ECG every few hours, as well as to document arrhythmias and similar factors as they occur. With the addition and use of the patient selector, the nurse is able to obtain a record from any patient simply by pressing the appropriate buttons.

In addition to the manual selection of data for any patient, the patient selector can be activated automatically in the event of an alarm from bedside (such as a sudden fast rate). When the patient selector is activated, it, in turn, activates the paper recorder for a permanent record of the event. Many ECG recorders also incorporate a delay of 6 to 10 seconds which allows the nurse to observe arrhythmia on the scope (e.g., a premature ventricular contraction, PVC). Then if the record button is pressed, the complex in question, and the electrical events immediately preceding it are captured. Some equipment will also identify on paper the bed number as well as whether the tracing was a manual selection or whether it was activated because of an alarm condition. Figure 11-5 shows two ECG strips showing bed identification as two short lines and indication for the automatic activation of the recorder. Some instruments will also print the patient's heart rate, name and the date.

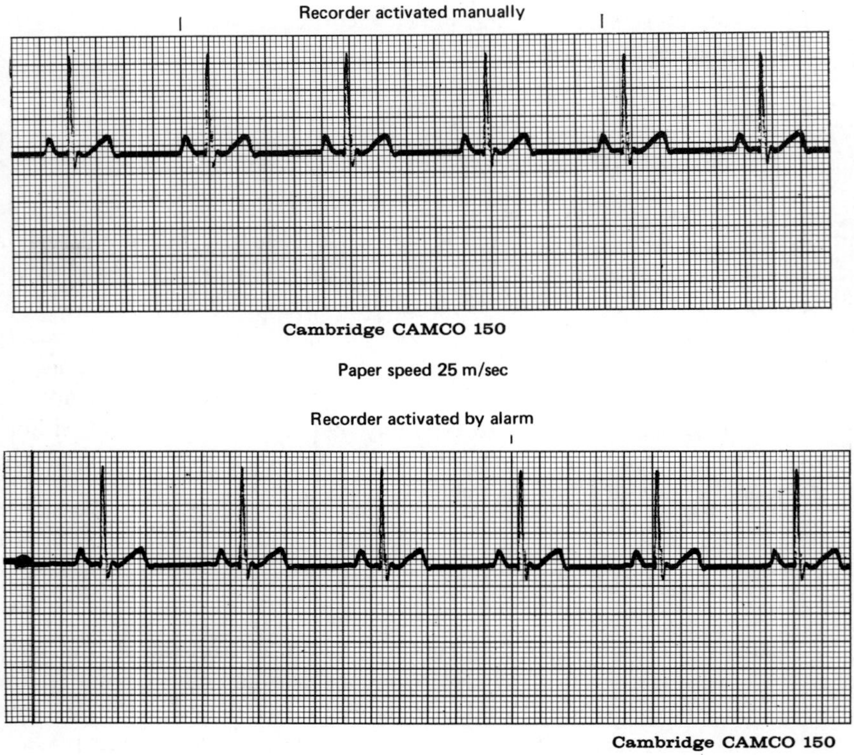

Fig. 11–5 ECG strips. (a) manual; (b) automatic. *(Courtesy of Cedars-Sinai Medical Center, Los Angeles, California.)*

11.4 Blood Pressure Monitoring

The subject of blood pressure monitoring and measurements was covered in detail in Chapter 9. However, it is important to be aware of the special considerations involved in blood pressure instrumentation in the critical care unit. In modern units it is common for a patient's hemodynamic function to be monitored, as well as the ECG and other parameters. Besides obtaining blood pressure values, it is becoming increasingly important to be able to observe blood pressure waveforms and their contours.

In addition to the blood pressure monitor, one of the more critical devices is the blood pressure transducer. This device is a small and delicate electromechanical instrument that converts a physical variable into an electrical signal. This signal, in turn, is fed to the blood pressure monitor for display and additional processing.

A typical bedside blood pressure monitor has several controls and adjustable characteristics that are necessary for proper measurements.

Pressure measurements are actually made with respect to the surrounding atmospheric (reference) pressure. Therefore some means must be provided for adjusting and correcting for differences between the reference pressure and a residual pressure that might exist for a given transducer.

In practice, two important adjustments are required in every blood pressure measurement system. First, there is a zero adjust, also known as the balance control. This adjustment allows the transducer-amplifier system to be set to display a reference zero when the reference pressure is zero. The second control is gain setting, sometimes known as sensitivity. This control permits adjustment of the system to indicate a given pressure value when that pressure is actually measured in the patient. On some instruments one or both adjustments may be automatic (built into the system). Most blood pressure amplifiers contain a special processing section that detects the maximum point of the pressure waveform and displays it as the systolic value. Similarly, another part of the processing section detects the minimum point of the waveform and displays that as the diastolic value. On certain instruments the average pressure value is obtained between the systolic and diastolic readings; it is displayed as the mean value. The systolic, diastolic, and mean values are generally displayed on an analog or digital (numerical) indicator.

11.5 Multichannel Displays

An increased understanding of human physiology and accompanying advances in medicine and technology have created the need for more sophisticated monitoring and display equipment. Such displays include multichannel cathode-ray tube (CRT) displays, multichannel paper recorders, and nonfade (also known as memory) displays. All these devices allow the staff to view several parameters or different views of one parameter simultaneously in true time perspective.

11.5.1 Multichannel CRT Displays

The most popular and most frequently used device is the multichannel CRT display. Usually it consists of a large cathode-ray tube (approximately 9 in. diagonally, although some are larger) that can display several traces. Each trace, in turn, has its own controls. The instrument can display many physiological parameters. In addition to the multitraces, these monitors possess the feature that all the displayed information is synchronized in time. For example, if a blood pressure waveform is displayed simultaneously with the ECG, the timing relationship between the two parameters will be a true indication of what is happening to both variables at any instant of time.

11.5.2 Multichannel Recorders

As with the multichannel CRT display, the multichannel recorder is also a useful medical instrument. Here also the timing between the various parameters has proper and accurate correlation. For simplicity, a typical two-channel recording of a patient's ECG and blood pressure is shown in Figure 9-7 in Chapter 9.

The advantage of the multichannel recorder over the multichannel CRT display is its ability to provide a permanent record. One of the channels is always used to record the patient's ECG; the other channels may be used for various parameters, such as blood pressure and respiration. Up to eight individual channels for simultaneous display are in current use. As stated, one of the most important features of the multichannel recorder is its ability to preserve true timing information among all the channels. Therefore since the paper moves at a precisely known rate, it is possible to make accurate timing measurements.

11.6 Fade and Nonfade Displays

Referring to the explanation of CRT displays in Section 4.6, it should be clear that the display of an ECG or any other waveform consists of a single dot that moves across the screen at a predetermined rate (25 or 50 mm/s). As the electron beam strikes the inner face of the CRT, that portion becomes brightly illuminated and appears as a continuous line to the human eye.

In early monitoring equipment all displays would fade, but modern technology has provided the nonfade display. The nonfade display is also known by other names, such as memory display, bright display, computer vision, and so on. In all cases, the idea is the same, but the trade names change from one manufacturer to the next. It is important to be able to distinguish between the two types of display, for the difference is significant in terms of visibility.

The fade or bouncing ball display will be explained first, followed by the principles of nonfade display.

11.6.1 The Bouncing Ball Display

As the electron beam moves across and writes a pattern on the face of the CRT, the earlier portion of the trace begins to fade away and finally disappears. The ability of the trace to remain visible on the face of the CRT is known as *persistence*. The duration of this persistence is determined by the phosphor (coating) inside the CRT. The longest persistence tubes that are available allow the trace to be visible for approximately 1 second. In the case of patterns like the ECG or blood pressure waveforms, for example, which may occur at a rate of 60 events per minute, the persistence of the tube will allow the viewer to see only one waveform. In addition, this displayed waveform will not be uniformly bright. The early portion of the display will always be dimmer than the more current portion. Such a "temporary display" has great limitations for the observer, who may need to evaluate the waveform for diagnostic purposes. Doing so becomes an almost impossible task. When it is necessary to perform any analysis on such waveforms, the waveforms must be permanently recorded on paper. Any event that might have occurred unseen may be lost within a second and cannot be documented on paper even with a time lag or delay between the CRT and writeout device.

For years the bouncing-ball display was the only means for waveform display, and it was useful despite its limitations.

11.6.2 The Nonfade Display

With the advancement and development of digital electronics, the nature of CRT displays has changed for the better. The term *digital electronics* applies to that phase of electronics that deals with the presence or absence of electronic pulses. An electronic pulse is known as a *bit,* and electronic signals are converted into a combination of these bits, which are further processed into special codes according to need. The nonfade display utilizes this technique of digital electronics. (See Chapter 19 for a further explanation of bits.)

First, the incoming signal is amplified as necessary to a level that permits easy and accurate conversion to a group of digital bits. A typical ECG waveform, when converted to digital bits, may consist of several thousand such bits. The more bits used, the more accurate the conversion. Once converted to digital bits, the information is stored in special electronic circuits. The bits can be stored indefinitely. For display purposes, they can be recalled from storage and displayed on the CRT without losing the original bits. This type of display is not a continuous line, as in the normal CRT display, but consists of closely spaced dots as shown in Figure 11-6 (the dots are spaced farther apart for illustration).

The electron beam in the CRT moves across the screen at a very fast rate instead of the slower rate of 25 or 50 mm/s. Every time it becomes necessary to display a dot, the beam is turned on; and in between dots the beam is turned off. Thus a pattern can be displayed on the CRT screen

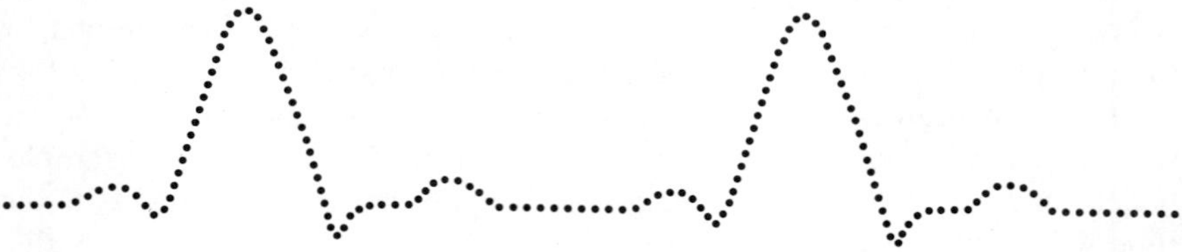

Fig. 11–6 ECG pattern made up of dots.

that consists of a group of dots resulting from bits that have been recalled from the electronic storage. Since the bits are recalled, the process can be repeated many times, with the same information repeated over and over again.

Each time the group of bits is recalled for display, the dots are moved very slightly to one side or another, thus making the trace appear as if it were moving when actually only the dots are moving. The rate at which the dots are made to move across is set to a low speed, such as 25 or 50 mm/s. This speed permits a continuous display of the waveform. In practice, several waveforms are converted to bits and displayed simultaneously. The storage elements are programmed in such a way as to allow information to be stored from 2 seconds up to 16 seconds and more. Slowly the old information in the storage elements is continuously replaced with fresh information, thereby providing a "history" of the waveform being displayed.

11.7 Neonatal Intensive Care Units

Neonatal critical care instrumentation is similar to that already discussed with the exception that different instruments are used for the purpose of monitoring slightly different parameters, which are of special importance to the high risk newborn or infant.

11.7.1 Respiratory Measurements

One of the more commonly monitored parameters is respiration, including rate and the respiratory waveform. The monitoring of respiration is important on the neonate because it provides necessary information regarding inspiratory and expiratory conditions and alerts the staff when an apnea period extends beyond a predetermined time period. In most instances, this instrument operates by measuring the variation in chest impedance. The measurement is accomplished via the ECG electrodes, thus eliminating another set of electrodes. When ECG and respiration are measured at the same time, it becomes extremely important that the electrodes be properly placed.

11.7.2 Temperature

Another measurement that is necessary for the neonate is temperature. Temperature measurements may include body surface temperature and core temperature, which indicates the temperature inside the body. Core temperature is normally measured rectally.

Temperature measurements can be displayed in analog or digital form. Since variations are small and the rate of change is relatively slow, a waveform display of temperature is seldom required.

11.8 Coronary Care Units

In conclusion, a typical coronary care unit is described. As might be expected, many different room and facility layouts for intensive coronary care units are in use. One type that is quite popular is a U-shaped design in which six or eight cubicles or rooms with windows surround the nurses' central monitoring station. Although the optimum number of stations per central console has not been established, a group of six or eight seems most efficient. For larger hospitals, monitoring of 16 to 24 beds can be accomplished by two or three central stations. The exact number depends on the individual hospital, its procedures, and the physical layout of the patient-care area. In certain areas in which recruitment of trained nurses is difficult, this factor could also be considered in selecting of the best design.

A central nurses' station in a coronary care unit is shown in Figure 11-7.

A coronary care unit usually includes the following components:

1. Skin electrodes used to sense ECG potentials. These electrodes are described in Chapter 6.
2. Amplification equipment.
3. An oscilloscope display that permits direct observation of the ECG waveforms. The bedside monitors normally contain medium-sized cathode-ray tube screens (5 to 9 in. in diameter), and each displays at least the ECG waveform from one patient. The central nurses' station generally has a larger oscilloscope screen on which electrocardiograms from several patients are displayed simultaneously.
4. A rate meter used to indicate the average number of heartbeats per minute and to provide a continuous indication of the heart rate.

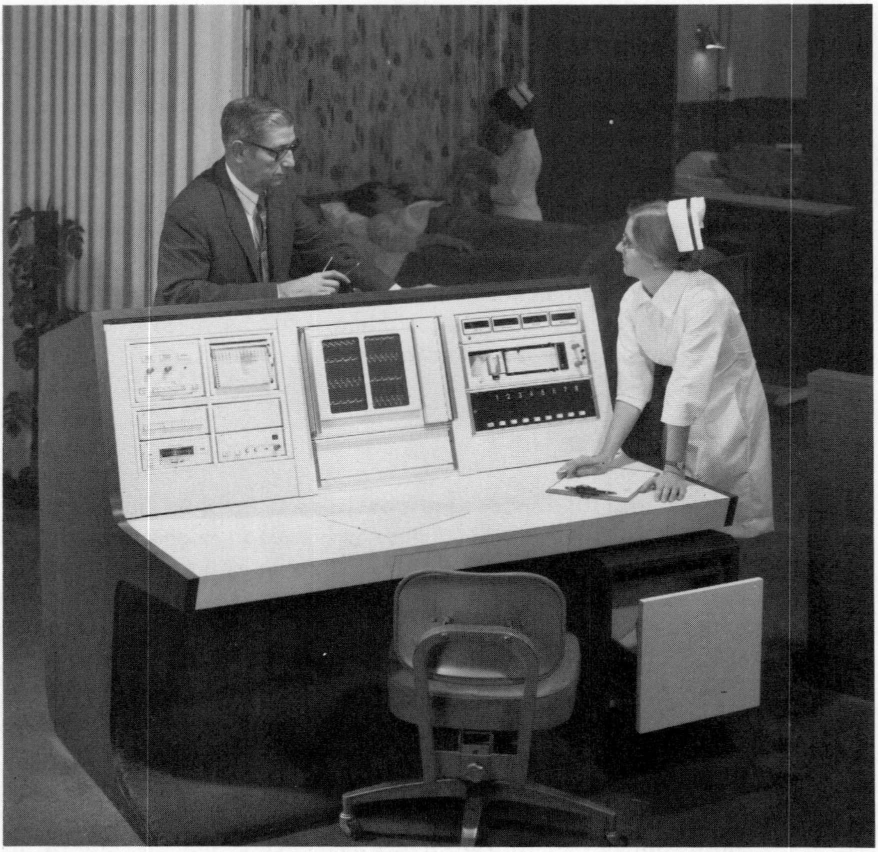

Fig. 11–7 (a) Central nurses station; (b) companion bedside unit (*see* page 229). *(Courtesy of Hewlett-Packard Company.)*

On most units, an audible beep or flashing light (or both) occurs with each heartbeat.

5. An alarm system, actuated by the heart rate meter, to alert the nurse or other observer by audible or visible signals whenever the rate falls below or exceeds some adjustable preset range.

In addition to these basic components, the following elements are useful and are often found in cardiac-monitoring systems.

1. A direct writeout device (an electrocardiograph) to obtain, on demand or automatically, a permanent record of the electrocardiogram seen on the oscilloscope. Such documentation is

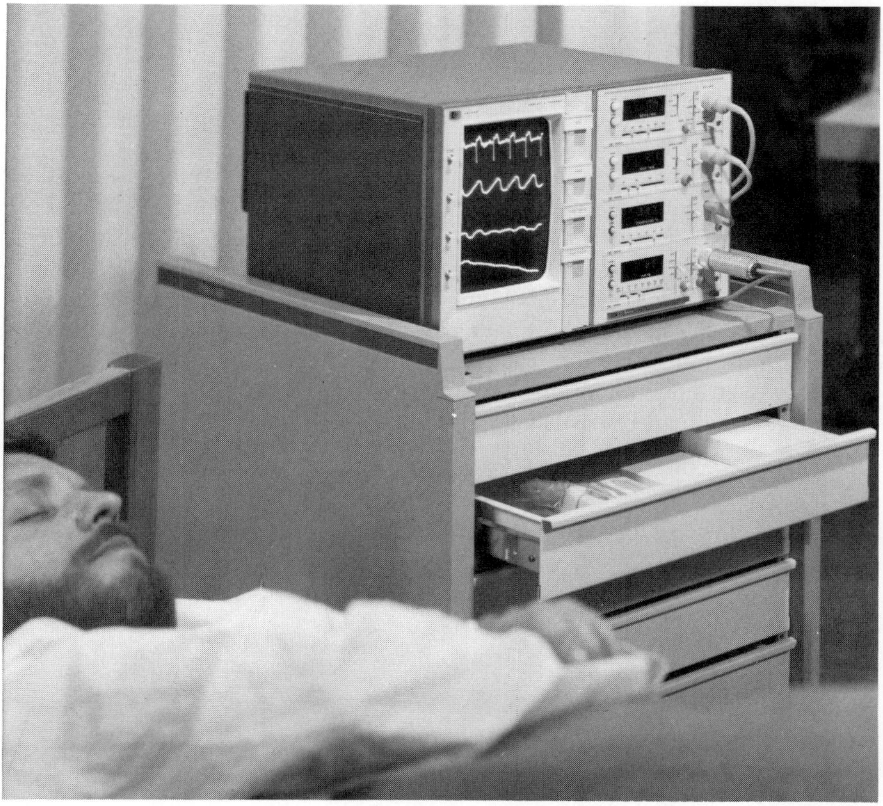

Fig. 11–7 (Continued.)

valuable for comparative purposes and is usually required in the event of an alarm condition.

2. A memory-tape loop to record and play back the electrocardiogram for the 10 seconds or more just prior to an alarm condition. Recording of the ECG may continue until the system is reset. In this way, the electrical events associated with the heart immediately before, during, and following an alarm situation can be displayed if the nurse or some other observer was not present at the time of the occurrence.
3. Additional alarm systems triggered by ECG parameters other than the heart rate. These alarms may be activated by premature ventricular contractions or by widening of the QRS complex in the ECG. Either situation may provide advance indication of a more serious problem.

4. Electrical circuits to indicate that an electrode has become disconnected or that a failure has occurred somewhere else in the monitoring system. Such a lead failure alarm permits instrumentation problems to be distinguished from true clinical emergencies.

Although the thrust of this chapter relates primarily to the hospital situation, the reader is encouraged to view the information presented here within the broader context of the "life-support" effort. The equipment, personnel, and philosophy of the paramedic team defibrillating the coronary patient on his living room floor are not essentially different from that encountered in the hospital coronary care unit that will admit that patient at a later point. In truth, the critical care unit that is composed of its often portable instrumentation and its well-prepared staff are providing life-support services wherever they are needed.

12

Blood Flow and Volume and Cardiac Output

Adequate blood supply is necessary for all organs of the body; in fact, an impaired supply of blood is the cause of various diseases. The ability to measure blood flow in the vessel that supplies a particular organ would therefore be of great help in diagnosing such diseases. Unfortunately, blood flow is a rather elusive variable that cannot be measured easily.

The rate of flow of a liquid or gas in a pipe is expressed as the volume of the substance that passes through the pipe in a given unit of time. Flow rates are therefore usually expressed in liters per minute or milliliters per minute (cm^3/min).

In order to measure the flow rate in a water pipe, a *flow meter* is connected into the pipeline. Obviously, a direct method of this type is not suitable for measurement of flow in a blood vessel, and so, indirect methods must be used. Three basically different techniques of indirect flow measurement are used to measure the blood flow in various parts of the body.

The *indicator dilution* method is one of the oldest methods and is used mainly to determine the blood flow in the aorta, also called the *cardiac output*. The principle of indicator dilution can also be employed to measure the *circulating blood volume*.

Magnetic and *ultrasonic blood flow meters* actually measure the *velocity* of the bloodstream. Because these techniques require that a transducer surround an excised blood vessel, they are mainly used during surgery. Ultrasound, however, can be used transcutaneously to detect obstructions of blood vessels where quantitative blood flow measurements are not required.

A *plethysmograph,* which actually indicates volume changes in body segments, can be used to measure the flow of blood in the limbs.

12.1 Principle of Indicator Dilution Measurements

The principle of the indicator dilution methods can be understood easily with the help of Figure 12-1. Here 8 oz of sugar (about one cup) is dissolved in the contents of each pitcher. The pitcher on the left contains 4 qt of water; the one on the right contains only one quart. When the sugar has dissolved completely, the solution at the right is obviously sweeter than the one at the left. To be precise, the solution at the right has a concentration of 8 oz/qt of sugar, while the one at the left has a concentration of 2 oz/qt, only one-fourth as much. Because the amount of sugar originally added was known, it is only necessary to measure the con-

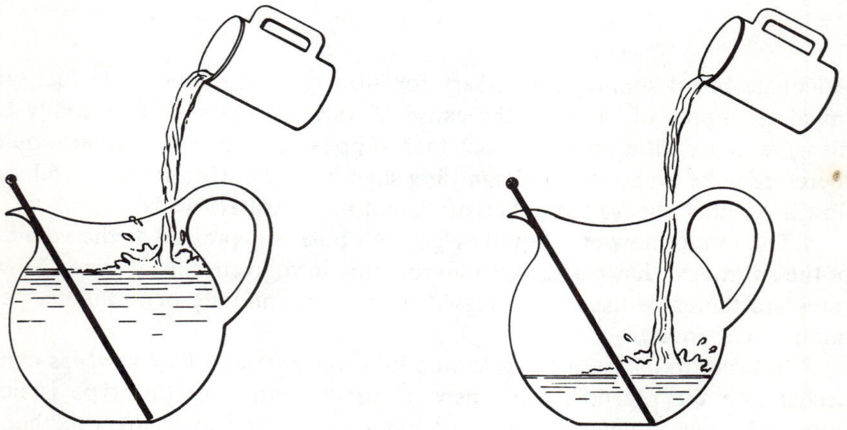

Fig. 12–1 Principle of volume determination by the indicator-dilution method: The same amount of sugar is added to both pitchers. The right pitcher contains less water than the one on the left. After the sugar has dissolved, the solution in the right pitcher, therefore, is sweeter than that in the left pitcher.

centration of the solution in ounces per quart in order to calculate the amount of water that was in each pitcher. The formula for doing this calculation is as follows:

$$\text{Amount of water in quarts} = \frac{\text{sugar added in ounces}}{\text{concentration in ounces per quart}}.$$

Note that the higher the concentration of the sugar solution, the smaller the volume of water in the pitcher.

This method is used to determine both the blood volume and the cardiac output in the human body. The sugar in the example served as an *indicator*. For blood flow and volume determinations, of course, other substances have to be used. The type of substance actually used as an indicator does not really matter, provided that it is not harmful to the human body and its concentration can be determined after it has been diluted in the bloodstream.

12.2 Blood Volume Determination

Measurement of the total volume of circulating blood is important in detecting internal hemorrhaging after surgery. The absolute volume measurement is not very meaningful for this purpose, but a decreasing volume during repeated measurements is indicative of internal hemorrhaging.

The indicator normally used for the determination of circulating blood volume is a *radioactive iodine isotope,* I_{131}, which is injected in the form of *iodated human serum albumen* (RIHSA). After it has been mixed with the blood by natural circulation, a blood sample is withdrawn. The concentration of the RIHSA in the sample can be determined from the radioactivity of the sample, using radioactivity counting methods. If the blood volume determination is to be repeated, however, the blood of the patient will still contain some amount of indicator from the previous determination or determinations. This residual concentration must be taken into account. Also, the radioactive strength of the RIHSA decreases slowly, due to the radioactive decay of the isotope, and some of the indicator may be retained in the syringe. Both effects require corrections in the calculation of the blood volume. This rather complicated computation is performed automatically in the device shown in Figure 12-2.

This instrument not only contains a simple computer to perform the calculations necessary, but it also has a number of lamps that indicate to the operator which step of the procedure should be performed next, a feature designed to reduce the likelihood of error.

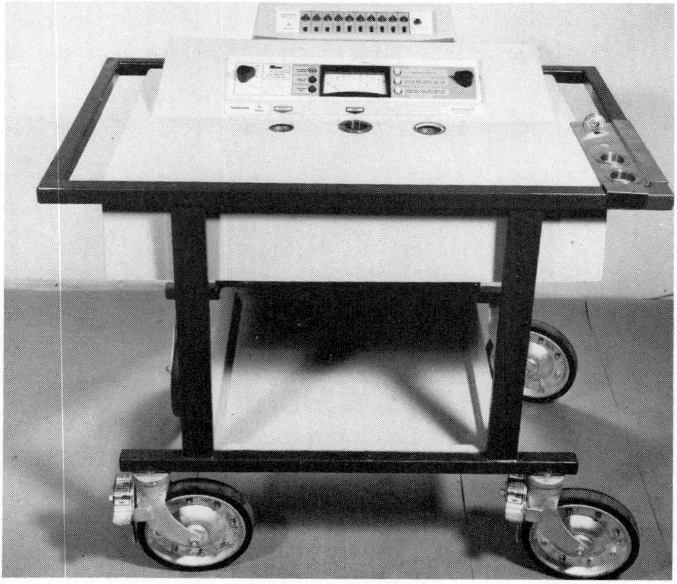

Fig. 12–2 Semi-automatic blood-volume measuring device. *(Courtesy of Ames Company, Division of Miles Laboratories, Inc., Elkhart, Indiana.)*

12.3 Determination of Cardiac Output Using Indicator Dilution

The indicator dilution method for the determination of cardiac output can be understood best with the help of Figure 12-3. The drawing at the upper left shows a fluid flow from the reservoir at the left through the pump in the center and out of the pipeline at the right. An indicator is infused upstream from the pump with a constant rate of infusion, measured, for example, in ounces per minute. The indicator is mixed with the fluid, and a detector downstream from the pump measures the indicator concentration in ounces per quart. The infusion of the indicator begins at the time marked *i* in Figure 12-3(a), and the concentration reading soon assumes a steady value as shown in that figure. From the indicator infusion rate and the measured concentration, the flow rate can be calculated as follows:

$$\text{Flow rate in quarts per minute} = \frac{\text{infusion rate in ounces per minute.}}{\text{concentration in ounces per quart}}.$$

The higher the measured indicator concentration, the lower is the flow rate and vice versa.

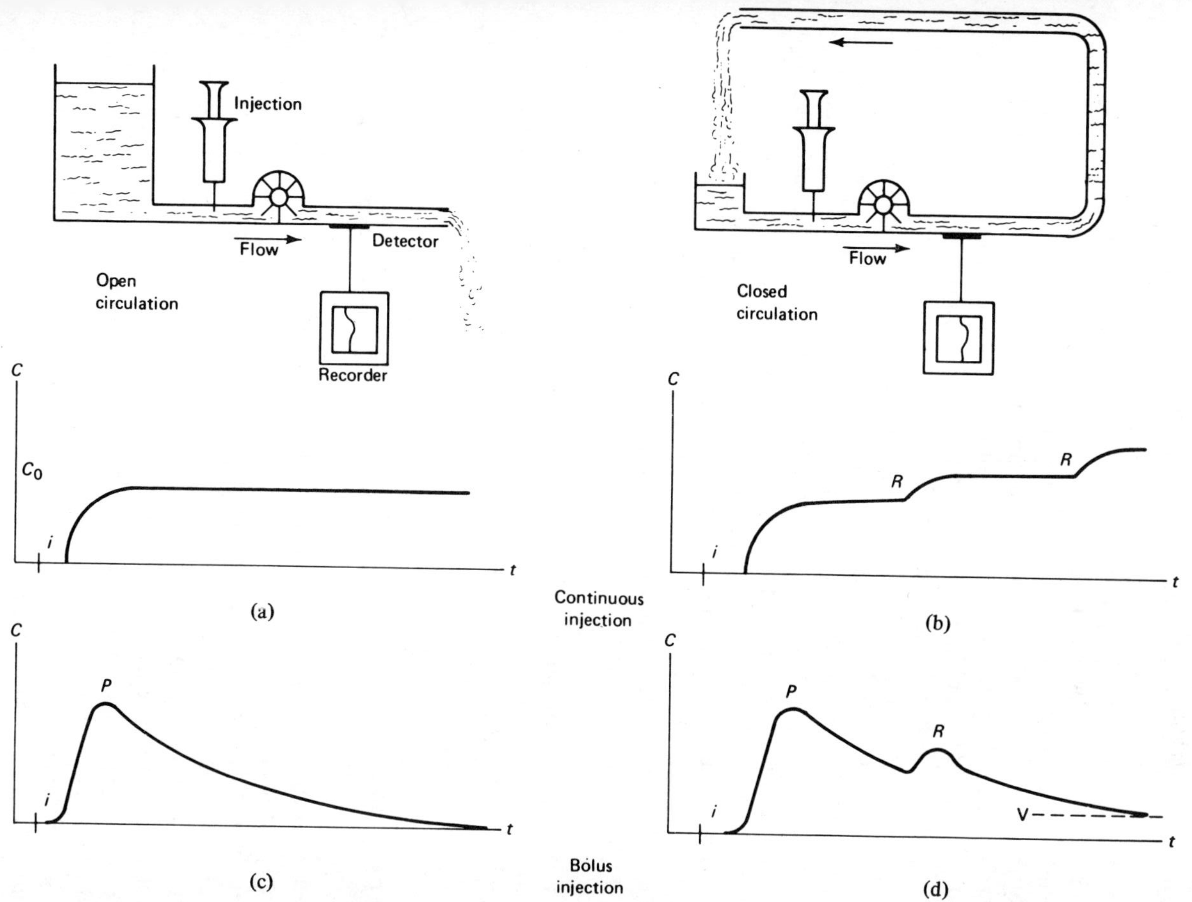

Fig. 12–3 Principle of flow measurements using the indicator dilution method.

The drawing at the left in Figure 12-3, however, resembles the blood circulation only superficially. A more accurate model is shown in the drawing at the right, in which the fluid is returned to the reservoir, as it is in the case of circulating blood. Indicator infusion and concentration measurements are the same as described before. However, the concentration reading for this case is shown in Figure 12-3(b). The infusion again starts at time *i*. The concentration increases and assumes a steady value but not for long. At the point marked R, the infused indicator has circulated completely through the system and is passing the detector a second time. The concentration reading therefore increases and will continue to do so every time the indicator recirculates. Because this recirculation "bump" can occur before the concentration assumes its steady "plateau," the indicator infusion method is generally not used for the determination of blood flow or cardiac output. The preferred method is one in which a measured amount of the indicator is injected as a *bolus* rather than infused at a constant rate. Assuming again the simplified case of the open circulation, the concentration reading is as shown in Figure 12-3(c). Shortly after the bolus of indicator substance has been injected, the concentration begins to increase, reaches a peak, and then declines slowly in a characteristic curve, sometimes called a *washout curve* or *exponential curve*. In order to use this curve to calculate the fluid flow, one must first determine the area under the curve or, more precisely, the area between the curve and the baseline. Because the two axes of the diagram are time (in minutes) and concentration (in ounces per quart), the area under the curve has the dimension minutes-ounces/quart. From this area and the amount of indicator that has been injected, the fluid flow can be calculated as follows:

$$\text{Flow rate in quarts per minute} = \frac{\text{injected indicator in ounces}}{\text{area under curve in minutes-ounces per quart.}}$$

As can be seen, the larger the area under the curve, the smaller the flow rate and vice versa.

In Figure 12-3(d) the concentration reading is shown again for the case of closed circulation. The recirculation of the indicator manifests itself in the form of a pronounced bump at the point R. Because of certain characteristics of the exponential washout curve, however, it is possible to extrapolate (predict) mathematically how the curve would have continued if the recirculation had not occurred.

Two different substances are currently favored as indicators for the determination of the cardiac output. One is a green dye (*cardiogreen®*), which is injected in quantities of between 1.25 and 5 mg. The concentration of the dye can be determined with a *densitometer,* which shines a light beam through a thin layer of the dye-containing blood and measures the amount of light absorption. For this purpose, blood is withdrawn continuously from an inserted catheter. The indicator dye is injected through a second catheter. Both catheters are usually placed with the help of a fluoroscope. Thus a cardiac output determination by this technique is normally performed in the cardiac catheterization room. Although the green dye is eventually excreted by the kidneys, the recirculation bump is very pronounced. The extrapolation and determination of the area under the curve are usually performed by a so-called *cardiac output computer,* one type of which is shown in Figure 12-4. The computer itself is shown on the console; the device on the left contains the densitometer and the withdrawal pump.

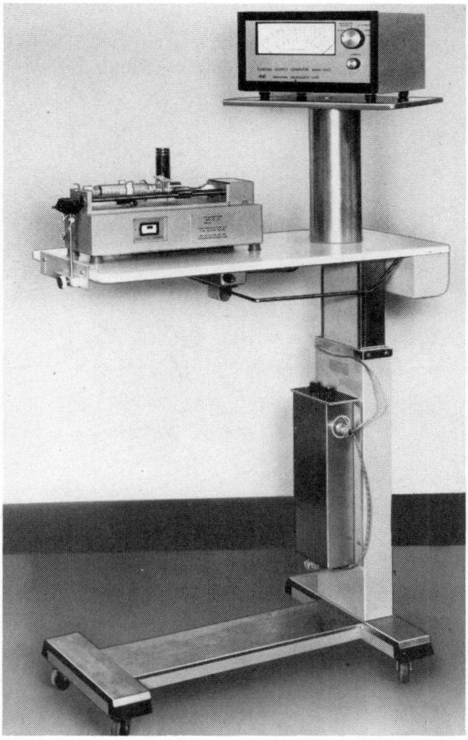

Fig. 12–4 Cardiac output computer (on column) with withdrawal pump in foreground and densitometer (dark) mounted on syringe of withdrawal pump. *(Courtesy of Lexington Instruments Corporation, Waltham, Massachusetts.)*

Another indicator substance used clinically is saline, which is injected after having been chilled in an ice bath. The concentration of this indicator can be determined simply by recording the temperature of the blood downstream from the injection point. Because the volume injected is normally only 10 ml, the circulating blood is rewarmed rapidly and no recirculation is visible on the concentration curve. Injection of the iced saline and measurement of the blood temperature are frequently performed with a single catheter of special design. This device is called the *Swan-Ganz® catheter,* the principle of which is shown in Figure 12-5. It is a special adaptation of the PA floatation catheter. This catheter contains four separate lumens. One lumen terminates about 30 cm (12 in.) from the tip and is used to inject the iced saline. The second lumen contains two thin wires that lead to a tiny electrical temperature sensor close to

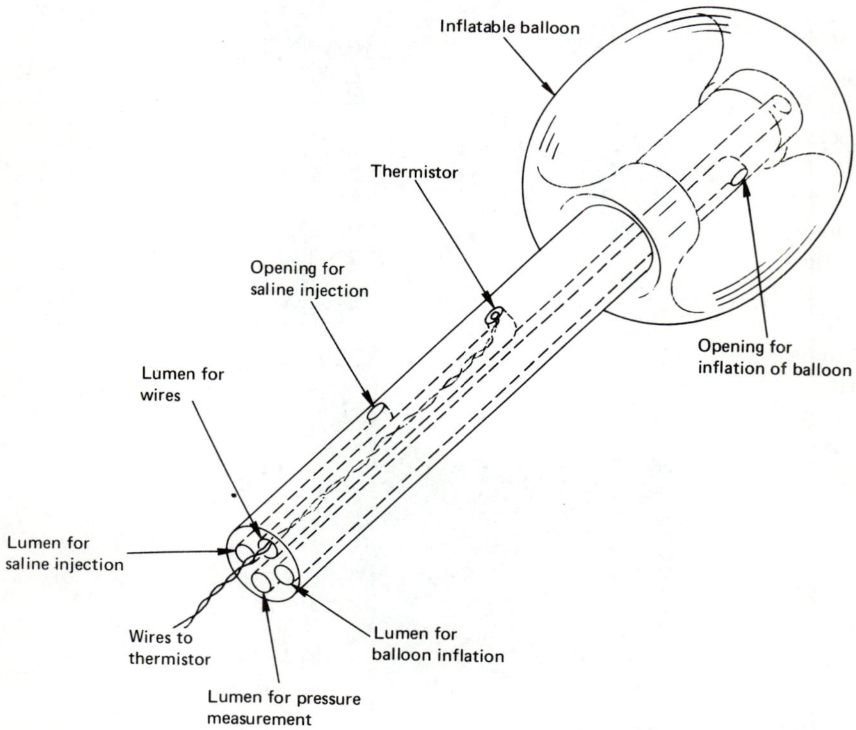

Fig. 12–5 Swan-Ganz® catheter for the measurement of cardiac output by the thermal dilution method. (Not drawn to scale). The opening for saline injection is actually located 30 cm distal from the catheter tip and the lumens vary in diameter.

the tip of the catheter. The third lumen ends at the catheter tip and can be used to measure the blood pressure at this point with one of the pressure transducers described in Chapter 9. The fourth lumen is used to inflate a small rubber ballon at the tip of the catheter. Once the catheter has been inserted into a vein, the ballon is inflated and the returning venous blood carries the catheter until its tip is positioned in the pulmonary artery. The position of the catheter can be checked by measuring the pressure at its tip. Thus the catheter can, if necessary, be inserted without fluoroscopic control. The cardiac output determination requires that the temperature sensor be connected to a suitable measuring circuit that allows the determination of the area under the temperature curve. The temperature rise of the cold saline during injection is compensated for by a correction factor in the calculation.

12.4 Ultrasonic Blood Flow Determination

The methods and instrumentation described in Section 12.3 are used to measure the total output of the heart. Other devices can be used to measure the flow of blood in a given vessel. One such type of instrument utilizes *ultrasonic energy,* sound energy far above the audible range. Most ultrasonic devices for the determination of blood flow are based on the principle of the *Doppler effect*. This effect can be experienced by any person standing at the curb while a car passes. The motor noise appears to change its pitch and becomes deeper at the instant of passing. Unlike the car in this example, the bloodstream does not emit sound of its own, and a slightly different version of the Doppler effect must be utilized. As shown in Figure 12-6, a crystal transmitter, similar to a loudspeaker, is used to send a beam of ultrasonic energy toward the blood vessel in which the blood flow is to be determined. The cells in the flowing blood reflect back some of the ultrasound, which is picked up by a crystal receiver, similar to a microphone. Because the reflecting blood cells are moving, the received signal has a slightly different frequency or pitch than the transmitted signal. Although the transmitted and received frequencies are both far above the range of human hearing, the frequency difference is conveniently within the audio range. This frequency actually depends on the velocity of the moving blood cells; thus ultrasonic devices actually measure the velocity of the blood rather than the flow rate. Nevertheless, if the diameter of the blood vessel is known, the device can be calibrated in flow rate. In clinical applications, ultrasonic blood flow meters are more frequently utilized to detect the presence or location of blood flow rather than to measure its magnitude accurately. For this purpose, the difference frequency is made

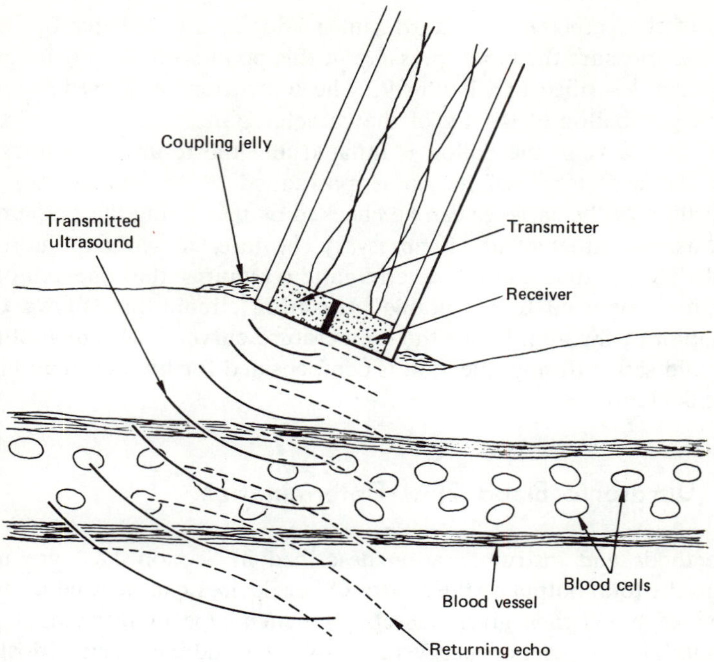

Fig. 12–6 Principle of percutaneous Doppler device for the detection of blood flow in superficial blood vessels. The probe, coated with coupling jelly, is held at an angle to pick up the signals reflected by the moving blood cells.

audible with a loudspeaker or earphones, as illustrated by the device shown in Figure 12-7. The sound heard is not a pure tone but is a characteristic "swish-swish-swish" in the rhythm of the pulse, because the blood cells from which the transmitted signal is reflected do not all have the same velocity.

Ultrasonic effects are now also used in fetal monitoring and blood pressure measurements, as mentioned in Chapters 8 and 17.

12.5 Magnetic Blood Flow Meters

Another type of instrument used to measure the flow of blood in a given vessel is the *magnetic blood flow meter*. These meters utilize the same basic principle as electrical generators except that the column of flowing blood itself acts as an electrical conductor. Consequently, a magnet must be applied around the flowing column of blood and two electrodes must make contact with the blood in order to pick up the electrical signal. In extra-

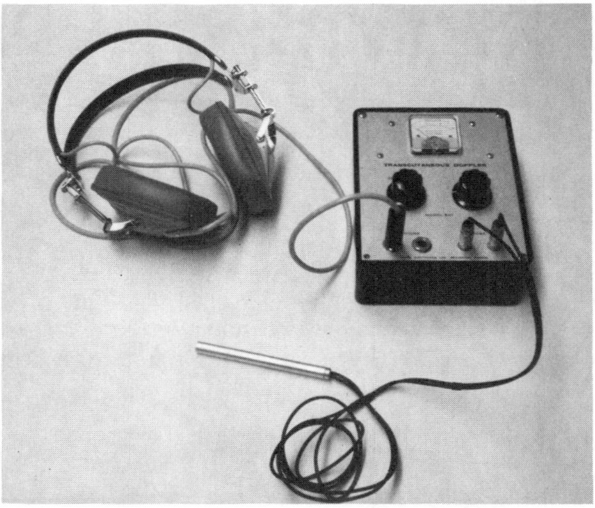

Fig. 12–7 Percutaneous Doppler device with probe and earphones. *(Courtesy of Veterans Administration Biomedical Engineering and Computing Center, Sepulveda, California.)*

corporeal blood flow meters, which are used to measure the blood flow in heart-lung machines and dialyzers, this requirement poses no problem. Blood flow probes for this application, as shown in Figure 12-8, are simply inserted at a convenient place in the tubing that carries the blood. Measur-

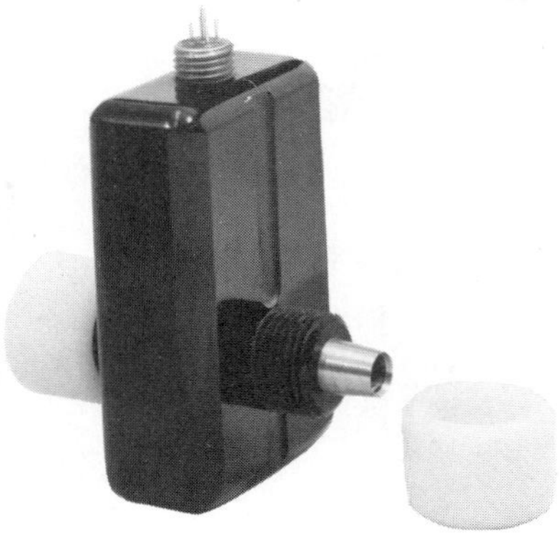

Fig. 12–8 Extracorporeal blood flow probe for insertion into blood lines. *(Courtesy of Biotronex, Silver Springs, Maryland.)*

ing blood flow in an intact blood vessel via this method, however, requires that the vessel be excised and slipped into a flow probe that has to have an orifice that matches the diameter of the blood vessel. Electrical contact with the flowing blood is established through electrodes that touch the walls of the vessel. Blood flow meters of this type are therefore normally used only during surgical procedures in which the blood vessels are exposed anyway. A flow probe of this type on a handle that can be clipped over a blood vessel is shown in Figure 12-9. Like the ultrasonic blood flow meters described earlier, magnetic blood flow meters actually measure the velocity of the blood rather than the flow rate. Because the diameter of the blood column at the place of measurement is defined by the diameter of the flow probe, however, devices of this type can be calibrated to read the flow rate.

12.6 Blood Flow Determination by Plethysmography

A *plethysmograph* (Greek: *Plethysmos* = enlargement) is a device to measure volume changes in parts of the body or even the whole body. Through such volume measurements, plethysmography can be used to determine the blood flow in an arm or a leg. For this purpose, an occluding cuff proximal to the plethysmograph is suddenly inflated to a pressure that

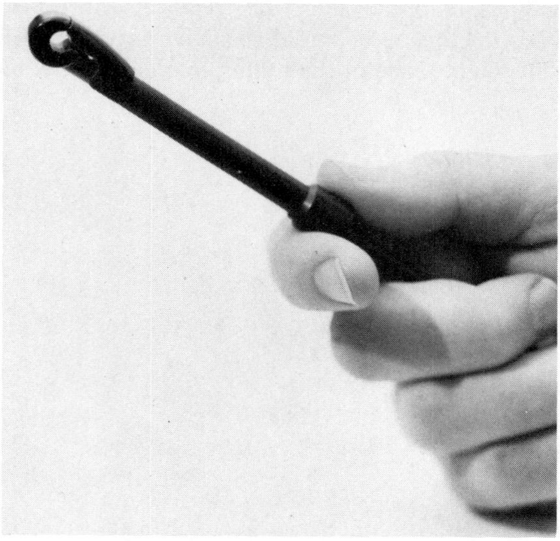

Fig. 12–9 Blood flow probe, clip-on-type for use during surgery. *(Courtesy of Biotronex, Silver Springs, Maryland.)*

occludes the venous return without impeding the arterial blood flow. This process causes the volume of the extremity to increase for some time until eventually the counterpressure of the occlusion cuff is overcome. The rate of blood inflow can be calculated from the rate of volume increase.

A "true" plethysmograph is one that actually responds to changes in volume. Such an instrument consists of a rigid cup or chamber placed over the limb or digit in which the volume changes are to be measured. The cup is tightly sealed to the member to be measured so that any changes of volume in the limb or digit reflect as pressure changes inside the chamber. Either fluid or air can be used to fill the chamber. A pressure transducer measures the pressure changes, which are read out as volume changes.

Several devices, although called plethysmographs, actually measure some variable related to volume rather than volume itself. One class of these instruments measures changes in diameter at a certain cross section of a finger, toe, arm, leg, or other segment of the body. Since volume is related to diameter, this type of device is sufficiently accurate for many purposes. The diameter is measured by means of a thin rubber tube filled with mercury that is wrapped around the limb or digit. As the diameter of the limb increases, the mercury column in the rubber tube becomes longer and thinner, resulting in a change in its electrical resistance.

Other devices used in indirect measurement of volume changes in a limb include the *impedance plethysmograph,* which measures the electrical impedance changes that result from the volume changes, and a so-called *photoelectric* or *optical* plethysmograph, which measures changes in the amount of light that can be transmitted through a vascular region, such as a fingertip or earlobe. The ability to transmit light varies with each pulse beat as the vascular region fills with blood. Both devices are extremely difficult to calibrate for quantitative measurement of blood volume or flow; however, both provide output patterns from which the pulse rate can easily be determined.

13

Telemetry in Health Care

Under certain circumstances it is advantageous, and sometimes necessary, to monitor physiological events without having to connect patients directly to a monitoring system. Such is the case in extended coronary care where patients must be monitored even though they can be allowed a certain amount of mobility. Similarly, it is desirable to obtain electrocardiograms during exercise without the encumbrance of connecting wires. To eliminate the need for connecting wires, electrical signals representing physiological variables are transmitted by radio from their point of origin to the location of the monitoring equipment. The distance of transmission may be just across the room, or it may be many miles. This process of performing measurements over a distance by radio is known as *radiotelemetry,* usually referred to by the shorter term, *telemetry.* Where biomedical information is involved, it is often called *biotelemetry.*

Literally, the word telemetry means "measurement from afar." It therefore applies to any method of transmitting information over a distance, including telephone lines. However, the use of telephone lines to transmit physiological data is not generally considered telemetry. On the other hand, a telemetry system may include both radio and telephone-line transmission. In such a system, information is transmitted from a patient to a nearby receiver, from which it is then carried to its final destination (which might be a computer) by telephone lines.

This chapter is concerned with transmission of physiological data by both radiotelemetry and telephone lines. The basic principles involved in both types of transmission are discussed, along with applications in clinical patient care.

13.1 Telephone-Line Transmission of Physiological Variables

Historically, Einthoven, the originator of the electrocardiogram as a means of analyzing the electrical activity of the heart, transmitted electrocardiograms from a hospital to his laboratory many miles away as early as 1903. The rather crude immersion electrodes were connected to a remote galvanometer directly by telephone lines. The telephone lines in this instance were merely used as conductors for the current produced by the biopotentials. In modern telephone-line transmission of the ECG, the biopotentials are amplified and processed by electronic equipment before they are transmitted.

Physiological signals can be transmitted by telephone lines in two different forms. Where the signal waveforms themselves are transmitted, the data are retained in *analog* form, the varying voltage being an analogy of the physiological variable its represents. The ECG waveform is an example of analog data. If an electrocardiogram is to be transmitted to some location to be interpreted by a cardiologist, it will most likely be transmitted in its original analog form.

Physiological data can also be transmitted in *digital* form. Here information is represented by a sequence of numbers or letters of the alphabet. Data entered into a digital computer must be in this form (see Chapter 19). If a physiological variable is to be transmitted in digital form, it must first be converted into a sequence of numerical values. This process, called *analog-to-digital conversion,* is discussed in Chapter 19. Where ECG waveforms are to be transmitted to a computer location for automatic screening or analysis, they may either be sent in analog form and converted at the computer location or converted into digital form before transmission.

In either form, transmission of physiological data by telephone lines requires special equipment at both the transmitting and receiving ends of the line. Where the telephone line is devoted exclusively to the transmission of data, the equipment is permanently connected at both ends. In cases where a special line is not justified, physiological data can be sent over conventional telephone equipment. In order to do so, the physiological information, whether analog or digital, is converted into an audible tone that varies according to the impressed information. A special device is provided to accept the standard telephone receiver and produce the varying tone in front of the mouthpiece. A similar device at the receiving end picks up the tone from the earpiece and retrieves the information that was transmitted.

Telephone-line transmission is generally used where physiological data must be transmitted over long distances for analysis or interpretation. Transmission of electrocardiograms and other physiological waveforms from homes or physicians' offices to a central location where they can be interpreted by specialists is routinely done in many parts of the country. Similarly, ECGs can be sent from hospitals and clinics throughout the United States to certain computer centers for analysis or screening.

13.2 Radiotelemetry

Although several different types of radiotelemetry equipment are used in patient care, a basic instrumentation system that includes telemetry consists of the components shown in Figure 13-1. The transducers and signal-conditioning equipment are no different from those introduced in Chapter 2 and described in the chapters 7, 8, 9, 12, and 17. Similarly, the display or readout equipment is the same as in a similar instrument that does not incorporate telemetry. The difference is that after some amplification, and possibly some other form of signal conditioning, the signal is applied to a *transmitter,* which impresses it on a *carrier,* a high-frequency ac voltage, which is fed to a transmitting *antenna* and propagated in the form of electromagnetic (radio) waves. At the receiving end, the electromagnetic waves are picked up by a receiving antenna, which is connected to a

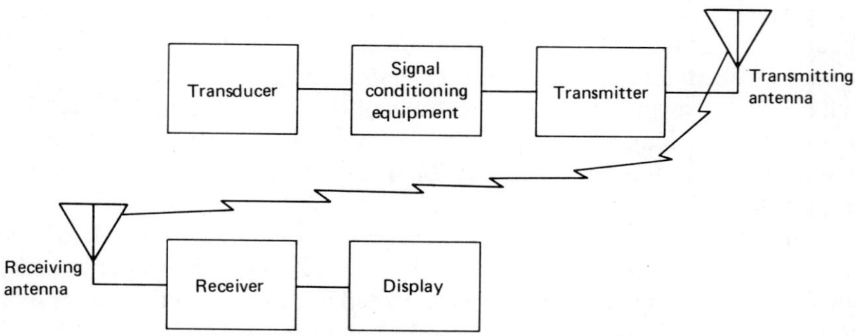

Fig. 13–1 Instrumentation system incorporating telemetry.

receiver that contains circuitry to retrieve the signal from the carrier. This signal is then amplified and applied to the appropriate display equipment.

The physiological signal is impressed on the carrier by a process known as *modulation.* If the amplitude of the carrier voltage is made to vary with the physiological signal, the process is called *amplitude modulation,* abbreviated AM. Standard broadcast radio stations and the video (picture) signal of television utilize this method of modulation. If, on the other hand, the frequency of the carrier is made to vary with the information to be transmitted, the result is *frequency modulation* (FM). FM radio stations and television sound utilize frequency modulation. Amplitude and frequency modulation are illustrated in Figure 13-2. Both types of modulation can be used for telemetry, although FM is used more frequently because it is less susceptible to some forms of interference. A third type of modulation, called *pulse modulation,* is also used in some telemetry

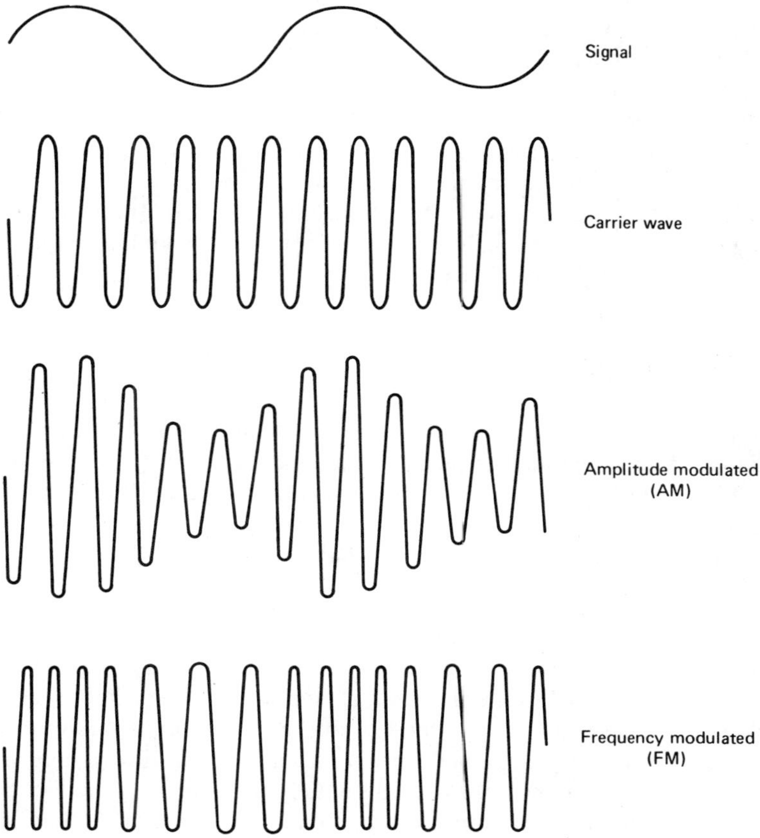

Fig. 13–2 Types of modulation.

systems. In this process, the height, width, or spacing of pulses is varied to represent the signal information.

In some telemetry systems two or more physiological signals can be broadcast on the same carrier at the same time. The process by which this feat is accomplished is called *frequency multiplexing.* Each of the physiological waveforms is called a *channel* of information. For multiplexing, each channel is impressed on a low-frequency carrier, called a *subcarrier*. Each subcarrier is of a different frequency. The subcarriers are then mixed together and all are impressed on the main radio-frequency (RF) carrier of the transmitter. Either frequency or amplitude modulation can be used for impressing data on the subcarriers, and this may or may not be the same modulation method that is used to place the subcarriers on the RF carrier. In describing this type of system, a designation is given in which the method of modulating the subcarriers is followed by the method of modulating the RF carrier. For example, a system in which the subcarriers are frequency modulated and the RF carrier is amplitude modulated is designated as FM/AM. An FM/FM designation means that both the subcarriers and the RF carrier are frequency modulated. Both FM/AM and FM/FM systems are used in biotelemetry.

The process of retrieving the information from the carrier is called *demodulation*. The telemetry receiver must be capable of accommodating the type of modulation used by the transmitter. Where frequency multiplexing is employed, the receiver must be able to demodulate each of the subcarriers as well as the main carrier.

13.3 Applications of Telemetry in Patient Care

There are a limited number of situations in which telemetry is practical in the diagnosis and treatment of hospital patients. Most involve measurement of the electrocardiogram. Some common applications are described below.

13.3.1 Telemetry of ECGs from Extended Coronary Care Patients

Cardiac patients must often be observed for rhythm disturbances for a period of time following intensive coronary care. Such patients are generally allowed a certain amount of mobility. To make monitoring possible, some hospitals have extended coronary care units equipped with patient monitoring systems that include telemetry. In this arrangement, each patient has ECG electrodes taped securely to his chest. The electrodes are connected to a small transmitter unit that also contains the signal-conditioning equipment. The transmitter unit, which is about the size of a king-size package of cigarettes, is fastened to a special belt worn around the patient's waist. Figure 13-3 shows a typical unit. Batteries for powering the signal-conditioning equipment and transmitter are also included in the transmitter package. These batteries must be replaced periodically. Some systems include provisions for easy testing of the transmitter batteries.

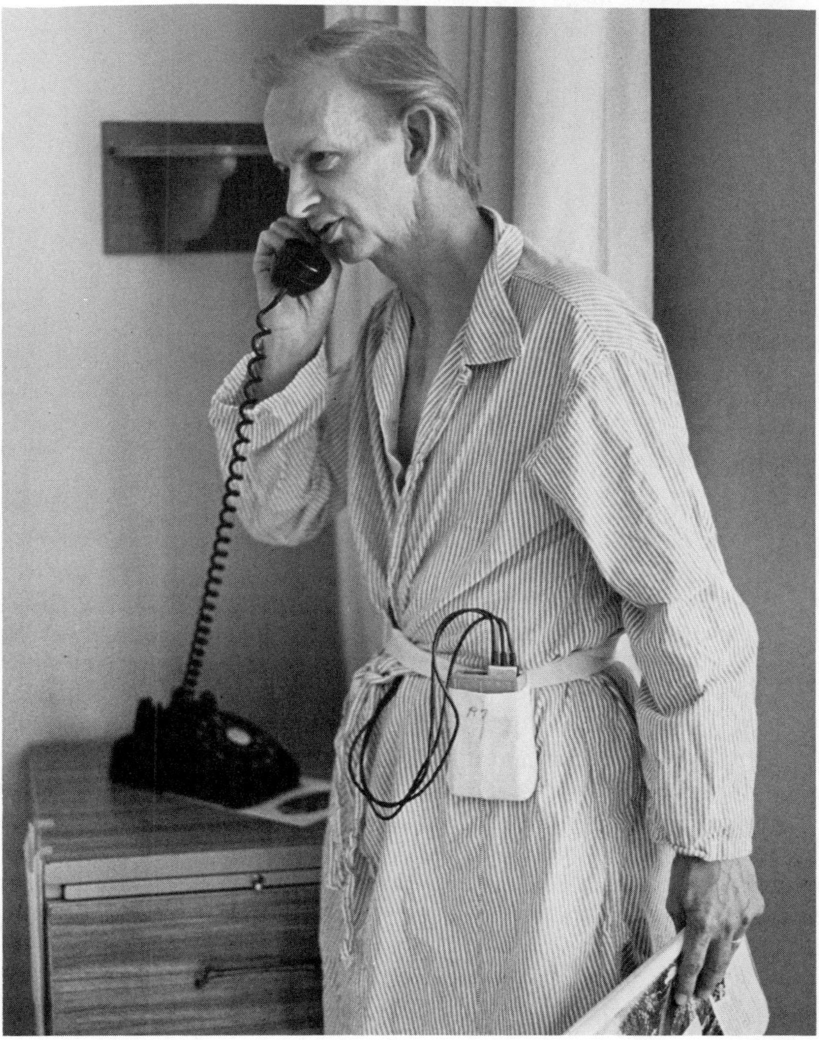

Fig. 13–3 ECG telemetry transmitter: (a) Hewlett-Packard Type 78100A in hospital use (*Courtesy of Hewlett-Packard Company, Waltham, Massachusetts*); (b) Electrode placement for telemetered ECG.

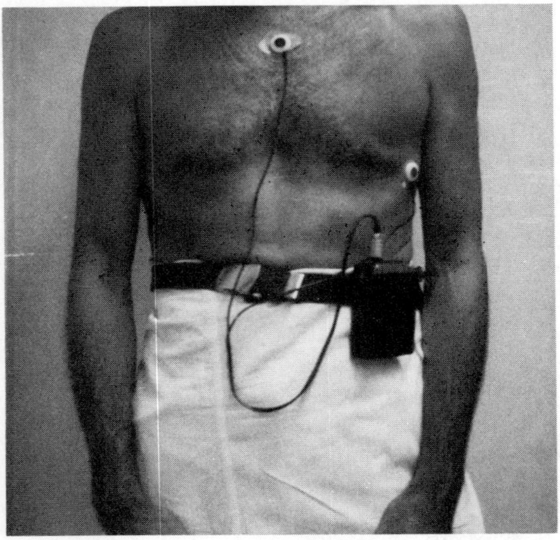

Fig. 13–3 (Continued.)

In other cases, the batteries must be replaced at some predetermined interval.

A telemetry receiver for each monitored patient is usually included as part of the monitoring system. The output of each receiver is connected to one of the ECG channels of the patient monitor. A potential problem in the use of telemetry with free-roaming patients concerns being able to locate a patient in case his alarm should sound. Telemetry equipment has no provision for indicating the location of a transmitter. The area in which the patients are allowed to move must be limited. There may also be a problem if patients are able to venture beyond the range of the telemetry transmitter. Most modern hospitals are constructed in such a way that radio waves cannot pass through the walls. Thus unless special antennas are provided in hallways, reception may be confined to the ward itself or to a very small portion of the hospital. If a patient wanders beyond the range of the system, his ECG can no longer be monitored and the purpose of the telemetry is defeated.

13.3.2 Telemetry for ECG Measurements During Exercise

For certain cardiac abnormalities, such as ischemic coronary artery disease, diagnostic procedures require measurement of the electrocardiogram while the patient is exercising, usually on a treadmill or a set of steps (see Chapter 7). Although such measurements can be made with direct wire connections from the patient to nearby instrumentation, the connecting cables are frequently in the way and may interfere with the performance of the patient. For this reason, telemetry is often used in conjunction with exercise ECG measurements. The transmitter unit used for this purpose is similar to that described earlier for extended coronary care and is normally worn on the belt. Care must be taken to ensure that the electrodes and all wires are securely fastened to the patient, to prevent their swinging during the movement of the patient. In most ECG telemetry systems movement of the wiring with respect to the body results in artifact on the ECG tracing. However, with proper equipment and with the wiring skillfully tied down, excellent results can be obtained. If other physiological variables in addition to the ECG are to be measured from the exercising patient, suitable transducers and signal-conditioning equipment must be included in the transmitter unit, along with the provision for multiplexing to accommodate the additional channels. In general, the receiver and other equipment used for conditioning and displaying the signals received from the exercising patient are located very near the patient. Thus the transmitter can operate with low power. The receiver must be able to retrieve the ECG and any other information transmitted, in addition to providing appropriate signals to the remainder of the instrumentation system.

13.3.3 Telemetry for Emergency Patient Monitoring

In many areas ambulances and emergency rescue teams are equipped with telemetry equipment to allow electrocardiograms and other physiological data to be transmitted to a nearby hospital for interpretation. Two-way voice transmission is normally used in conjunction with the telemetry to facilitate identification of the telemetered information and to provide instructions for treatment. Through the use of such equipment, ECGs can be interpreted and treatment begun before the patient arrives at the hospital.

Telemetry of this type requires a much more powerful transmitter than the two applications previously described. Often the data must be transmitted many miles and sometimes from a moving vehicle. To be effective, the system must be capable of providing reliable reception and reproduction of the transmitted signals regardless of conditions. In some cases, an emergency rescue squad can transmit physiological information from a portable transmitter to a receiver in their vehicle. The vehicle, which contains a more powerful transmitter and better antenna system, is able to retransmit the data to the hospital. This process of *retransmission* is necessary in cases where the emergency team might be working in some location from which they are unable to maintain direct communication with the hospital.

One type of system in use is illustrated in Figures 13-4 and 13-5.

Figure 13-4 shows the unit that is carried on the paramedic emergency ambulance or the fire department emergency vehicle. It is a completely portable medical communication system that allows paramedics to work closely with hospital personnel. Two-way voice communication and ECG telemetry transmissions are broadcast simultaneously. It is battery powered, can transmit over UHF radio or any telephone, and since the paramedic units frequently use defibrillators along with this equipment, it is defibrillator protected.

The ECG capability is for the full 12-lead system, although in emergency situations only the three primary lead signals are transmitted unless otherwise requested by the hospital. There is built-in test circuitry for electrodes, cables and calibration.

The transmitter is able to transmit on six channels at different frequencies. Each hospital in a local area is assigned a frequency in the 450-

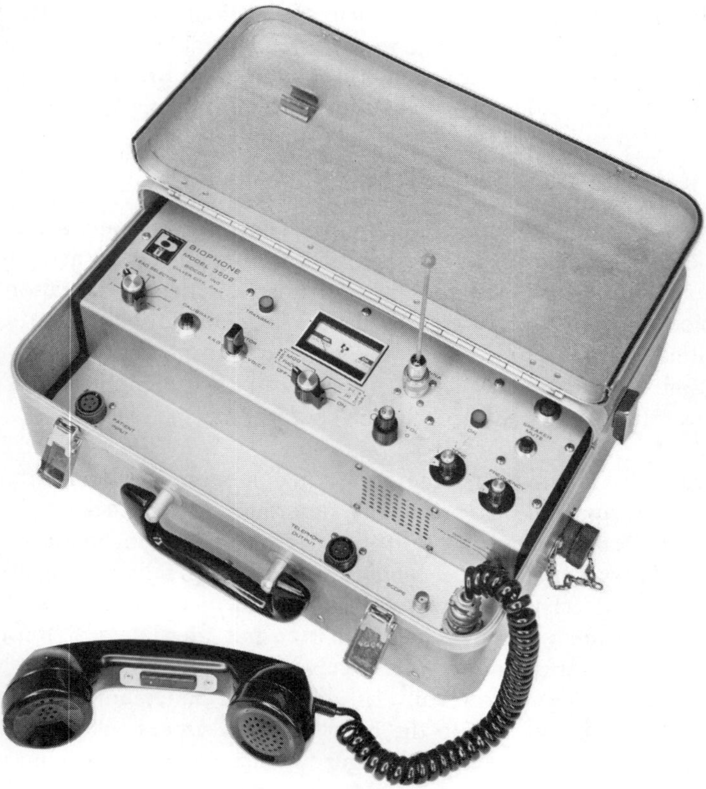

Fig. 13–4 Emergency medical communication system (Model 3502 Biophone). *(Courtesy of BIOCOM, Inc., Culver City, California.)*

to 470-mHz range, and so the emergency crew is capable of reaching a choice of hospitals. The power output is 12 W. However, 38 W of effective power can be obtained with a high-gain antenna.

A command station console (Figure 13-5) is installed at the hospital. It interfaces with the emergency medical communication system to display and record ECGs on an oscilloscope or a strip-chart recorder. It includes a cardiac rate meter and magnetic tape recording of all voice and ECG transmissions. Information can be stored on tape cassettes for later use. It also contains a loudspeaker so that hospital personnel can hear the paramedic transmissions from a distance. A voice-priority circuit quiets displays during voice transmission and mutes the speaker during ECG transmission.

13.4 Percutaneous Transmission

Radio transmission is sometimes used to obtain physiological measurements from within the gastrointestinal tract or other internal locations

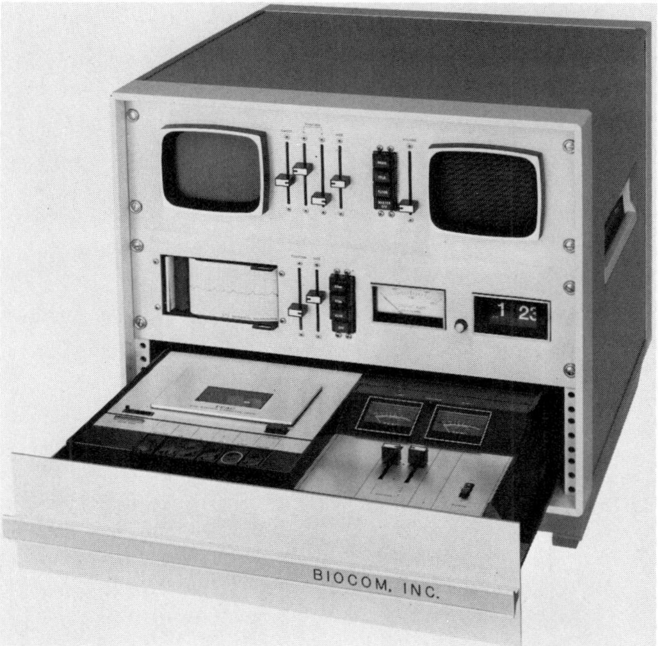

Fig. 13–5 Hospital telemetry command console (Model 4000 Biophone Command Console). *(Courtesy of BIOCOM, Inc., Culver City, California.)*

without the necessity of interconnecting wires. For example, a capsule containing a miniature sensing element and radio transmitter can be swallowed by a patient to permit measurement of pressures or the pH of fluids encountered all along its journey through the gastrointestinal tract. This device is sometimes called an *endoradiosonde*. A receiver outside the body picks up the radio signals for display and recording.

A reverse situation is also possible. By implanting a miniature receiver subcutaneously and locating a transmitter on the surface of the body with its antenna over the receiver location, signals can be transmitted percutaneously to control stimulation of motor nerves or muscles where a normal physiological function has been lost. Such stimulation can, for example, be used to lift the toe of a stroke patient who has a condition called "footdrop," in which the reflex that normally lifts the toe while walking is inoperative. By stimulating the motor nerve at the appropriate portion of the walking cycle, a near-normal gait can be achieved.

This method may find future applications in newer prosthetic devices to replace normal body functions, such as the micturition process.

14

Respiratory Measurements and Instrumentation

The term *respiration* covers the entire process of obtaining oxygen from the atmosphere, delivering it to all the cells of the body, removing carbon dioxide from the cells, and exhausting waste gases into the atmosphere. To assess the various functions involved in the respiratory process and to diagnose and treat respiratory disorders, a large and varied assortment of medical instrumentation is required. However, these instruments can easily be separated into two basic categories: *diagnostic instrumentation* and *respiratory therapy equipment.*

Diagnostic tests of the respiratory system are called *pulmonary function tests.* Instrumentation used for pulmonary function tests is of two distinct types. One set is used for tests related to the mechanics of breathing and the physical characteristics of the lungs. The second type includes instrumentation for measurement of the diffusion of gases in the lungs, the distribution of oxygen to the cells, and the collection of carbon dioxide.

Apparatus for respiratory therapy includes equipment to administer oxygen, assist or control breathing, humidify the air or oxygen, and administer therapeutic agents through nebulization.

Following a description of the diagnostic tests employed in measuring the mechanics of breathing, this chapter describes the instruments associated with those tests and the principles on which they are based. Some precautions pertaining to their use are then given. This information is followed by a description of instrumentation used clinically for measuring the diffusion of oxygen and carbon dioxide in the lungs and their concentrations in the blood. The chapter closes with a discussion of the various types of respiratory therapy equipment.

14.1 Tests and Instrumentation for the Mechanics of Breathing

The mechanics of breathing concern the ability of a person to bring air into his lungs from the outside atmosphere and to exhaust air from the lungs. This ability is affected by the various components of the air passage, the diaphragm and associated muscles, the rib cage and associated musculature, and the characteristics of the lungs themselves. Tests can be performed to assess each of these factors, but no one measurement has been devised that can adequately evaluate the overall performance of the breathing mechanism.

14.1.1 Lung Volumes and Capacities

Among the basic pulmonary tests are those designed for determination of lung volumes and capacities. These parameters, which are a function of an individual's physical characteristics and the condition of his breathing mechanism, are illustrated in Figure 14-1. This figure shows a graphic representation of respiration, with time moving from right to left. Inspiration is upward and expiration downward. A number of cycles of quiet breathing at rest are followed by a maximal expiration and then a maximal inspiration, after which the subject resumes quiet breathing. From the breathing levels thus attained, the various volumes and capacities can be defined as follows:

The *tidal volume* (TV), or normal depth of breathing, is the volume of gas inspired or expired during each normal, quiet, respiration cycle.

Inspiratory reserve volume (IRV) is the extra volume of gas that a person can inspire with maximal effort after reaching the normal end inspiratory level. The *end inspiratory level* is the level reached at the end of a normal, quiet inspiration.

The *expiratory reserve volume* (ERV) is that extra volume of gas that can be expired with maximum effort beyond the end expiratory level. The *end expiratory level* is the level reached at the end of a normal, quiet expiration.

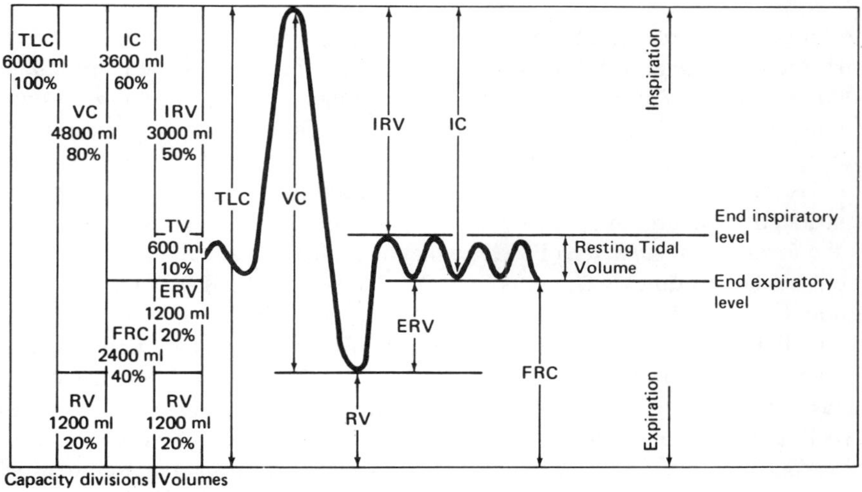

Fig. 14–1 Lung volumes and capacities. (From W. F. Evans, *Anatomy and Physiology, The Basic Principles*. Englewood Cliffs, N.J.: Prentice-Hall, Inc.)

The *residual volume* (RV) is the volume of gas remaining in the lungs at the end of a maximal expiration.

The *vital capacity* (VC) is the maximum volume of gas that can be expelled from the lungs by forceful effort after a maximum inspiration. It is actually the difference between the level of maximum inspiration and the residual volume, and it is measured without respect to time. The vital capacity is also the sum of the tidal volume, inspiratory reserve volume, and expiratory reserve volume.

The *total lung capacity* (TLC) is the amount of gas contained in the lungs at the end of a maximum inspiration. It is the sum of the vital capacity and residual volume. Total lung capacity is also the sum of the tidal volume, inspiratory reserve volume, expiratory reserve volume, and residual volume.

The *inspiratory capacity* (IC) is the maximum amount of gas that can be inspired after reaching the end expiratory level. It is the sum of the tidal volume and the inspiratory reserve volume.

The functional residual capacity, often referred to by its abbreviation, FRC, is the volume of gas remaining in the lungs at the end expiratory level. It is the sum of the residual volume and the expiratory reserve volume. The FRC can also be calculated as the total lung capacity minus the inspiratory capacity, and it is often regarded as the baseline from which other volumes and capacities are determined, for it seems to be more stable than the end inspiratory level.

In addition to these volumes and capacities, several related measures are used in assessing the breathing mechanism. For example, a useful measure of the overall capacity of the breathing apparatus is the *respiratory minute volume.* This is a measure of the amount of air inspired during one minute at rest. It is obtained by multiplying the tidal volume by the number of respiratory cycles per minute.

A number of forced breathing tests are used to assess the muscle power associated with breathing and the resistance of the airway. Among them is the *forced vital capacity* (FVC), which is really a vital capacity measurement taken as quickly as possible. By definition, the FVC is the total amount of air that can forcibly be expired as quickly as possible after taking the deepest possible breath. If the measurement is made with respect to the time required for the maneuver, it is called a *timed vital capacity* measurement. A measure of the maximum amount of gas that can be expelled in a given number of seconds is called the *forced expiratory volume* (FEV). This is usually given with a subscript indicating the number of seconds over which the measurement is made. For example, FEV_1 indicates the maximum amount of air that can be blown out in one second following a maximum inspiration, while FEV_3 is the maximum amount of air that can be expired in 3 seconds. Sometimes FEV is given as a percentage of the forced vital capacity.

Since forced vital capacity measurements are often encumbered by patient hesitation and the inertia of the instrument, a measure of the *maximum midexpiratory flow* (MMF) is taken. This is flow measured over the middle half of the forced vital capacity (from the 25% level to the 75% level). The corresponding FEV measurement is called $FEV_{25\%-75\%}$.

Another important flow measurement is the *maximal expiration flow* (MEF) rate, which is the rate during the first liter expired after 200 ml have been exhausted at the beginning of the FEV. It differs from the *peak flow,* which is the maximum rate of airflow attained at any time during a forced expiration.

Another useful measurement for assessing the integrity of the breathing mechanism is the *maximal breathing capacity* (MBC) or *maximal voluntary ventilation* (MVV). This is a measure of the maximum amount of air that can be breathed in and blown out over a sustained interval, such as 15 or 20 seconds. A ratio of the maximal breathing capacity to the vital capacity is also of clinical interest.

14.1.2 Compliance and Airway Resistance

The volume and capacity measurements just described, particularly the forced measurements, are a good indication of the *compliance* of the lungs and rib cage and the resistance of the air passages. However, direct measurement of these parameters is also possible and is often used in the measurement of pulmonary function.

Determination of *compliance,* which is defined as the volume increase in the lungs per unit increase in lung pressure, requires measurement of an inspired or expired volume of gas and of intrathoracic pressure. Compliance values are given as liters per centimeter H_2O.

Airway resistance is a ratio of pressure to flow. Thus for the determination of airway resistance, intra-alveolar pressure and airflow measurements are required. The intra-alveolar pressure is given in centimeters H_2O and the flow in liters per second; the airway resistance is expressed in centimeters H_2O per liter per second. Most airway resistance measurements are made at or near the functional residual capacity (end expiratory) level.

14.1.3 The Spirometer

The most widely used laboratory instrument for respiratory volume measurements is the *recording spirometer,* an example of which is shown in Figure 14-2. All lung volumes and capacities that can be determined by measuring the amount of gas expired under a given set of conditions or

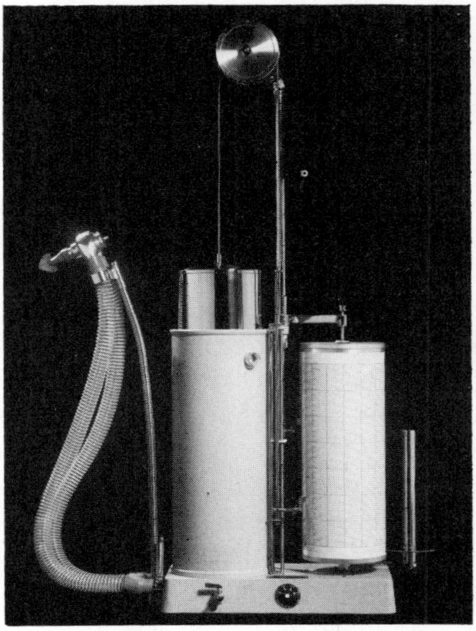

Fig. 14–2 Spirometer. *(Courtesy of Warren E. Collins, Inc., Braintree, Massachusetts.)*

during a specified time interval can be obtained by use of the spirometer. Included are the timed vital capacity and forced expiratory volume measurements. The only volume and capacity measurements that cannot be obtained with a spirometer are those requiring measurement of the gas that cannot be expelled from the lungs under any conditions. Such measurements include the residual volume, functional residual capacity, and total lung capacity.

The common spirometer consists of a movable bell inverted over a chamber of water. Inside the bell, above the water line, is the gas that is to be breathed. The bell is counterbalanced by a weight to maintain the gas inside at atmospheric pressure so that its height above the water is proportional to the amount of gas in the bell. A breathing tube connects the mouth of the patient with the gas under the bell. As the patient breathes into the tube, the bell moves up and down with each inspiration and expiration in proportion to the amount of air breathed in or out. Attached to the bell or the counterbalancing mechanism is a pen that writes on an adjacent drum recorder, called a *kymograph.* As the kymograph rotates, the pen traces the breathing pattern of the patient.

Various bell volumes are available, but 9 and 13.5 liters are most common. A well-designed spirometer offers little resistance to the airflow, and the bell has little inertia. Various paper speeds are available for the kymograph, with 32, 160, 300, and 1920 mm/min most common. The instrument directly records basal minute volume, exercise ventilation, or maximum breathing capacity. The ventilation equivalent for oxygen may be calculated directly from the spirogram slope lines for ventilation and oxygen uptake.

Waterless spirometers, which are also used clinically, operate on a principle similar to that of the spirometer just described. One type, called the *wedge spirometer,* is shown in Figure 14-3. In this instrument the air to be breathed is held in a chamber enclosed by two parallel metal pans hinged to each other along one edge. The space between the two pans is enclosed by a flexible bellows (like a fireplace bellows) to form the chamber. One of the pans, which contains an inlet tube, is fixed to a stand and the other swings freely with respect to it. As air is introduced into the chamber or withdrawn from it, the moving pan changes its position to compensate for the volume changes. Construction is such that the pan moves in response to very slight changes in volume. A well-designed wedge spirometer imposes an almost undetectable amount of air pressure on the patient's lungs. The instrument provides electrical outputs proportional to both volume and airflow, from which the required determinations can be obtained.

In a similar type of waterless spirometer, the volume of the chamber is varied by means of a lightweight piston that moves freely in a cylinder as air is withdrawn and replaced in breathing. A silastic® rubber seal

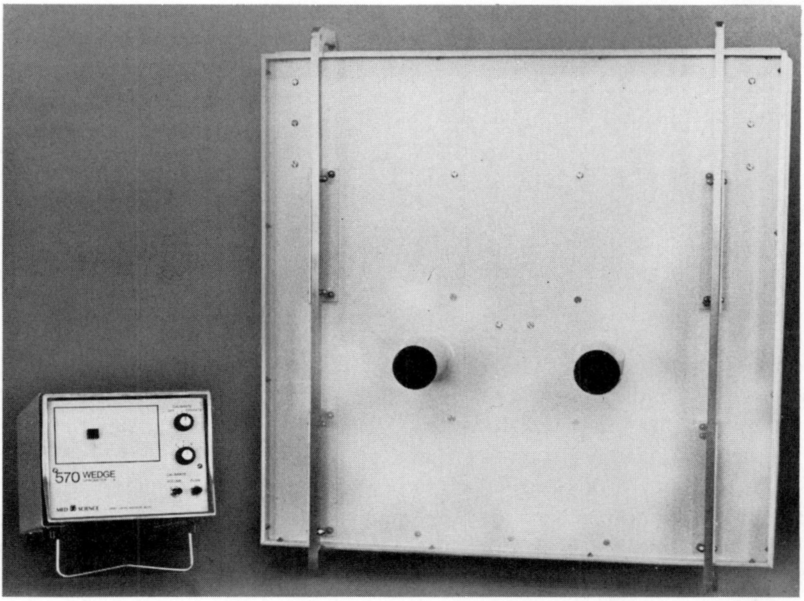

Fig. 14–3 Wedge spirometer. *(Courtesy of Med Science Electronics, St. Louis, Missouri.)*

between the piston and the cylinder wall keeps the chamber airtight. Instruments of this type have characteristics similar to those of the wedge spirometer.

Another group of instruments, sometimes called *electronic spirometers,* measures airflow and, by use of electronic circuitry, calculates the various volumes and capacities. Such a device is shown in Figure 14-4. This

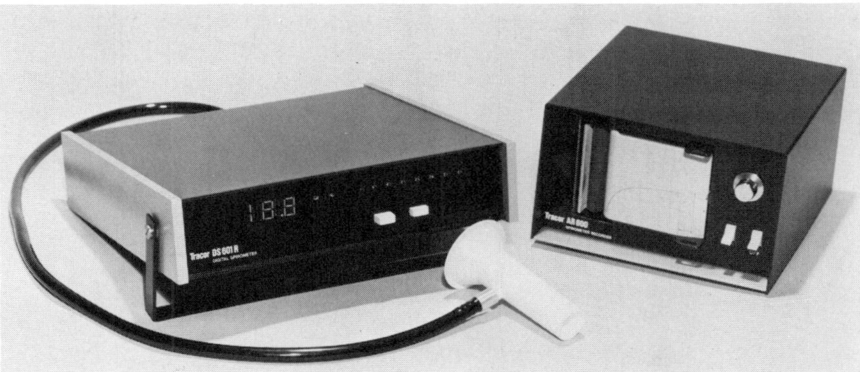

Fig. 14–4 Electronic spirometer with digital readout. *(Courtesy of Tracor Instruments, Austin, Texas.)*

instrument provides both a graphic output similar to that of a standard spirometer and a digital readout of the desired parameters. Various types of airflow transducers are used, utilizing such devices as small breath-driven turbines and heated wires that are cooled by the breath.

A *broncho-spirometer* is a dual spirometer that measures the volumes and capacities of each lung individually. The air input device is a double-lumen tube that divides for entry into the airway to each lung and thus provides isolation for differential measurement. The main function of the broncho-spirometer is the preoperative evaluation of oxygen consumption of each lung.

The usual output of a spirometer is the *spirogram*. An example is shown in Figure 14-5. The recording is read from right to left. In this particular example, inspiration moves the pen toward the bottom of the chart and expiration toward the top. Some spirometers, however, provide spirograms with inspiration toward the top.

In order to produce a spirogram, the patient is instructed to breathe through the mouthpiece of the spirometer. His nose is blocked with a clip so that all breathing is through the mouth. The recorder is first set to a slow speed to measure vital capacity (typically, 32 mm/min). To produce the spirogram shown in the figure, the patient breathed quietly for a short time at rest so as to provide a baseline. He was then instructed to exhale completely and then to inhale as much as he could. This process produced

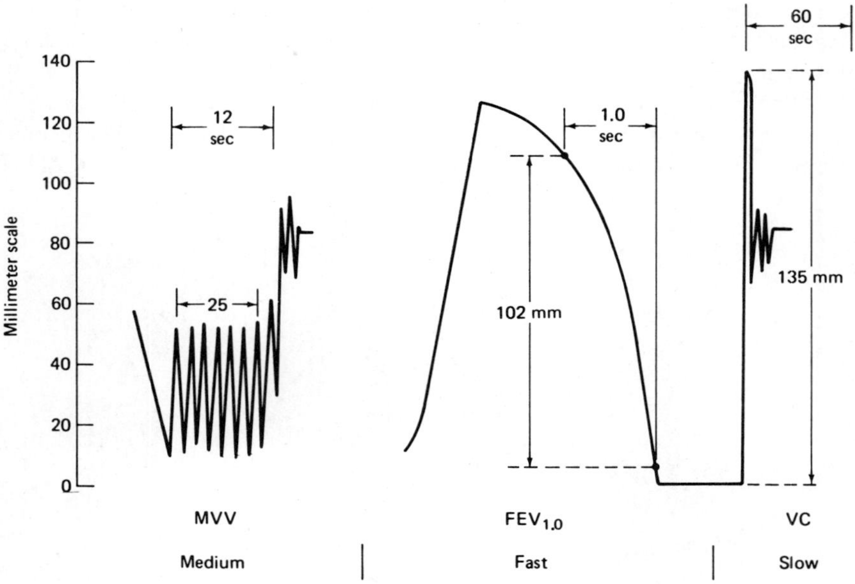

Fig. 14–5 Typical spirogram, read right to left. (See text for explanation.)

the vital capacity record at the extreme right of the figure. With his lungs at the maximal inspirational level, the patient held his breath a short time while the recorder was shifted to a higher chart speed (e.g., 1920 mm/per). The patient was then instructed to blow out all the air he could as quickly as possible to produce the FEV_1 curve on the record. To calculate the FEV_1, a 1-second interval was measured from the beginning of the maximum slope. Sometimes it is necessary to determine the beginning point by extending the maximum slope to the level of maximum inspiration. This step ensures that the initial friction and inertia of the spirometer have been overcome and compensates for error on the part of the patient in performing the test as instructed.

The spirogram in Figure 14-5 also shows a maximal voluntary ventilation (MVV) record. For this determination, the recorder is set at an intermediate speed. After a short rest, a few cycles of resting respiration were recorded. The patient was then instructed to breathe in and out as rapidly as possible for about 10 seconds, producing the MVV record in the figure.

Most spirometry tests are repeated two or three times, and the maximum values are used to ensure that the patient performed the test to the best of his ability. Although some instruments are calibrated for direct readout, others require that the height of the tracings be converted to liters by use of a calibration factor for the instrument, called the *spirometer factor*. This calibration factor can be obtained from a table or chart.

Although the usual output for a spirometer is the spirogram, other types of output, including digital readouts, are available, particularly from the waterless and electronic types of spirometers. Some instruments even have built-in computational capability to calculate automatically the required volumes and capacities from the basic measurements.

The most frequent difficulties associated with the use of the spirometer (and most of the special pulmonary function testing instruments described below) involve patient performance. An FEV test, for example, is not valid unless the patient tries his best to blow out all the air he can as quickly as possible. An important part of the technique of administering these tests is explaining the procedure to the patient and gaining his full cooperation. With practice and experience, the nurse, therapist, or technician administering the tests can usually tell if the patient is doing his best by carefully watching both the patient and the spirogram as it is recorded. For instance, the presence of steps or interruptions in an FEV curve indicates that the patient did not exert sustained effort throughout the test.

Air leaks are another possible source of trouble in spirometry measurements. During the time of quiet breathing at the beginning of a test, a check should be made to ensure that the average level of the tidal volume variations is not gradually drifting. Such drifting is an indication that air is escaping from the closed breathing chamber or associated tubing. The leak must be located and repaired in order to obtain valid measurements.

14.1.4 Other Instruments for Pulmonary Function Tests

A number of other commercially available instruments that perform some of the functions of a spirometer are used clinically. An example is the *Pulmonary Function Indicator* shown in Figure 14-6. From a single forced expiration through a heated-wire transducer (of the type used in some electronic spirometers), the instrument calculates peak airflow, FEV_1, FEV_3, vital capacity, and each of the FEVs as percentages of vital capacity. The results are displayed on a meter.

Other instruments of this type print out the readings to provide a permanent record. An alternate method of measuring the maximum voluntary ventilation (MVV) utilizes a tube through which the patient breathes rapidly from a rubber balloon filled with a measured amount of air. As the patient breathes, air is removed from the balloon for 15 seconds, and the change in volume is measured. Rough values for MVV can be obtained from a table provided with the equipment.

14.1.5 Measurement of Residual Volume

From the spirogram and the outputs of some of the other instruments described, all the lung volumes and capacities can be determined except

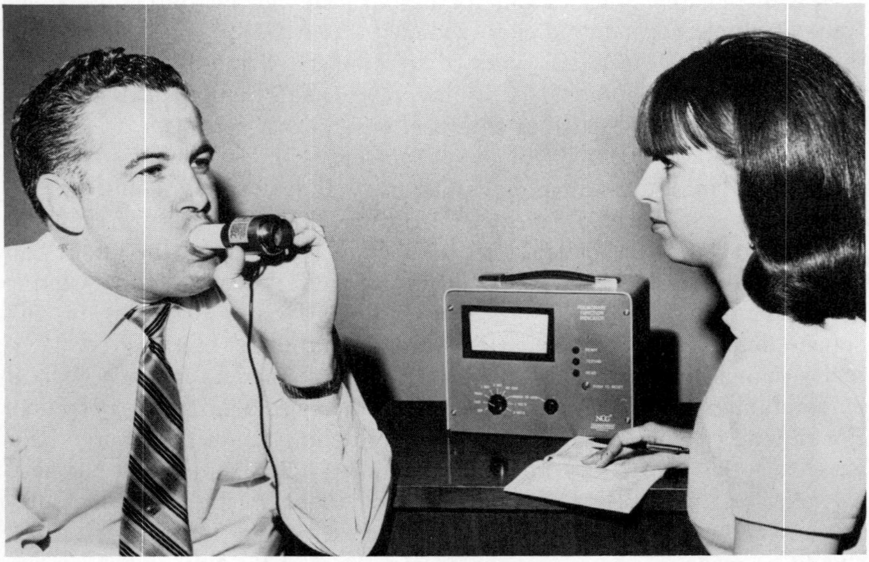

Fig. 14–6 Pulmonary function indicator in use. *(Courtesy of National Cylinder Gas Division of Chemetron Corporation, Chicago, Illinois.)*

those that require measurement of the air still remaining in the lungs and airways after maximum expiration. These parameters include the residual volume, FRC, and total lung capacity.

Residual volume measurements can be obtained through use of foreign gas mixtures. A gas analyzer is required for these tests.

The *closed-circuit* technique involves rebreathing from a spirometer charged with a known volume and concentration of a marker gas, such as hydrogen or helium. Helium is usually used. After several minutes of breathing, complete mixing of the spirometer and pulmonary gases is assumed, and the residual volume is calculated by a simple proportion of gas volumes and concentrations.

The *open-circuit* or *nitrogen washout method* involves the inspiration of pure oxygen and expiration into an oxygen-purged spirometer. If the patient has been breathing air, the gas remaining in his lungs is 78% nitrogen. As he begins to breathe the pure oxygen, it will mix with the gas still in his lungs, and a certain amount of nitrogen will "wash out" with each breath. By measuring the amount of nitrogen in each expired breath, a washout curve is obtained from which the volume of air initially in the lungs can readily be calculated. The preferred breathing level for beginning this measurement is the end of normal expiration, which is the functional residual capacity.

The functional residual capacity (FRC) (from which residual volume can also be calculated by subtracting the expiratory reserve volume) can be measured by using a *body plethysmograph*. This instrument, shown in Figure 14-7, is an airtight box in which the patient is seated. The patient breathes air from within the box through a tube containing an airflow transducer and a shutter to close off the tube for certain portions of the test. Pressure transducers measure the air pressure in the breathing tube on the patient's side of the shutter and inside the box. The amount of air in the box, including that in the patient's lungs, remains constant, since there is no way for air to enter or escape. However, when the patient compresses the air in his lungs during expiration, his total body volume is reduced, thus reducing the pressure in the box. Conversely, when the patient inhales by reducing the pressure in his thoracic region, his body volume increases and increases the box pressure. The FRC is measured with the shutter in the breathing tube closed. With no air allowed to flow, the mouth pressure (sensed by the transducer in the tube) can be assumed to equal the alveolar pressure. The patient is instructed to pant at a slow rate against the closed shutter. As he does so, he alternately expands and compresses the air in his lungs. By measuring the changes in mouth pressure and corresponding changes in intrathoracic volume (equal and opposite to changes in box volume outside the patient), it is possible to calculate the intrathoracic volume. If the test is performed at the end expiratory level, the intrathoracic volume is equal to the FRC.

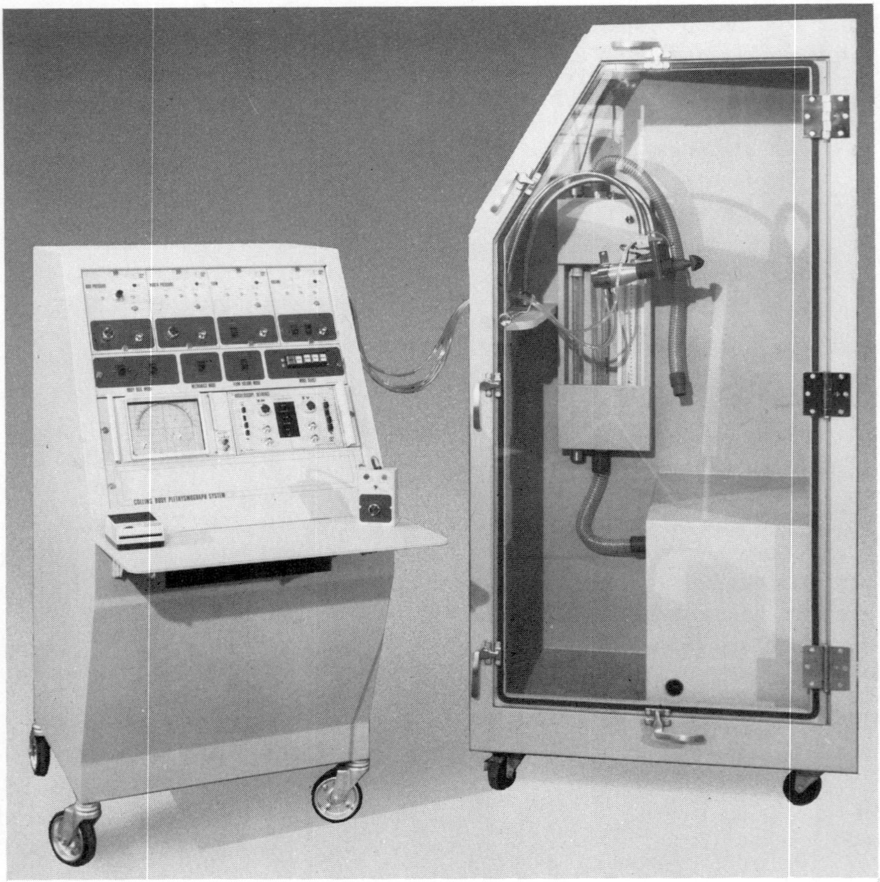

Fig. 14–7 Body plethysmograph. *(Courtesy of Warren E. Collins, Inc., Braintree, Massachusetts.)*

In using the body plethysmograph, care must be taken to ensure that the patient performs as instructed. When the patient first enters the box, a few minutes must be allowed for the air inside to warm up to body temperature. The pressure inside the plethysmograph must also be equilibrated to atmospheric pressure by means of a solenoid valve that can be operated momentarily to vent the box to the outside. Calibration must be carefully performed according to the manufacturer's instructions before the test is begun. The person using the body plethysmograph must also be familiar with the operation of associated recording and display equipment in order to obtain valid results.

14.1.6 Measurement of Airway Resistance and Lung Compliance

Since pressure measurements are required for both compliance and airway resistance determinations, methods of measuring intra-alveolar and pleural pressures are important in pulmonary function laboratories where such determinations are performed. Unfortunately, measurement of these pressures presents some problems, primarily because of the inaccessibility of the chambers in which the measurements are to be made. For this reason, indirect methods have been developed.

The body plethysmograph, described in the previous section and shown in Figure 14-7, can be used for measuring intra-alveolar pressure. For this measurement, the shutter in the breathing tube is opened. As air is breathed from within the box, the pressure or volume variations in the box are the inverse of pressure variations in the lungs. Since the mouth pressure and intra-alveolar pressure are the same when the breathing tube is closed, data are obtained for calibration by having the patient pant a few seconds against a closed shutter at the beginning of the test.

Airway resistance can be determined by simultaneously measuring the intra-alveolar pressure and airflow in the body plethysmograph. Any of the airflow transducers mentioned in Sections 14.1.3 and 14.1.4 can be placed in the breathing tube. However, the most widely used device for airflow measurement is the *pneumotachometer,* sometimes called a *pneumotachograph.* This device, shown in Figure 14-8, utilizes the principle that air

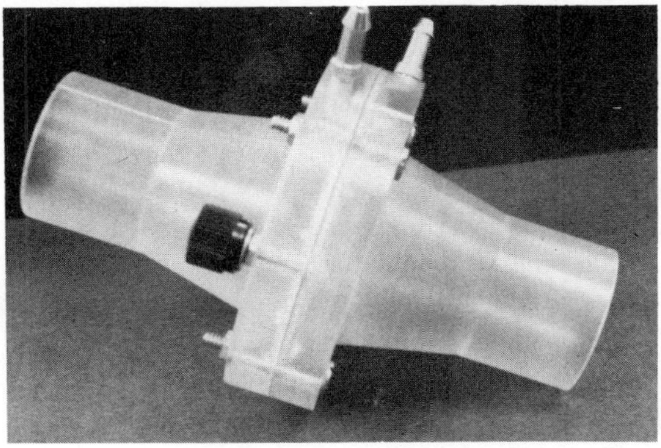

Fig. 14–8 Pneumotachometer. Air inlet and outlet are at left and right. Connections at top are for pressure transducer. Black "knob" is a heating element. *(Courtesy of Veterans Administration Hospital, Sepulveda, California.)*

flowing through an orifice produces a pressure difference across the orifice that is a function of the velocity of the air. In the more common pneumotachometer, the orifice consists of a set of capillaries or a metal screen. Since the cross section of the orifice is fixed, the pressure difference can be calibrated to represent flow. Two pressure transducers or a differential pressure transducer can be used to measure the pressure difference.

For measurement of intrathoracic pressures, a balloon is placed in the patient's esophagus, which is within the thoracic cage. Since the balloon is exposed to the intrathoracic pressure, the pressure, measured with respect to mouth pressure by using some form of differential pressure transducer, represents the difference between pressures.

14.1.7 Measurement of Closing Volume

In detecting obstruction of the small airways in the lungs, a procedure involving measurement of the *closing volume* is often used. The closing volume level is the volume at which certain zones within the lung cease to ventilate, presumably as the result of airway closure. Two techniques can be used to determine this level. In the *bolus method,* a bolus of a marker gas (usually argon, xenon, or helium) is inspired at the residual volume level. The patient is then instructed to inhale air until he reaches his maximal inspirational level and then *slowly* expire as much as he possibly can. A person with average lung volume should complete this expiration in about 8 to 10 seconds. During the expiration, the concentration of the marker gas is monitored at the mouthpiece and plotted against the lung volume level.

In the second method of measuring closing volume, the residual nitrogen in the lungs is used as the marker gas. To perform the measurement, the patient fills his lungs with pure oxygen and exhausts all the air he possibly can. The nitrogen concentration of the exhausted air is plotted against lung volume level. At the closing volume level, the nitrogen concentration suddenly begins to increase at a more rapid rate. The *closing volume* is the difference between that level and the residual volume level and is usually expressed as a percentage of the patient's vital capacity.

14.2 Measurement of Gas Exchange and Distribution

Once air is in the lungs, oxygen and carbon dioxide must be exchanged between the air and the blood in the lungs and between the blood and the cells in the body tissues. In addition, the gases must be transported between the lungs and the tissues by the blood. The mixing of gases within the lungs, the ventilation of the alveoli, and the exchange of oxygen and carbon dioxide between the air and blood in the lungs all take place through a process called *diffusion*. Diffusion is the movement of gas molecules from a point of higher concentration to a point of lower concentration to equalize the concentration difference. This process can occur when the gas is unequally distributed in a chamber or wherever a concentration difference exists in the gas on two sides of a membrane permeable to that gas. To determine the effectiveness of gaseous exchange and diffusion, it is necessary to measure the quantity of the respiratory gases (oxygen and carbon dioxide) in both expired air and blood.

The amount of oxygen or carbon dioxide in the expired air can be measured by various types of *gas analyzers*. A device commonly used for this purpose in the hospital is the *Scholander gas analyzer* shown in Figure 14-9. A small sample of the gas mixture to be analyzed is introduced into a chamber in which its volume can be measured. A fluid that absorbs one of the respiratory gases (e.g., oxygen) is then introduced into the chamber. As the oxygen is absorbed by the fluid, the volume of the gas sample is reduced accordingly. The difference in volume before and after the oxygen is absorbed is equal to the amount of oxygen that was in the sample. The process is repeated but this time with a fluid that absorbs the carbon dioxide.

The quantities of various gases in the expired air can also be determined by a *gas chromatograph* in which the gases are separated as they flow through a column containing various substances that interact with the gases. The quantity of each gas present is measured as it emerges from the tube.

The amount of oxygen and carbon dioxide in the blood provides a good indication of the effectiveness of both the respiratory and cardiovascular systems. For this reason, blood gas measurements are important diagnostic procedures. The quantities are usually given as *partial pressures* which are directly related to concentration levels and are expressed in millimeters of mercury (mm Hg). The partial pressure of any dissolved gas is the contribution of that gas to the total dissolved gases in the blood. The partial pressure of oxygen is written P_{O_2} and the partial pressure of carbon dioxide is P_{CO_2}.

Closely related to the P_{CO_2} is the pH of the blood. The pH indicates the acidity or alkalinity of a solution and is related to the hydrogen ion concentration in the solution. An acid has a low pH value, whereas a base has a high pH. A neutral solution has a pH of 7. Most human body fluids are slightly basic. The pH of normal arterial blood ranges between 7.38 and 7.42. Venous blood has a pH around 7.35, due to its higher CO_2

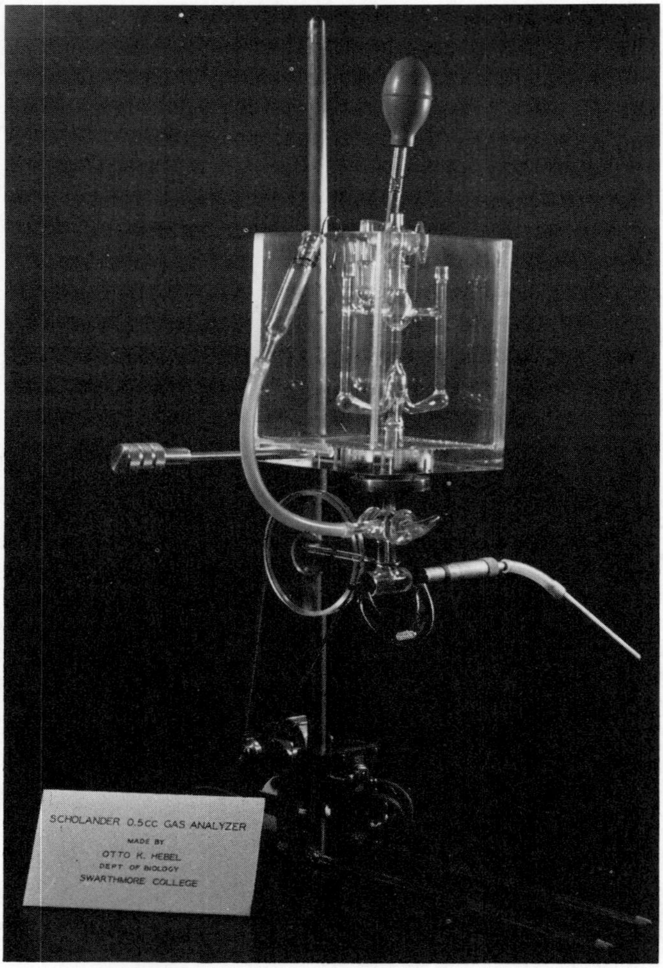

Fig. 14–9 Scholander gas analyzer. *(Courtesy of Otto K. Hebel Scientific Instruments, Rutledge, Pennsylvania.)*

concentration. Because of its relationship to the CO_2 in the blood and because it is involved in a number of the regulatory processes in the body, the pH is a very important physiological variable.

The pH of body fluids can be measured both in vivo and in vitro. It is measured by a *pH electrode* placed in the fluid. This type of electrode is called a *glass electrode* because of a special thin glass membrane across which a voltage is developed that varies with the pH of the fluid. This voltage can be measured between the pH electrode and a *reference electrode*.

The reference electrode (see Chapter 6) is a second electrode placed in the fluid along with the measuring electrode in order to provide a complete circuit for voltage measurement. Unlike the measuring electrode, the reference electrode does not respond to changes in the entity being measured (in this case, pH).

The P_{CO_2} of a fluid directly affects its pH. Thus if a pH electrode is surrounded by a membrane that allows the dissolved carbon dioxide to pass through it, but blocks any other substance that might affect the pH, a P_{CO_2} electrode is formed. One widely used type of P_{CO_2} electrode is the *Severinghaus electrode,* named after its inventor. This electrode has been especially designed to provide a stable reading of the carbon dioxide level in a shorter time than its more conventional counterparts.

A different type of electrode is used for measuring P_{O_2}. One version of the P_{O_2} electrode is based on the principle that when a small electric voltage (about 0.7 V) is applied between a piece of platinum wire and a reference electrode in the blood, with the platinum wire negative, current will flow in proportion to the amount of oxygen in the blood. A single electrode that combines both the platinum wire and the reference electrode in a single unit is called a *Clark* electrode.

Figure 14-10 shows a diagram of a *flow-through* electrode that combines the glass electrode for measurement of P_{CO_2}, the platinum wire for P_{O_2}, and the reference electrode all in one unit. The flow-through feature makes such an electrode suitable for measuring the respiratory gases in circulating blood.

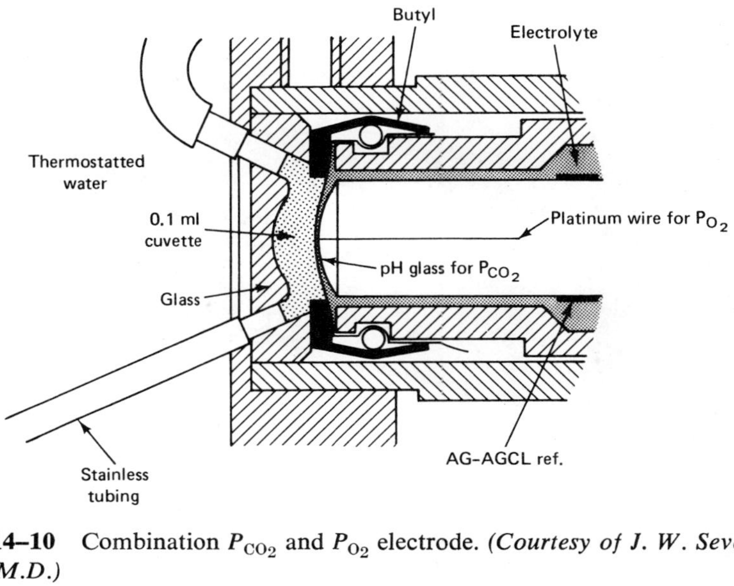

Fig. 14–10 Combination P_{CO_2} and P_{O_2} electrode. *(Courtesy of J. W. Severinghaus, M.D.)*

The blood gas analyzer shown in Figure 14-11 utilizes electrodes of the types described above. It is a complete unit that provides a digital readout of pH, P_{CO_2} and P_{O_2}. The instrument includes a water-bath temperature controller and other features to ensure accurate measurements. Other types of blood gas analyzers that use absorption techniques to measure P_{CO_2} and P_{O_2} are also available.

An important test in indicating the ability of the lungs to diffuse or transfer gases between air and blood is the determination of the *diffusing capacity*. In this test carbon monoxide (CO) is used as a marker gas. A low concentration of CO is inhaled, and the amount taken into the blood is estimated by measuring the amount of CO remaining in the expired air. This air-CO mixture is analyzed by means of an *infrared carbon monoxide analyzer,* an instrument in which a beam of infrared energy is directed through a gas sample. The amount of infrared energy absorbed is proportional to the CO concentration. The diffusing capacity is the ratio of the number of milliliters of CO taken up per minute to the concentration of CO in the lungs.

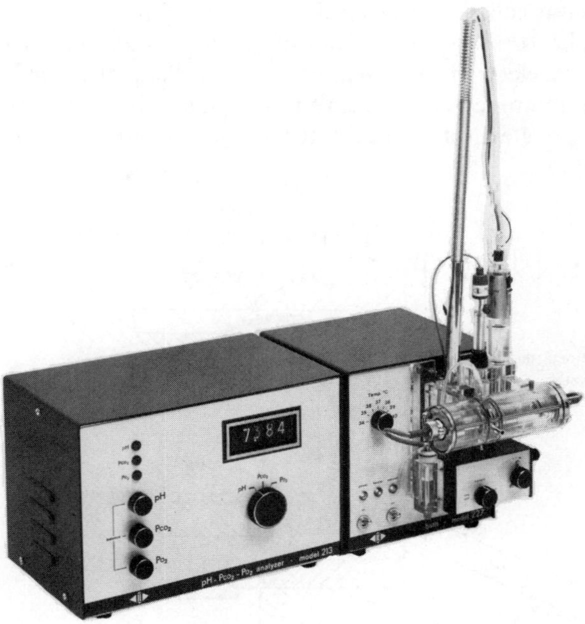

Fig. 14–11 Digital blood gas analyzer. *(Courtesy of Instrumentation Laboratory, Inc., Lexington, Massachusetts.)*

14.3 Respiratory Therapy Equipment

When a patient is incapable of adequate ventilation by natural processes, mechanical assistance must be provided so that sufficient oxygen is delivered to the organs and tissues of the body and excessive levels of carbon dioxide are not permitted to accumulate. The procedures and instrumentation involved in providing mechanical assistance in respiration and in supplying hypoxic patients with higher-than-normal concentrations of oxygen or other therapeutic gases or medications constitute a field known as *respiratory therapy*. Until the past few years, this field was known as *inhalation therapy,* but since it covers much more than inhalation, the more encompassing term is preferred. Instruments for respiratory therapy include such devices as inhalators, ventilators, respirators, resuscitators, positive-pressure breathing apparatus, humidifiers, and nebulizers. Many of these instruments, however, have overlapping functions, and the name used for a particular device may vary among manufacturers.

14.3.1 Inhalators

The term *inhalator* generally indicates a device used to supply oxygen or some other therapeutic gas to a patient who is able to breathe spontaneously without assistance. As a rule, inhalators are used when a concentration of oxygen higher than that of air is required. The inhalator consists of a source of the therapeutic gas, equipment for reducing the pressure and controlling the flow of the gas, and a device for administering the gas. Devices for administering oxygen to patients include nasal cannulae and catheters, face masks that cover the nose and mouth, and, in certain settings, such as pediatrics, oxygen tents. Figure 14-12 shows the use of a portable inhalator with a face mask. The oxygen concentration presented to the patient is controlled by adjusting the flow of gas into the mask.

The nurse, respiratory therapist, or anyone else who uses an inhalator to administer oxygen or some other therapeutic gas must be familiar with the specific apparatus involved and must be properly trained in its use. The hazards of an oxygen atmosphere require special precautions. Smoking in the vicinity must be strictly prohibited, and care must be taken that no other possible source of flame or sparking (such as sparking toys in a pediatrics ward) is present. It is also important that all nondisposable equipment be properly cleaned and that fittings be free of grease before each use, in accordance with manufacturers' instructions.

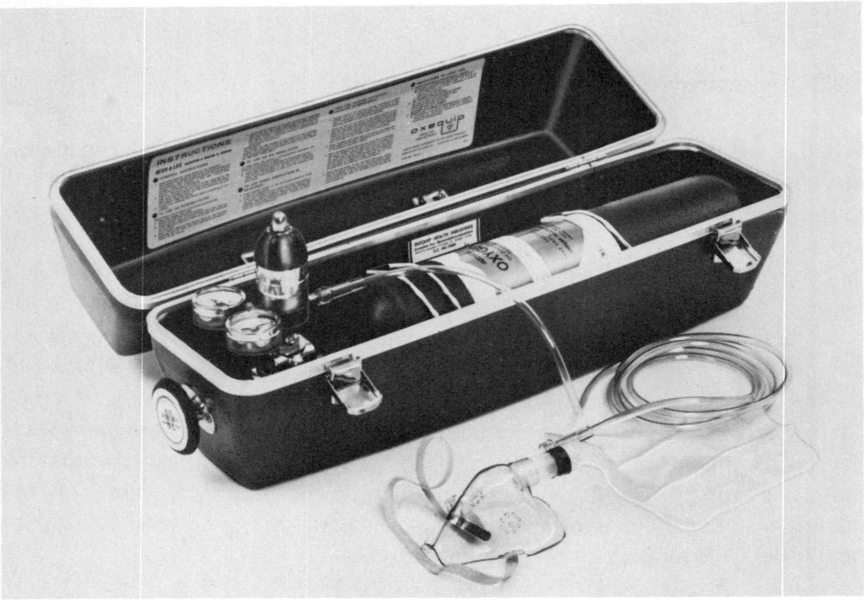

Fig. 14–12 Portable inhalator with face mask. *(Courtesy of Oxequip Health Industries, Chicago, Illinois.)*

14.3.2 Ventilators and Respirators

The terms *ventilator* and *respirator* are used interchangeably to describe equipment that may be employed continuously or intermittently to improve ventilation of the lungs and to supply humidity or aerosol medications to the pulmonary tree. Most ventilators in clinical settings use positive pressure during inhalation to inflate the lungs with various gases or mixtures of gases (air, oxygen, carbon dioxide, helium, etc.). Expiration is usually passive, although under certain conditions pressure may be applied during the expiratory phase as well, in order to improve arterial oxygen tension. Such conditions include the application of continuous positive airway pressure (CPAP) to the infant with hyaline membrane disease or positive end expiratory pressure (PEEP) to certain adult patients in respiratory failure. Only under rare circumstances is negative airway pressure utilized during expiration.

Most respirators in common use are classified as assistor-controllers, and can be operated in any of three different modes. These modes differ in the method by which inspiration is initiated.

1. In the *assist* mode inspiration is triggered by the patient. A pressure sensor responds to the slight negative pressure that occurs

each time the patient attempts to inhale and triggers the apparatus to begin inflating the lungs. Thus the respirator helps the patient inspire when he wants to breathe. A sensitivity adjustment is provided to select the amount of patient effort required to trigger the machine. The assist mode is used for patients who are able to control their breathing but are unable to inhale a sufficient amount of air without assistance or for whom breathing requires too much effort.

2. In the *control* mode breathing is controlled by a timer set to provide the desired respiration rate. Controlled ventilation is required for patients who are unable to breathe on their own. In this mode the respirator has complete control over the patient's respiration and does not respond to any respiratory effort on the part of the patient.
3. In the *assist-control* mode the apparatus is normally triggered by the patient's attempts to breathe, as in the assist mode. However, if the patient fails to breathe within a predetermined time, a timer automatically triggers the device to inflate the lungs. Thus the patient controls his own breathing as long as he can, but if he should fail to do so, the machine is able to take over for him. This mode is most frequently used in critical care settings.

In addition to the three modes described, many respirators can be triggered manually by means of a control on the panel.

Once inspiration has been triggered, inflation of the lungs continues until one of the following conditions occurs:

1. The delivered gas reaches a predetermined pressure in the proximal or upper airways. A ventilator that operates primarily in this manner is said to be *pressure cycled.*
2. A predetermined volume of gas has been delivered to the patient. This is the primary mode of operation of *volume-cycled ventilators.*
3. The air or oxygen has been applied for a predetermined period of time. This is the characteristic mode of operation for *time-cycled ventilators.*

The various types of ventilators in clinical use can be categorized by two basic types. The first is a *pressure-cycled,* positive-pressure *assistor-controller.* An example of this type of respirator is shown in Figure 14-13. The device is powered pneumatically from a source of gas and requires no electrical power. Devices in this category may contain an electrically powered compressor or can be used with a separate compressor to permit ventilation with ambient air.

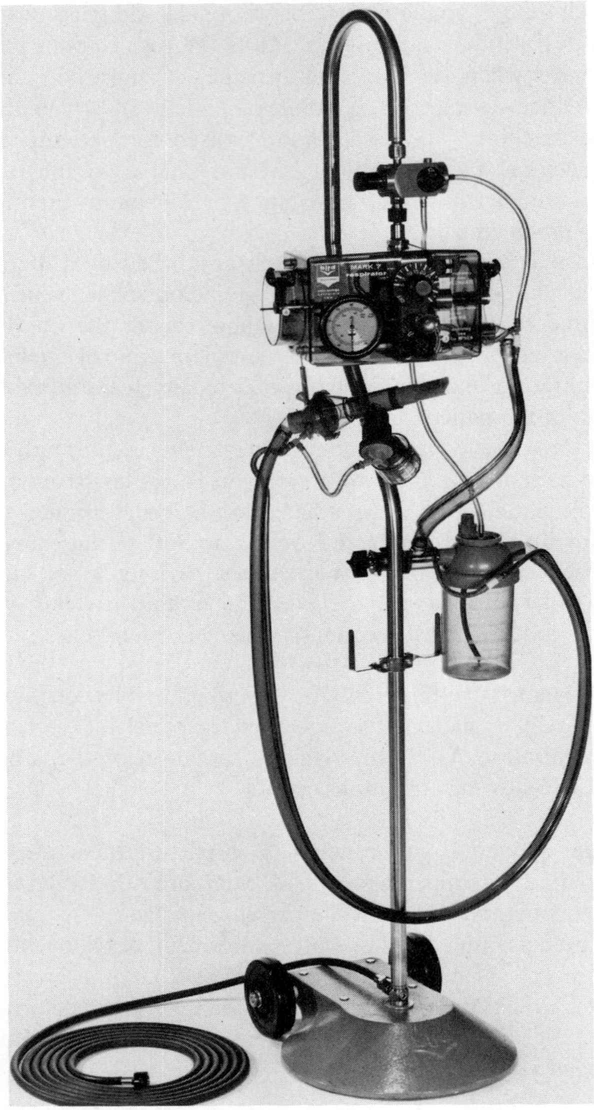

Fig. 14–13 Mark 7 respirator, an example of a pressure-cycled, positive-pressure, assistor-controller. *(Courtesy of Bird Corporation, Palm Springs, California.)*

Although a ventilator of the type shown in Figure 14-13 is quite small, it includes all the necessary equipment to control the flow of gas, mix air and oxygen, sense the patient's effort to inspire, terminate the inspiration when the desired pressure is reached, permit adjustment of the sensitivity of the triggering mechanism and the desired pressure level, and even generate a negative pressure to assist expiration on some devices. A special type of valve that incorporates a magnet senses the small negative pressure created by a patient when he attempts to inhale. Timing for operation in the controlled mode is accomplished by filling a chamber with gas and letting it bleed off through an adjustable needle valve. In the prescribed time, the pressure drops to a level at which a spring-loaded valve can operate. One widely used respirator in this category includes three pneumatic timing devices of a somewhat different type to provide time cycling as well as pressure cycling.

A form of volume-controlled respiration is possible with the type of pneumatically-operated respirator that permits time cycling. This flexibility is based on the premise that a given amount of airflow for a specified time duration results in a controlled volume. Such time cycling, however, is safe and effective only with patients whose respiratory status is stable and who do not experience minute-to-minute changes in lung compliance, due to airway obstruction from mucous, for example. Under these circumstances insufficient gas would be delivered to the patient, a highly dangerous situation in critical care. Constant observation by means of a spirometer connected to the patient's outflow valve and skillful adjustment of the controls may overcome this danger in situations where a volume-cycled ventilator is not available.

The second category of respirator is the *volume-cycled ventilator,* often called a *volume respirator.* This type of device, an example of which is shown in Figure 14-14, uses either a piston or bellows to dispense a precisely controlled volume for each breath. In the critical care setting where patients have pulmonary abnormalities and require predictable volumes and concentrations of gas, this type of ventilator is preferred. It is much larger than the pneumatically-operated units, and most units stand on the floor beside the patient's bed. Volume respirators are electrically operated and provide a much greater degree of control over the ventilation than the pressure-cycled types.

Most devices of this type have adjustable pressure limits and alarms for safety. Also, their provision for adjusting pressure limits and both inspiratory and expiratory times can be used in conjunction with the volume setting to ensure therapeutic pulmonary function in the patient who needs it most.

Volume-cycled ventilators used in critical patient care are always supplied with a spirometer to permit accurate monitoring of the patient's ventilation. Other available features include a heated humidifier and optional capabilities for negative pressure and positive end expiratory pressure (PEEP).

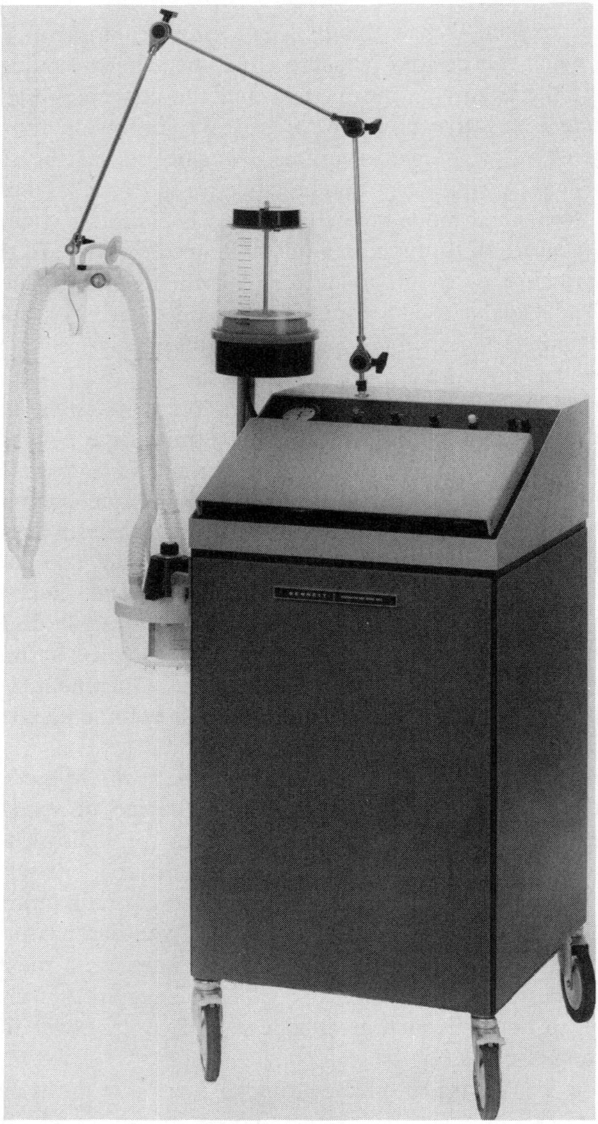

Fig. 14–14 Volume-cycled respirator. *(Courtesy of Bennett Respiration Products, Inc., Santa Monica, California.)*

Ventilation of a patient by either pressure-cycled or volume-cycled equipment requires that the system be leakproof. The only exception to this rule is a deliberate leakage of gas in patients who require *intubation,* the passing of a tube into the trachea via the nose or mouth or through tracheotomy. This procedure is required to reduce dead space and provide ventilation to a person who is critically ill or under the effects of anesthesia. In such situations, a specified volume of leakage around the tube prevents tracheal damage due to pressure on the mucous membrane and hypoxia in that area. The use of volume-cycled ventilators typically requires patient intubation. Pressure-cycled ventilators may also be used with intubated patients, but their primary use is with patients who require intermittent therapy using a mask or mouthpiece. Because significant leaks may occur with masks or mouthpieces, considerable skill is required on the part of the practitioner to ensure the desired therapeutic effect.

Because the consequences of error are so serious, it is extremely important that only well-trained personnel be permitted to apply ventilators to patients or to adjust their controls. This textbook makes no attempt to describe the operation of any of these devices in sufficient detail to serve as an operation manual. Such information can be obtained from the references given for this chapter and from manuals published by the manufacturers of the specific equipment.

Whenever a ventilator is used, its mode of operation and the settings of the various controls must be adjusted to the specific needs of the patient. Patient cooperation is essential for effective use of the equipment in any mode. When a machine is to be used in the assist or assist-control mode, the patient must be taught to work with the machine. In the control mode, any effort on the part of the patient to breathe may be detrimental. In all circumstances, care must be taken to avoid undesirable leaks. Excessive pressure should also be avoided, especially in the neonatal setting. The patient should be carefully observed so as to detect any problems that might arise. His chest should rise and fall rhythmically with the ventilatory cycle. His color and other physical assessment parameters must be monitored, and he should not demonstrate excessive fatigue following intermittent therapy, nor excessive restlessness during continuous therapy. Under no circumstances should an acutely ill patient be left alone during respiratory therapy of any kind. Adequate sterilization is also important to prevent cross-contamination among patients. Because a ventilator or respirator is a vital life-sustaining device, it is very important that a manually operated bag-mask combination and someone capable of operating it be available in case of equipment failure or electrical power outage.

14.3.3 *Intermittent Positive Pressure Breathing (IPPB)*

In the broad sense, *intermittent positive pressure breathing (IPPB)* is any form of assisted or controlled breathing in which air or some other gas is administered under positive pressure, but only during the inspiration portion of a patient's respiratory cycle. More specifically, the term IPPB is used to indicate a short-term treatment in the assist or assist-control mode, often including the administration of medication by nebulization (see Section 14.3.5). Although most respirators of the type described in the previous section are suitable for IPPB, pressure-cycled respirators are usually used for this purpose because of their portability and fitness for use with comparatively well patients. Some ventilators, especially those designed for home use, are intended for intermittent therapy only.

14.3.4 The Incentive Spirometer

The *incentive spirometer,* or *"yawn box"* as it is frequently called, operates on a very different although more physiological principle than the intermittent positive pressure breathing (IPPB) devices discussed previously. It has been suggested that IPPB often causes special difficulties in that secretions may be forced deeper into the lungs, thus further diminishing the available pulmonary tissue and promoting *atelectasis,* in which areas of the lung collapse. While IPPB equipment forces gas into the lungs, the incentive spirometer allows the patient to inhale room air (usually) through a mouthpiece against relatively low resistance, using his muscles of respiration normally to expand his thorax until a certain preset volume is inhaled and an indicator light signals a successful "yawn." At this point, exhalation can begin. Several "yawns" every hour will usually prevent the most obvious pulmonary complications, and most patients can work their own devices with only a minimum of help. The successful use and control of this device by a relatively immobilized patient must also be rewarding in terms of his active participation in his therapy and ultimate improvement. It is anticipated that the cheaper, more effective incentive spirometer will replace intermittent positive pressure breathing for a high percentage of patients presently needing such assistance.

14.3.5 Resuscitators

Resuscitation is defined as the act of reviving or restoring to life or consciousness. Thus a resuscitator is an emergency device designed to apply oxygen or to assist breathing on a temporary basis until the patient is able to breathe spontaneously. Although any of the inhalators or respirators in the hospital can be used for resuscitation if necessary, special equipment of this type has been designed for emergency use. The distinction lies in its portability and ease of use under emergency conditions. In the absence of any specially designated resuscitation equipment, mouth-to-mouth resuscitation or, better, a manually operated bag-mask combination connected to an oxygen source will serve the purpose.

A special type of resuscitator, called a *heart-lung resuscitator (HLR)* or *cardiopulmonary resuscitator,* provides emergency ventilation while simultaneously applying mechanical heart massage. This equipment is described in Chapter 10.

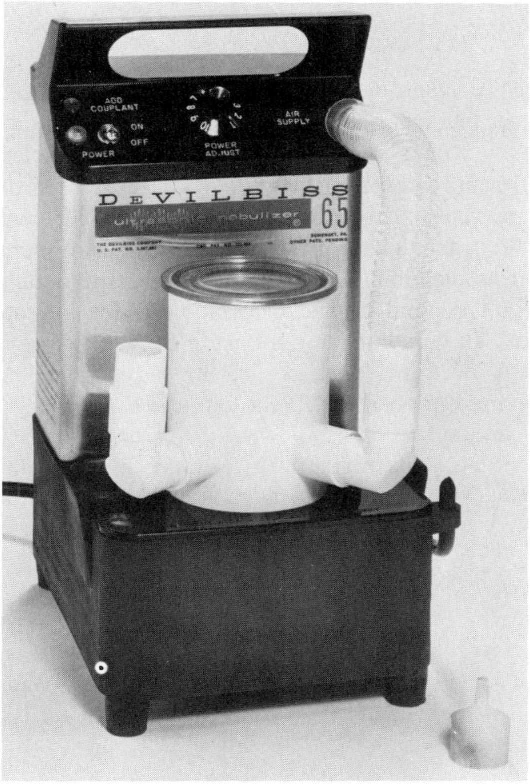

Fig. 14–15 Ultrasonic nebulizer. *(Courtesy of the DeVilbiss Company, Medical Products Division, Somerset, Pennsylvania.)*

14.3.6 Humidifiers, Nebulizers, and Aspirators

In order to prevent damage to the patient's lungs, the air or oxygen applied during respiratory therapy must be humidified. Thus virtually all inhalators, ventilators, and respirators include equipment to humidify the air, either by heat vaporization (steam) or by bubbling an air stream through a jar of water.

When therapy requires that water or some type of medication be suspended in the inspired air as an aerosol, a device called a *nebulizer* is used. In a nebulizer the water or medication is picked up by a high-velocity jet of oxygen (or some other gas) and thrown against one or more baffles or other surfaces to break the substance into controllable-sized droplets or particles, which are then applied to the patient via a respirator. (See Sections 14.2 and 14.3.)

A more effective (but also more expensive) type of nebulizer is the *ultrasonic nebulizer,* shown in Figure 14-15. This electronic device produces high-intensity sound energy well above the audible range. When applied to water or medication, the ultrasonic energy vibrates the substance with such intensity that a high volume of minute particles is produced. Such equipment usually consists of two parts, a generator that produces a radio-frequency current to drive the ultrasonic transducer, and the nebulizer itself, in which the transducer generates the ultrasound energy and applies it to the water or medication. Unlike the conventional nebulizer, the ultrasonic unit does not depend on the breathing gas for operation. Thus the therapeutic agent can be administered during oxygen therapy or a mechanical ventilation procedure. Because of its advantages, the ultrasonic nebulizer is often used in place of IPPB treatment.

Aspiration and other types of *suction apparatus* are often included as part of a ventilator or inhalator to remove mucous and other fluids from the airways. Where the aspirator is not provided as part of the respiratory therapy equipment, a separate suction device may be utilized.

15

X-Ray Equipment

In 1895 Wilhelm Conrad Röntgen, a German physicist, discovered a previously unknown type of radiation. He found that this radiation could actually penetrate nontransparent objects and provide an image of their inner structure. Because of these mysterious properties, he called his discovery *X rays.* In many countries, however, X rays are referred to as *Röntgen rays* in honor of their discoverer, who received the Nobel Prize in 1901 for his work.

Soon after the discovery of X rays, their importance as a tool for medical diagnosis was recognized. Later it was found that X rays could also be used for therapeutic purposes. Both applications of X rays are the domain of the medical specialty known as *radiology.* X-ray machines were the first widely used electrical instruments in medicine. In fact, hospitals still spend more money for the purchase of X-ray equipment than for any other type of medical instrumentation.

15.1 X rays

X rays are actually a form of electromagnetic radiation like radio waves or visible light except that their wavelength is much shorter. At the short end of the visible spectrum, radiation is perceived by the human eye as violet light. Radiation with an even shorter wavelength is not visible, but such *ultraviolet radiation* can cause skin burns and eye damage. It is beyond the range of the ultraviolet light that the X rays begin. X rays, in fact, cover quite a range of wavelength. The shorter the wavelength, the *harder* the X rays and the stronger is their penetration power. Like light, X rays normally move in a straight line. When they travel through an object, such as the body of a patient, however, not all the rays entering the object emerge from the other side. A portion of the entering X rays will either be absorbed in the object or will be *scattered,* which means that they change their direction of travel. The amount of absorption and scattering depends on the density of the medium. It is greater in metal than in bone, greater in bone than in soft tissue, and greater in soft tissue than in air. The use of X rays for medical diagnostics is based on this effect.

The X rays that are absorbed or scattered do not leave the medium in which this effect occurs unchanged but interact with the atoms of the matter and dislodge electrons. This process is called *ionization,* and X rays are therefore sometimes referred to as *ionizing radiation.* It is the ionization caused by X rays that accounts for their therapeutic effect.

15.2 Generation of X rays

X rays are generated in an X-ray tube, the principle of which is shown in Figure 15-1. This tube consists of an evacuated glass envelope with two

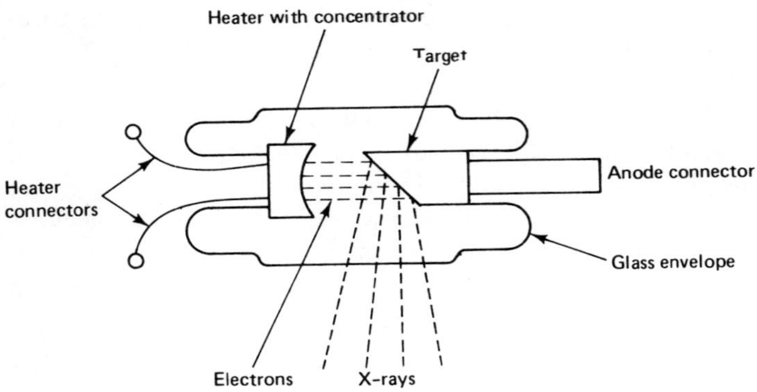

Fig. 15–1 X-ray tube, principle of operation.

metal electrodes. One of these electrodes, called the *cathode,* consists of a metal filament that is heated to a dark red glow by an electrical current. A voltage applied between the cathode and the other electrode, the *anode,* sends a stream of electrons through the vacuum. When these electrons strike the part of the anode called the *target,* they interact with the metal atoms and X rays are released in all directions. The voltage between the electrodes is very high (thousands of volts), and the higher the voltage, the harder (more penetrating) the X rays that are generated. The amount of X rays, on the other hand, depends on the number of electrons striking the target or on the current that flows through the tube. This current can be varied by varying the temperature of the heater, which, in turn, is done by changing the heater voltage.

15.3 Visualization of X rays

X rays normally cannot be detected directly by the human senses; thus indirect methods of visualization must be used in order to give an image of the intensity distribution of the X rays that have passed through the body of a patient. Three different techniques are in common use.

15.3.1 Fluoroscopy

Röntgen actually discovered X rays when he noticed that certain metal salts glowed in the dark when struck by the radiation. The brightness of this *fluorescence* is a function of the radiation intensity, and cardboard pieces coated with such metal salts were first used exclusively to visualize X-ray images. Early *fluoroscopes* were simply cardboard funnels, open at the narrow end for the eyes of the observer, while the wide end was closed with a thin cardboard piece that had been coated on the inside with a layer of a fluorescent metal salt. The fluoroscopic image obtained in this way is rather faint, however, and the X-ray intensity necessary to obtain a reasonably bright image is of such a magnitude that it can be harmful to both the patient and the observer. If the radiation intensity is reduced to a safer level, the fluoroscopic image becomes so faint that it must be observed in a completely darkened room and after the eyes of the observer have adapted to the dark for 10 to 20 minutes. Because of these inconveniences, direct fluoroscopy now has only limited use.

15.3.2 X-ray Films

Although X rays have a much shorter wavelength than visible light, they react with photographic emulsions in a similar fashion. After processing in a developing solution, therefore, a film that has been exposed to

X rays shows an image of the X-ray intensity. The sensitivity of this effect can be increased by the use of *intensifying screens,* which are similar to the fluoroscopic screens described above. The screen is brought into close contact with the film surface so that the film is exposed to the X rays as well as to the light from the fluorescence of the screen. X-ray films, with or without intensifying screens, are packaged in light-tight *cassettes* in which one side is made of thin plastic that can easily be penetrated by the X rays.

15.3.3 Image Intensifiers

The faint image of a fluoroscopic screen can be made brighter with the help of an electronic *image intensifier*. For this purpose, the screen is located at one end of a huge electronic tube; at the other end is a smaller screen of a type similar to a TV screen. This device provides an increase in brightness of several hundredfold and not only allows the X-ray intensity to be decreased but makes it possible to observe the image in a normally illuminated room. The intensifying tube, however, is rather heavy and requires a special suspension. For chest or pelvic examinations with the patient in a supine position, the screen on which the intensified image appears is high above the patient and requires a system of lenses and mirrors to present the image to the radiologist, who normally stands right next to the patient. For this reason, a TV camera is now used frequently to pick up the intensified image, which can then be observed on conveniently placed TV monitors. This TV picture can also be recorded on a TV tape recorder. Similarly, a movie camera can be used to record directly the intensified X-ray image during an examination.

15.4 X-ray Machines

In order to obtain an X-ray image from a certain part of the body, the region to be examined must be positioned between the X-ray tube and the imaging device, as shown in Figure 15-2 for a chest X ray. Similar to a light that throws the shadow of an object on a wall, the X-ray tube projects the "shadow" of the structures inside the body on the imaging device. In order for the X-ray image to be a sharp and well-defined replica of these structures, the part of the body being X rayed must be as close as possible to the imaging device. The X-ray tube, on the other hand, should be as far away as possible.

With mobile X-ray machines, such as the one shown in Figure 15-3, the cassette with the X-ray film is usually placed directly beneath the patient. The X-ray tube is mounted on an arm and can be adjusted to the desired height. "Aiming" of the tube is simplified by a small light that

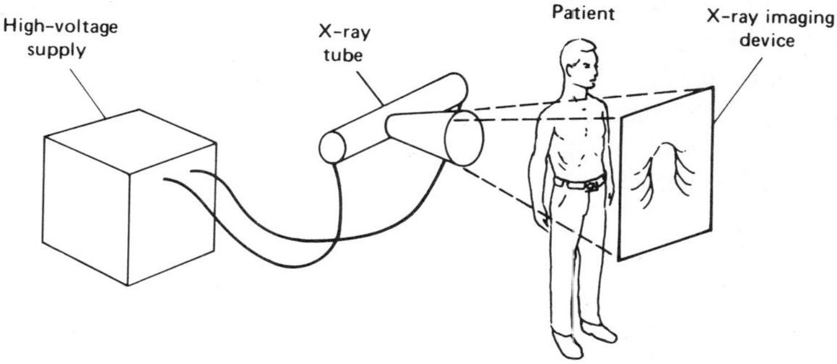

Fig. 15–2 Use of X rays to visualize the inner structure of the body.

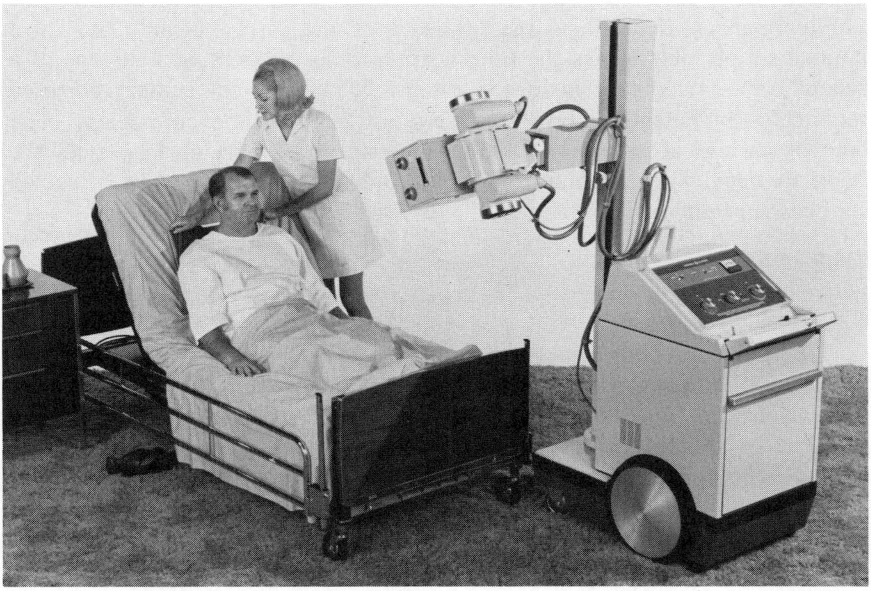

Fig. 15–3 Mobile X-ray machine. *(Courtesy of General Electric Company, Medical Systems Division, Milwaukee, Wisconsin.)*

projects the shadow of cross hairs along the axis of the X-ray beam. Mechanical shutters can be adjusted to limit the size of the beam to the area over which an X ray is to be taken.

In stationary X-ray machines the support arm for the X-ray tube is mounted on the wall or ceiling of the examination room in such a way that its height can be adjusted and the direction of the beam can be changed. For chest X rays, a holder for the film cassette is mounted adjustably on a wall of the room. For most other X rays, the cassette is inserted in the top of an adjustable table while the X-ray tube is placed above the patient, who lies on the table in a suitable position. With image intensifiers, however, the tube is normally below the table while the intensifier is positioned above the patient. In some X-ray machines the X-ray tube and image intensifier are mounted at either end of a C-shaped structure in such a way that they face each other. Figure 15-4 shows this arrangement in a mobile X-ray machine.

The high voltage for the operation of the X-ray tube is provided from a transformer, often mounted in an oil-filled enclosure, which is connected to the tube housing by a pair of heavy cables. The control panel of an X-ray machine normally provides for three different controls. The tube voltage, expressed in KVP (kilovolts-peak), determines the hardness or penetration power of the X-ray beam. The beam current, expressed in mA (milliamperes), determines the intensity of the X-ray beam. The third control simply determines the time (expressed in seconds or fractions of a second) that the beam is turned on for X-ray photos. Battery-powered mobile X-ray machines, however, may not have a time adjustment. The control settings necessary to obtain an X-ray photo of a given part of the body are usually determined from tables, but they may have to be corrected for obese or bony patients.

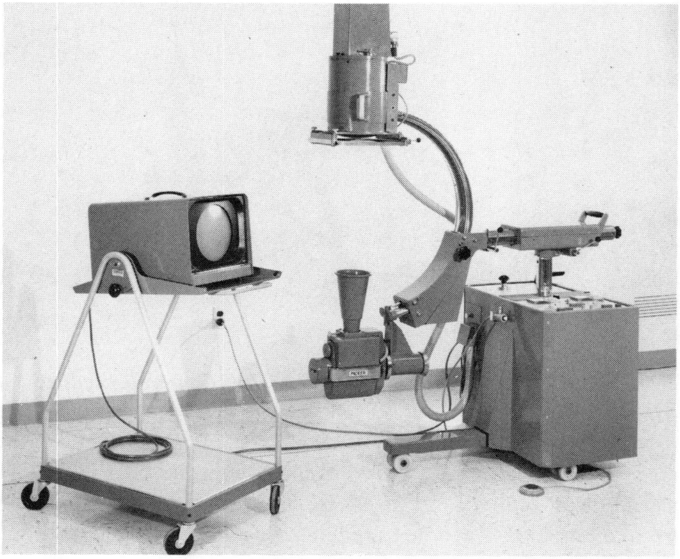

Fig. 15–4 Mobile X-ray unit (with image intensifier and television monitor). *(Courtesy of Picker Corporation, Cleveland, Ohio.)*

15.5 Special Techniques

The previous section described the general principle of obtaining X-ray images, but often special techniques must be used in order to obtain usable images from certain body structures.

15.5.1 Grids

As mentioned in Section 15.1, some of the X rays entering the body of a patient are actually scattered and no longer travel in a straight line. If the body section examined is very thick and if the X-rayed area is large, the scattered X rays can cause a blurring of the X-ray image. This effect can be reduced by the use of a so-called *grid* or a *Bucky diaphragm* (named after Gustav Bucky, its inventor). This device consists of a gridlike structure made of thin lead strips that is placed directly in front of the X-ray film. Like a venetian blind that lets sun rays through only when they strike parallel to the slats of the blind, the grid absorbs the scattered X rays while those traveling in straight lines can pass. In order to keep the grid from throwing its own shadow on the film, it may have to be moved by a motorized drive during the exposure of the film.

15.5.2 Contrast Media

While foreign bodies and bone absorb the X rays much more readily than soft tissue, the organs and soft tissue structures of the body show very little difference in X-ray absorption. In order to make their outlines visible on the X-ray image, it may be necessary to fill them with a *contrast medium* prior to taking the X-ray photo. In the *pneumoencephalogram,* the ventricles of the brain are made visible by filling them with air, which absorbs X rays less than the surrounding brain structures. Similarly, the structures of the gastrointestinal tract can be made visible with the help of *barium sulfate,* given orally or as an enema, which has a higher X-ray absorption than the surrounding tissue. Other body structures and organs can also be visualized by filling them with suitable contrast media.

15.5.3 Angiography

In angiographic procedures, the outlines of blood vessels are made visible on the X-ray image by injecting a bolus of contrast medium directly into the bloodstream in the region to be investigated. Because the contrast medium is rapidly diluted in the blood circulation, an X-ray photo or a series of such photos must be taken immediately after the injection. This procedure is often performed automatically with the help of a power-operated syringe and an electrical cassette changer.

15.5.4 Cardiac Catheterization

Cardiac catheterization is a technique used primarily to diagnose valve deficiencies, septal defects, and other conditions of the heart characterized by hemodynamic changes. For this purpose, a special catheter is inserted through an artery, vein, or, occasionally, directly through the chest wall into the heart. Under fluoroscopic control (with an image intensifier), the catheter is manipulated until its tip is in the desired position within the heart. By means of the catheter, intracardiac pressures can be measured in various parts of the heart that show characteristic changes if the heart valves are either narrowed or do not close completely. Septal defects can be detected by withdrawing blood samples from various heart chambers and measuring the oxygen concentration of the samples. Similarly, pumping efficiency can be assessed by measuring pressures within the ventricles at various points of the cardiac cycle. By injection of an indicator through the catheter (see Chapter 12), the cardiac output can be measured. By the injection of a contrast medium through a suitably placed cardiac catheter (*selective angiography*), the vascular structures of the heart, including the coronary arteries (*coronary arteriography*), can be visualized. Catheterization in general is discussed in more detail in Chapter 10.

15.5.5 Three-Dimensional Visualization

A basic limitation of X-ray images is the fact that they are two-dimensional presentations of three-dimensional structures. One organ located in front of or behind another organ therefore frequently obscures details in the image of the other organ. In *stereoradiography* two X-ray photos are taken from different angles, which, when viewed in a stereo viewer, give a three-dimensional X-ray image. In *tomography* (from the Greek word *tomos,* meaning slice or section) the X-ray photo shows the structure of only a thin slice or section of the body. Several photos representing slices taken at different levels permit three-dimensional visualization. Tomographic X-ray photos can be obtained by moving the X-ray tube and the film cassette in opposite directions during the exposure of the film. This procedure causes the image of the structures above and below a certain plane to be blurred by the motion, whereas structures in this plane are imaged without distortion. Special tomography machines that scan body sections with a thin X-ray beam and that determine the X-ray absorption with a radiation detector have been developed. The image of the section is reconstructed from a large number of such scans with the help of a digital computer (see Chapter 19).

15.6 Radiation Therapy

The ionizing effect of X rays is utilized in the treatment of certain diseases, especially of certain tumors. In dermatology very soft X rays that do not have enough penetration power to enter more deeply into the body are used for treatment of the skin. They are called *Grenz rays* (from the German word *Grenze,* meaning border) because in the spectrum they are actually at the border between the normally used X rays and the ultraviolet range (see Section 15.1). In the therapy of deep-seated tumors, on the other hand, very hard X rays that are generated with voltages much higher than those for diagnostic X rays are used. Sometimes *linear accelerators* or *betatrons* are used to obtain electrons with a very high voltage for this purpose. Changing the direction of entry of the beam in successive therapy sessions or rotating the patient during a session reduces the radiation damage to unafflicted body parts while concentrating the radiation at the site of the tumor.

15.7 Safety Precautions

The merits of X rays as a diagnostic tool have been appreciated since shortly after their discovery, but it took much longer for their potential dangers to the medical staff to be recognized completely. Radiation burns, tumors, and genetic damage were among the professional hazards associated with working in the field of radiology. Greatly improved equipment and strict safety precautions have made it possible to eliminate these hazards. Only if the equipment is maintained and used properly and if safety procedures are followed strictly, however, can the safety of the staff be ensured. It should always be kept in mind that a patient encounters only a few exposures to the X rays during an examination or while in the hospital. The physician, technician, or nurse who works with X-ray equipment day after day, on the other hand, can accumulate a dangerous level of radiation exposure, even if the individual dose by itself is harmless. The maximum dose that an employee may safely accumulate during certain time intervals is set forth in government regulations; and *radiation badges* (which contain envelopes with a special film) should be worn by all personnel working near X-ray equipment. X rays can reach a staff member either in the form of primary rays, emitted from the X-ray tube, or in the form of scattered radiation. In all modern equipment the X-ray tube is shielded in such a way that X rays are emitted only in the intended direction. Movable shutters that limit the size of the actual beam should always be adjusted to the smallest possible field. To avoid scattered radiation during the exposure of an X-ray photo, the staff member enters a small cubicle that is shielded with lead and that usually has a lead glass window to allow observation of the patient. With mobile X-ray machines, where this situation is not possible, the exposure switch is mounted at the end of a long cable, thus allowing the staff member to step back some distance from the exposure. In addition, personnel should also avoid standing in the direction of the beam when X-ray photos are taken with this kind of machine. In fluoroscopy and other procedures where the radiologist and other staff members must attend the patient, protective aprons and sometimes gloves are worn to protect them from the scattered radiation. These garments are made of rubber or plastic containing lead dust or of glass fiber made from lead glass.

16

The Surgical Suite

Today electronic instrumentation is used extensively in the operating room. With the aid of this equipment, which is similar to that already described in earlier chapters, the surgeon and anesthesiologist are able to improve their observation of the physiological condition of the patient and take the proper corrective steps when necessary. Instruments that can be found in the operating room include the ECG and blood pressure monitor, the patient temperature indicator, blood flow instrumentation, and sometimes blood gas instruments which are used during critical procedures.

Certain pieces of equipment used during surgery are not strictly instruments but can be considered to be in a similar category. The electrosurgical generator, also known as the electrosurgical unit (abbreviated ESU), differs from other equipment in that it performs not a monitoring function but rather an operating function. In a way, the ESU is considered an electronic scalpel. There is also one branch of surgery that is completely dependent on another piece of equipment. The heart–lung machine, or blood oxygenator, has made complex heart surgery possible by use of a cardiopulmonary bypass and associated equipment.

This chapter describes some aspects of monitoring unique to the surgical suite and introduces both the electrosurgical generator and the heart–lung machine.

16.1 Monitoring

The need for patient monitoring in surgery has become increasingly important. Initially only the patient's ECG and heart rate were monitored. Now, however, surgery is performed on critically ill infants as well as adults, partly as a result of improved monitoring techniques. With the development of new equipment, more complex and useful instruments have been introduced into the operating room. In the more complex surgical procedures it is common, for instance, to find a multichannel monitoring system.

The characteristics and operation of the various instruments are similar to those found in the critical care unit. Blood pressure is monitored more frequently in the operating room (see Chapter 9). Being able to observe instantaneous changes of blood pressure is now considered highly important.

The one major difference between patient monitoring in the operating room and patient monitoring elsewhere is the existence of some limitations that must be considered and overcome. For instance, in open-chest surgery no ECG electrodes can be placed on the chest of the patient. Therefore electrode location must be carefully selected in order to provide useful ECG readings. Posterior shoulder locations can be used, for example. An additional problem in the operating room is the electrical noise generated by the electrosurgical unit. The nature of this noise is such that it cannot be eliminated, and it appears as interference on the CRT display or any recording system. The problem is so severe at times that electrical noise from the ESU in one operating room may cause interference in an adjoining room.

A few less common types of instruments can also be found in the operating room. They are special instruments and are used in special cases. Fibrillators, for example, are used for the sole purpose of fibrillating the heart during open-chest surgery. This instrument is a simple source of alternating current that is connected directly to the patient's heart. The amount of current is increased until the heart fibrillates. At the end of the procedure it is necessary to defibrillate the heart in order to achieve normal heart function.

Special equipment to measure blood flow may also be found in the operating room. Ultrasonic and magnetic blood flow meters are described in Sections 12.4 and 12.5. Both types require exposure of the vessel in which blood flow is to be measured.

Temperature-measuring instruments are used to monitor patient temperature during some surgical procedures. Although simple, they provide relatively good accuracy. This type of instrument has a probe, which is attached to the patient. The tip of the probe is heat sensitive; thus it requires a good contact to the patient's skin for proper heat transfer between the patient and probe.

16.2 The Electrosurgical Generator

The *electrosurgical unit* (ESU) is perhaps one of the oldest electrically powered instruments used in the operating suite. In spite of the rapid expansion of modern electronic technology, some older units, dating back 20 to 30 years, are still used along with modern, compact instruments. Major differences between the old and the new have caused a certain amount of confusion, primarily because of the technical characteristics and clinical performances of these units. Because electrosurgical units are responsible for more injuries to patient and staff than any other electromedical instrument, the safety features of the newer units make them much more desirable.

The ESU is a high-power generator of high-frequency electrical energy. This energy, when applied to the tissue with a high-current density, causes localized dissolution of the tissue cells. By varying the waveform and duration of this energy, the instrument can be used to cut tissue or coagulate the severed ends of small blood vessels. Often a mixture or blend of the two waveforms is used to cut and coagulate simultaneously. Generally the only controls available on an ESU are for adjusting the amount of delivered energy, selecting the cut, coagulate or blend modes, and activating the instrument.

Figure 16-1 shows a typical modern solid-state electrosurgical unit.

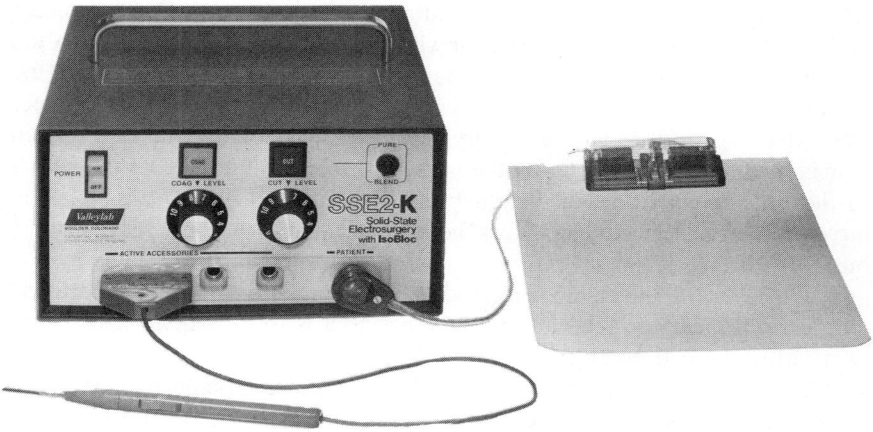

Fig. 16–1 Electrosurgical generator. *(Courtesy of Valleylab, Boulder, Colorado.)*

The front panel contains the ON–OFF switch, the coagulate or cut controls, and the blend control. In operation, two connections are made to the patient. One wire connects to what is called the *patient electrode,* a large metal plate that is placed under the patient's buttocks or stomach, depending on whether the patient is lying supine or prone. This electrode, which serves as a reference electrode, provides a large skin-contact area, to reduce heating. The patient electrode is frequently called the *ground plate,* since in some older instruments the plate is actually connected to ground through the instrument power cord. Also, the electrode is sometimes known as the *indifferent* or *dispersive electrode.* In all new instruments the electrode is not connected to ground; instead it is isolated from ground. A second wire from the instrument is connected to the active electrode known as the *pencil.* This pencil has a very small electrically conductive tip that causes high current densities at the tip-tissue interface, thus causing the necessary cutting of the tissue or coagulation of blood vessels.

Among the most common injuries for which the ESU is responsible are burns, which can occur easily if the instrument is not used properly. A burn may occur at the patient electrode as a result of poor electrical contact between the electrode and the patient. A burn is possible with any type of ESU—the isolated type (where the patient electrode is not grounded) and the nonisolated type. The only way in which burns can be prevented is by careful application of the patient electrode to the patient. A burn may also be caused by a poor electrical connection between the patient electrode and the ESU, but this type of burn will occur primarily at a site other than the patient electrode. It can happen when the ESU is the nonisolated type (patient electrode connected to ground), or when the unit is used on a patient who is also connected to another instrument that has a grounded electrode (such as an ECG monitor with a grounded RL electrode). An accidental burn resulting from the simultaneous use of such an ECG monitor and the ESU is caused by current flowing from one instrument through the patient to the other instrument. The patient electrode is applied to the patient as shown in Figure 16-2. The proper location for the patient electrode depends on the particular surgical needs. Normally, when the pencil comes in contact with the body, the electric current will flow from the pencil to the patient electrode, as shown by dashed line *A* in Figure 16-2. The large area of the electrode allows heat to dissipate, thereby preventing a burn.

However, if the patient electrode fails to make a good electrical contact with the skin surface, or if the contact area is too small, or if the wire connecting the patient electrode to the ESU is open (some instruments will shut off in the event that the wire opens), then the electric current will flow as shown by lines *B* and/or *C* or any combination of *A, B,* and *C.* ECG

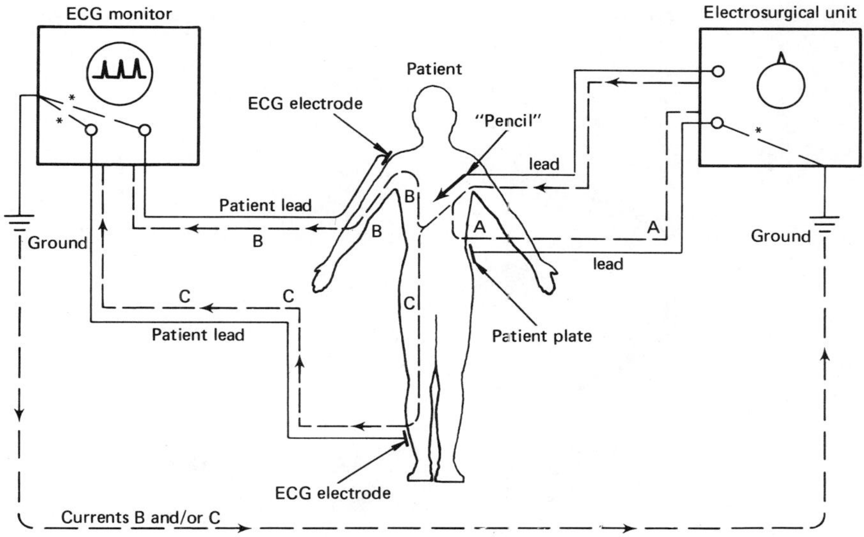

Notes:

1. * indicates internal connection, inside the instrument
2. For simplicity only two ECG electrodes are shown
3. Ground connection as shown is normal and proper. This connection is made through the electrical power cord.
4. Locations for all the electrodes are shown for reference only. Actual location may vary based on surgical requirement.
5. Dashed lines indicate electric current flow.

Fig. 16–2 Current flow between ESU and ECG monitor.

electrodes have a small conductive area in contact with the skin. Therefore any electric current that flows from the ESU through the ECG monitor will exit with high density at the ECG electrode site. This high current concentration will cause a burn at the electrode location. Such burns are not limited to an ESU–to–ECG monitor interconnection, but are also possible with any instrument that may provide an undesirable high current density path. This type of burn can be eliminated by the use of isolated equipment (ESU or other) and by careful application of the patient electrode.

Attempts to eliminate or reduce the problem of poor electrical connection between the patient electrode and patient have resulted in improved disposable patient electrodes that are sometimes called *pads* (Figure 16-3). These adhesive pre-jellied electrodes can be placed close to the point where the surgery is performed. They must be placed very carefully.

The ESU burns just described cannot occur when the intense light of a laser beam is used as a *laser scalpel*. This type of laser (*L*ight *A*mplification by *S*timulated *E*mission of *R*adiation) is able to coagulate (and seal) the

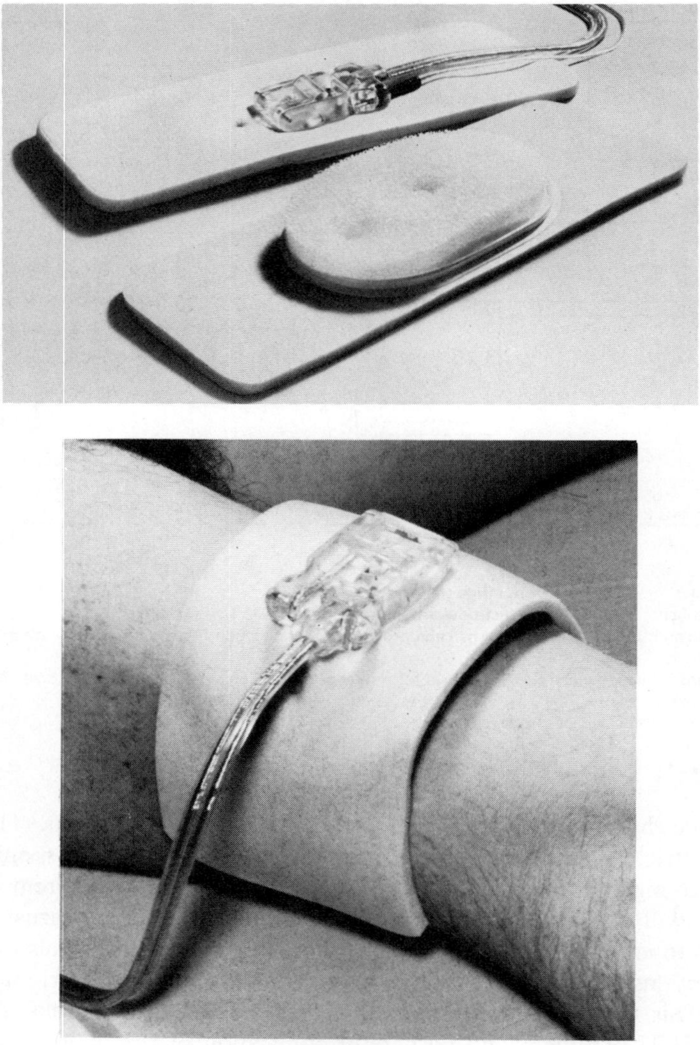

Fig. 16–3 Adhesive electrosurgical grounding plate: (a) electrode and pad; (b) positioned on patient. *(Courtesy of NDM Corporation, Dayton, Ohio.)*

ends of tiny blood vessels while cutting tissue. Thus, in cancer surgery, the spread of cancer cells to other body parts via the bloodstream is minimized. Because only the beam of light contacts the patient's skin, electrical burns are avoided.

16.3 The Heart–Lung Machine

The concept of extracorporeal circulation (heart–lung bypass) is not new; attempts had been made during the last century. However, the development of a reliable, safe heart–lung machine is a relatively recent innovation. During the 1960s advances were such that heart surgery is now almost a routine procedure in many hospitals.

The operating principle of this machine duplicates the real body system. Essentially, deoxygenated venous blood is pumped through an oxygenation process and returns to the cardiovascular system carrying the necessary oxygen for metabolism. The basic idea is to bypass the heart so that it can be immobilized in order for surgical procedures to be achieved, such as replacement of a valve, resection of a ventricular aneurysm, septal defects, and the myriad heart problems for which surgery is indicated.

Numerous heart–lung machines with different means of operation have been designed. However, two major types will be described. They can be categorized by the type of oxygenator used: the bubble oxygenator, and the membrane oxygenator. The former has been in general use for many years, but the latter, in improved form, is a comparatively recent addition.

The bubble oxygenator type consists of five major components: the oxygenating column, the debubbling chamber, the reservoir, the heat exchanger, and the pump. With the exception of the pump and the heat exchanger, the whole system is hung vertically from a movable metal frame. The tubes, through which the blood passes, are made of transparent plastic, which provides easy visibility.

Venous blood returning to the heart via the superior and inferior vena cavae is drained by gravity to the base of the oxygenating column. Raising or lowering the height of the frame can adjust blood flow rate by changing the vertical distance between the vena cavae level and the base of the oxygenating column. Blood is driven up the oxygenating column by the oxygen dispersion system as gas exchange takes place. The oxygenated blood passes over stainless steel sponges coated with high-viscosity silicon antifoam in the debubbling chamber. At this maximum-height point of the system, there is an outlet that allows carbon dioxide release from the blood and excess oxygen to escape. Blood then flows through a filter into an angulated reservoir. From the base of the reservoir, a roller pump forces blood through a heat exchanger, which maintains the blood at constant temperature, and a bubble trap. Oxygenated blood is then returned to the patient through the common femoral artery.

Coronary venous return and bronchial arterial blood is collected by a left ventricular sump and an intracardiac aspirator. The blood passes through a cardiotomy reservoir for defoaming and is also introduced into the base of the oxygenating column.

Figure 16-4 is a photograph of a bubble oxygenator of the type used in cardiac surgery. The pumps and heat exchanger are all of modular design so that they can be replaced rapidly. Pumps are available for ac or

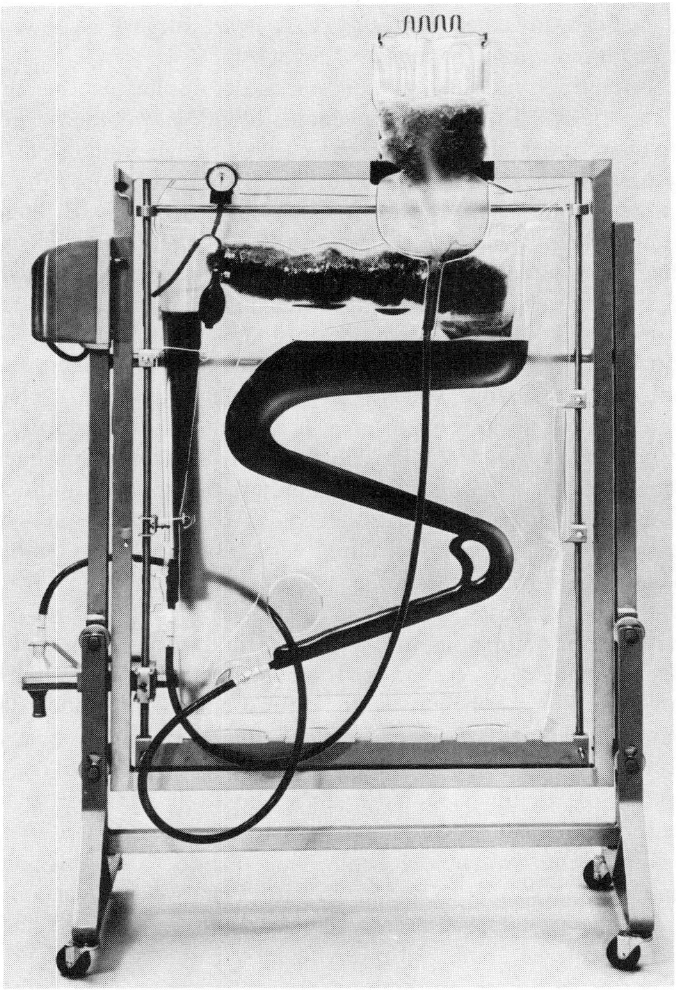

Fig. 16–4 Bubble oxygenator (heart–lung machine). *(Courtesy of the Artificial Organs Division of Travenol Laboratories, Inc., Morton Grove, Illinois.)*

dc power operation or for operation from a battery. The whole system can also be obtained as a mobile unit for emergency room use.

The process is capable of functioning for periods of up to several hours without changing the biologic properties of the blood. This situation implies, ideally, that no damage is done to the fragile red blood cells and that the numerous and delicate proteins constituting the blood plasma are not otherwise changed by exposure to foreign surfaces.

In practice, however, a certain amount of destruction of the red blood cells and other blood-formed elements is acceptable as long as this amount remains within the compensating capabilities of the patient. The most complex of the plasma proteins—for example, those connected with the coagulation process—can be protected by heparin, a compound that prevents blood clotting. All parts that come into contact with blood have rounded edges and are free from recesses where gas bubbles, cell clumps, or fibrin strands might accumulate.

It should be noted that the reason for the unusual-looking design of this system is that it must be fully visible at all times so that any change in blood level can be seen immediately. It must be capable of total body perfusion and oxygenation during cardiopulmonary bypass. It must be sterile and pyrogen-free. It should be fully collapsible so that there is no possibility of air embolism. Since hazards are possible with pooled donor-blood incompatibility, it should have the capability of a minimum amount of solution for a prime and also be capable of using solutions other than whole blood (e.g., 5% dextrose in water). And, finally, it must be safe, simple, and capable of handling large volumes with adequate speed. The system illustrated in Figure 16-5 meets all these requirements.

The *membrane oxygenator* type is replacing the bubble oxygenator type in some units. Figure 16-5 shows the Modulung-Teflo® Membrane Oxygenator System. An adapter system allows the oxygenator, heat exchanger, and oxygenator reservoir set to be used with any existing pump system. A two-pump mechanical speed synchronization control is used to operate the two pumps required for proper oxygenator use. It can be used with all existing pump console systems and modular pump systems, provided that the output of the two pumps is similar throughout the operating range. It is a single self-contained unit that incorporates 2.25 m^2 of membrane and is capable of total bypass on patients at flow rates up to 6 liters/minute.

This unit reduces hemolysis due to turbulence found in blood/gas interface oxygenator designs, reduces blood protein denaturation, since there is no blood/gas interface, and prevents oxygenator-produced microbubbles. The membrane itself serves as a barrier to particles larger than 0.5 μ.

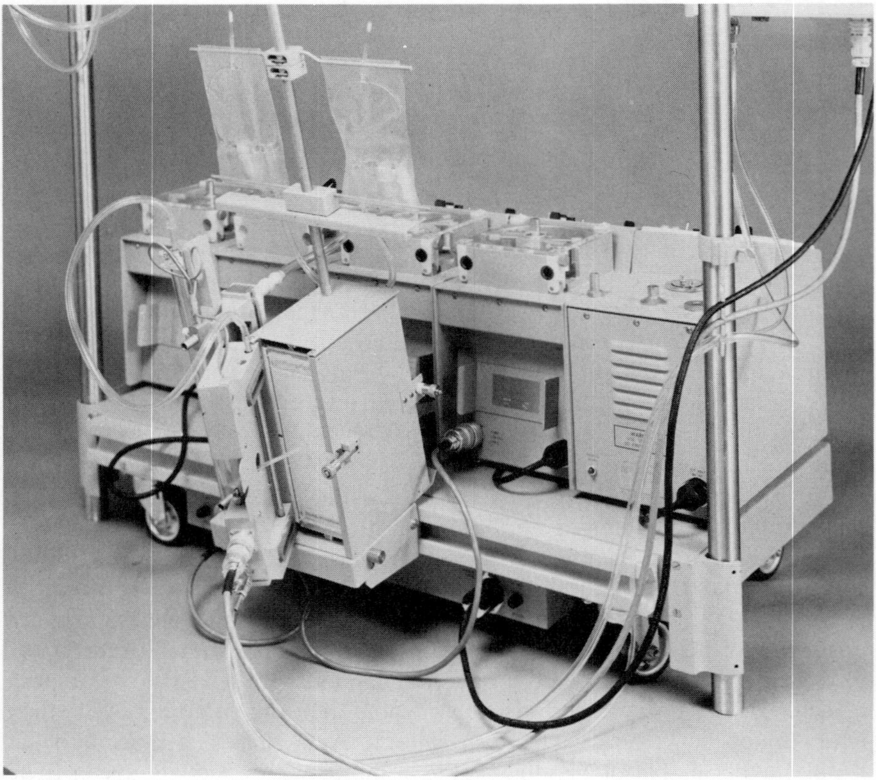

Fig. 16–5 Membrane oxygenator. *(Courtesy of Travenol Laboratories, Inc., Morton Grove, Illinois.)*

The circuit design includes a collapsible arterial reservoir, which reduces the chance of air embolism. Because the reservoir also acts as an efficient bubble trap and because the oxygenator produces no microbubbles, it is possible to eliminate a filter, used for that purpose, from the high-pressure arterial line.

The Modulung-Teflo unit requires no defoaming materials; circulating surfactants and defoaming sponge particles are eliminated.

17

Additional Types of Instrumentation

In addition to the instrumentation already described, several other devices used in certain patient-care situations should be considered in a textbook of this type. This chapter describes such instruments, which include the electroencephalograph, electromyograph, echoencephalograph, echocardiograph, fetal monitoring equipment, and instrumentation for measuring systemic and skin surface temperatures. Some of these devices have been in clinical use for a number of years; others have only recently found extensive use.

17.1 The Electroencephalograph (EEG)

Electroencephalography was introduced in Chapter 5 as the measurement of the electrical activity of the brain. Since clinical EEG measurements are obtained from electrodes placed on the surface of the scalp, these waveforms represent a very gross summation of potentials that originate from an extremely large number of neurons in the vicinity of the electrodes. As stated in Chapter 5, the electrical patterns obtained from the scalp are now believed to be the result of the graded potentials on the dendrites of neurons in the cerebral cortex and other parts of the brain, as they are influenced by the firing of other neurons that impinge on these dendrites.

EEG potentials have random (irregular)-appearing waveforms with peak-to-peak amplitudes ranging from less than 10 μV to over 100 μV. The frequency range for the EEG signal extends from below 1 Hz to over 100 Hz.

Electrodes for measurement of the EEG are described in Chapter 6. For clinical measurements, surface or subdermal needle electrodes are used. In some situations, surface electrodes are mounted in a headband for easy application. The ground reference electrode is often placed on the ear. As discussed in Chapter 6, a suitable electrolyte paste or jelly is used in conjunction with the electrodes to enhance coupling of the ionic potentials to the input of the measuring device. To reduce interference and minimize the effect of electrode movement, the resistance of the path through the scalp between electrodes must be kept as low as possible. Generally this resistance ranges from a few thousand ohms to nearly a hundred kilohms, depending on the type of electrodes used.

Placement of electrodes on the scalp is commonly dictated by the requirements of the measurement to be made. For diagnostic EEG measurement, a standard pattern, called the *10–20 Electrode Placement System,* is generally used. This system, devised by a committee of the International Federation of Societies for Electroencephalography, is so named because electrode spacing is based on intervals of 10 and 20% of the distance between specified points on the scalp. The 10–20 EEG electrode configuration is illustrated in Figure 17-1.

In addition to the electrodes, the measurement of the electroencephalogram requires a readout or recording device and sufficient amplification to drive the readout device from the microvolt-level signals obtained from the electrodes. Diagnostic electroencephalographs provide the capability of simultaneously recording EEG signals from several regions of the brain. For each signal, a complete channel of instrumentation is required. Thus electroencephalographs having as many as 16 channels are used. A typical diagnostic instrument with eight channels and a portable unit are shown in Figure 17-2.

Because of the low-level signals, the electroencephalograph must have high-quality differential amplifiers with good common-mode rejection (see Chapter 4). The differential preamplifier is followed by a power amplifier to drive the pen mechanism for each channel. Most EEG instruments permit selection of the appropriate upper- and lower-frequency limits for each channel. By properly setting these limits, the EEG technician is able

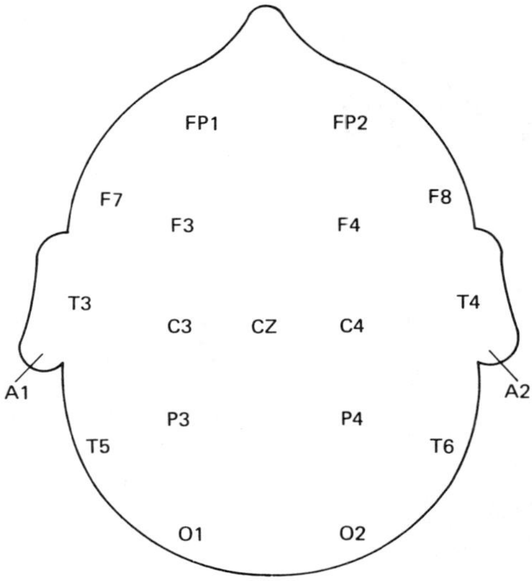

Fig. 17–1 10-20 EEG electrode configuration.

to reduce noise and interference from the recording. However, care must be taken to avoid excessive filtering that could distort the EEG waveform. In order to reduce the effect of electrode resistance changes, EEG amplifiers have very high input impedances, usually greater than 10 megohms.

An important feature of an electroencephalograph is its rather elaborate lead selector panel, which, in most cases, permits any two electrodes to be connected to any channel of the instrument. Either a bank of rotary switches or a panel of push buttons is used. The switch panel also permits one of several calibration signals to be applied to all channels for calibration of the entire instrument. A calibration signal is usually a dc voltage of a known number of microvolts, which appears on the EEG recording as a step followed by a gradual return to baseline.

The readout in a clinical electroencephalograph is a multichannel pen recorder with a pen for each channel. The standard chart speed is 30 mm/second, but most electroencephalographs also provide a speed of 60 mm/second for improved detail of higher-frequency signals. Some have a third speed of 15 mm/second to conserve paper during setup time. An oscilloscope presentation of the EEG is also possible, but it does not provide a permanent record.

As stated in Chapter 5, certain distinguishable EEG patterns usually precede and accompany epileptic seizures. Patterns indicating possible seizure activity can often be induced in patients who are susceptible to such

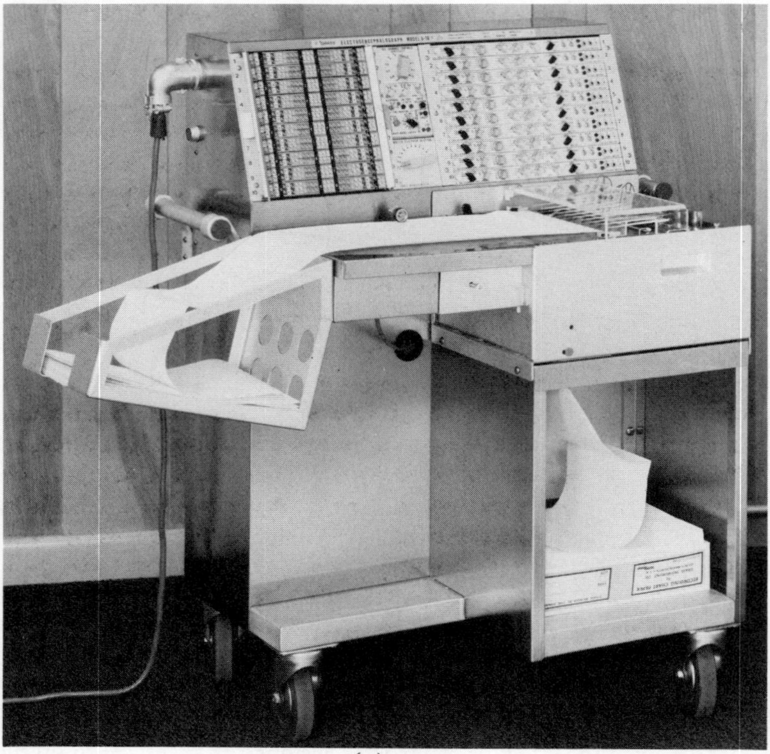

(a)

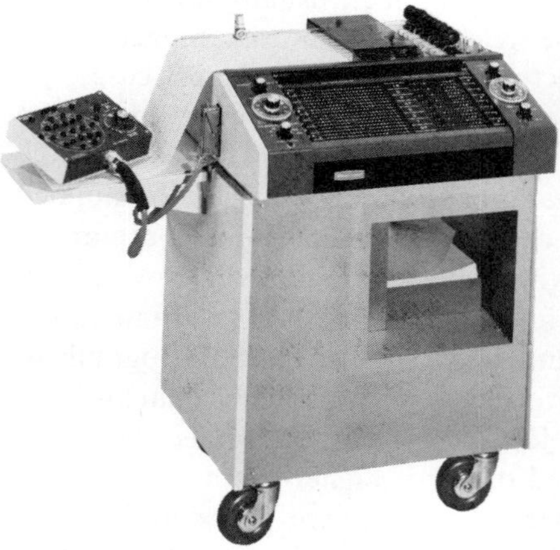

(b)

Fig. 17–2 Electroencephalographs: (a) Grass Model 8-10-10. *(Courtesy of Grass Instrument Company, Quincy, Massachusetts)*; (b) Beckman Portable Model. *(Courtesy of Beckman Instruments, Schiller Park, Illinois.)*

seizures by subjecting them to a flashing light. A *photic stimulator* of the type shown in Figure 17-3 usually serves as the source of the light flashes. This instrument produces short (about 10-μs duration), high-intensity (1.5 million candlepower at a distance of 2 ft from the glass face plate), blue-white flashes at a rate adjustable from about 2 to 45 per second. When used to produce EEG patterns indicative of possible seizure activity, the rate is set between 2 and 20 flashes per second. In some clinical settings, the flashes are applied in bursts of 10-second duration separated by 10-second periods in which the light remains off.

It has been determined that in some patients seizure activity is more likely to occur during sleep than during waking hours. For this reason, sleep is sometimes induced in order to study EEG patterns that might indicate a tendency toward seizures.

Hospital personnel using an electroencephalograph must be sure that electrodes are properly attached to the patient's head. The reference electrode(s) must be properly connected and the instrument grounded in order to obtain usable EEG tracings. Improper grounding generally results in an increased level of 60-Hz powerline interference. Also, the patient must be kept quiet, since movement frequently causes artifacts on the tracing.

The technician must continually watch for any indication of a malfunctioning electrode. Such a malfunction can be identified by a large artifact that periodically appears in the channels in which the faulty electrode is involved. A malfunctioning electrode should be replaced as soon as possible after discovery.

During the recording of EEG, the tracing should be watched very carefully for any indication of a possible seizure so that aid can be provided to the patient. Psychotic patients must be observed for signs of uneasiness that can cause movement artifacts. Care must also be taken to ensure that incontinent patients do not contact the metal bed rail or wheelchair, thereby creating interference on the tracing.

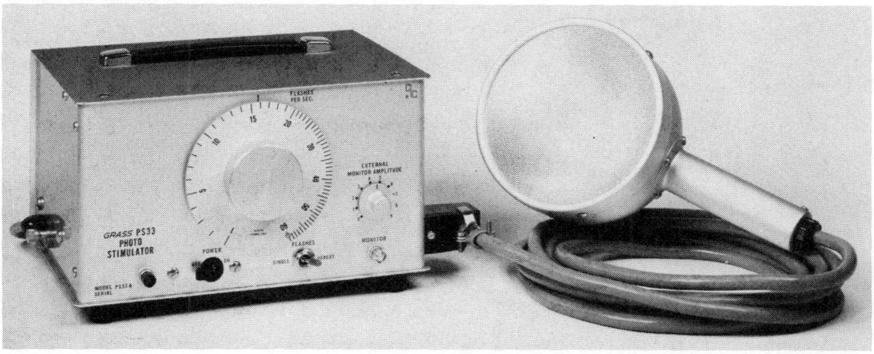

Fig. 17–3 Photic stimulator to induce EEG patterns related to epileptic seizures. *(Courtesy of Grass Instrument Company, Quincy, Massachusetts.)*

In stocky or obese patients, ECG potentials can often be picked up by the ear electrodes along with the EEG potentials. The ECG can easily be identified by its regular pattern, which occurs at the heart rate. Sometimes an extra ground electrode can be applied to the mastoid bone to eliminate this ECG artifact. Muscle potentials also appear as artifact on an EEG tracing as a result of facial, neck, or shoulder tenseness. Movement artifact can be caused by tremor of the patient.

17.2 The Electromyograph (EMG)

As introduced in Chapter 5, the *electromyogram* is a presentation of the electrical activity associated with the contraction of muscles. In clinical practice, the EMG is used primarily to analyze problems in motor neurons, neuromuscular junctions, and muscles. The instrument for measurement and observation of the EMG is the *electromyograph,* shown in Figure 17-4.

Unlike ECG and EEG equipment, the typical electromyograph has an oscilloscope readout instead of a graphic pen recorder. The reason for this is the higher frequency response required. Sometimes a *storage cathode-ray tube,* a special type of oscilloscope tube that retains a pattern for prolonged study, is provided for retention of data, or an oscilloscope camera is used to obtain a permanent visual record of data from the oscilloscope screen.

Most electromyographs also include an audio amplifier and loudspeaker in addition to the oscilloscope display to permit the operator to hear the "crackling" sounds of the EMG. This audio presentation is especially helpful in the placement of needle or wire electrodes into a muscle.

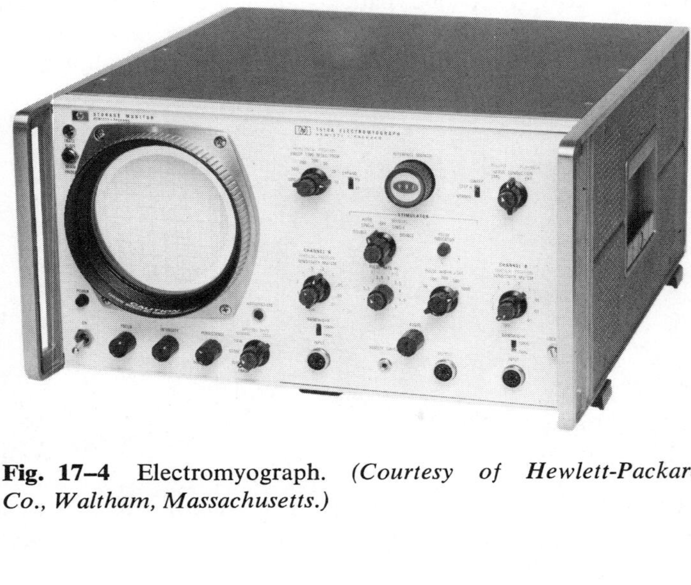

Fig. 17–4 Electromyograph. *(Courtesy of Hewlett-Packard Co., Waltham, Massachusetts.)*

A trained operator is able to tell from the sound when his electrodes are making good contact with a muscle and identify which of several adjacent muscles have been contacted.

Modern electromyographs generally incorporate provisions for measuring nerve conduction *latencies* and *velocities*. By stimulating a given nerve location and measuring the EMG downstream, a latency can be determined from the time difference displayed on the oscilloscope. By measuring the latencies from two different points along a given nerve and determining the difference between the two latencies, the *nerve conduction time* can be obtained. By dividing the physical distance along the nerve between the two points by the nerve conduction time, the *nerve conduction velocity* can be calculated. Latency and nerve conduction time are given in milliseconds, nerve conduction velocity is in meters per second.

Although action potentials from individual muscle fibers can be recorded under special conditions, it is the electrical activity of an entire muscle or group of muscles that is of primary clinical interest. In this case, the signal is a summation of all the action potentials within the range of the electrodes, the magnitude of each determined by its distance from the electrodes. Since the overall strength of muscular contraction depends on the number of fibers energized and the time of contraction, there is a correlation between the overall amount of EMG activity for the whole muscle and the strength of muscular contraction. There are also characteristic EMG patterns associated with fatigue and tremor.

The EMG potentials from a muscle or group of muscles produce a noiselike waveform that varies in amplitude with the amount of muscular activity. Peak amplitudes vary from 50 μV to about 1 mV, depending on the location of the measuring electrodes with respect to the muscle and the activity of the muscle. A frequency response from about 10 Hz to well over 3000 Hz is required for faithful reproduction.

In general, surface electrodes are unsuitable for clinical EMG measurements, for they produce potentials that are too small and susceptible to interference. Also, it is often difficult to obtain sufficient localization with surface electrodes. For these reasons, fine wire needle electrodes are generally used. They can be either *unipolar* or *bipolar*. A *unipolar* electrode, which consists of a single wire inserted into the muscle, measures the potentials from that location with respect to a reference electrode elsewhere on the body. Electrodes of this type are small, relatively inexpensive, and obtain potentials from a fairly large region, which may include other nearby muscles. In contrast, *bipolar* electrodes consist of two wires inserted into the muscle, or a coaxial electrode in which a fine wire is inserted into the muscle inside a hypodermic needle, which serves as the second electrode. Although larger and more expensive, bipolar electrodes provide better localization and are often able to obtain potentials from a single muscle.

In either case, the fine wire electrodes are insulated along their surfaces except at the very tip, which is sharpened to provide the point of contact.

Although not suitable for EMG potential measurements, surface electrodes can be used for nerve velocity and latency measurements as well as needle electrodes. Two sets of electrodes are required for these measurements, one set for application of the stimulus and a second set for obtaining the resultant EMG potentials. Placement of both sets of electrodes is critical for good results.

The amplifier for EMG measurements, like that for ECG and EEG, must have high gain, high input impedance and a differential input with good common-mode rejection (see Chapter 4). However, the EMG amplifier must accommodate higher frequencies. In many commercial electromyographs, the upper-frequency response can be varied by use of switchable lowpass filters.

Useful EMG measurements require proper application of electrodes. All electrodes must have good contact with the skin or muscle tissue. For surface electrodes, the same type of skin preparation and jelly used with ECG electrodes (see Chapter 7) is required. Care should be taken to avoid an excessive amount of jelly that may provide a short between adjacent electrodes. Before fine-wire needle electrodes are inserted into a muscle, the skin at the point of entry and the surface of the electrode must be properly sterilized.

Care must be taken in the use of needle electrodes to ensure that they are inserted into the muscle from which measurements are to be made. It is very easy to mistakenly place the electrodes into the wrong muscle. Proper electrode placement requires a good knowledge of anatomy. Because fine-wire needle electrodes are small and sharp, they cause little pain. However, patients must be kept from moving, to prevent tearing of tissue by the wires and to ensure proper contact of the wires with the muscle tissue.

17.3 Diagnostic Instrumentation Utilizing Ultrasound

Ultrasound is sound energy at frequencies above the audible range (higher than 20,000 Hz). When a source of ultrasound, called an *ultrasound transducer,* is placed against the skin, ultrasound waves enter the body, traveling in a relatively straight line through tissues, blood, and bone. Whenever the waves strike an interface between substances of two different densities, such as the blood inside the left ventricle and the tissue of the endocardium, a small portion of the energy is reflected back toward the transducer while the remainder continues on in about the same direction.

If the density difference is great, as in the case of an interface between soft tissue and bone, nearly all the energy is reflected and very little continues on. If the ultrasound energy is sent out in short bursts, called *pulses,* each transmitted pulse produces a reflected pulse, called an *echo,* to be sent back from each interface encountered in its travel through the body. Between transmitted pulses, the transducer can be used as a receiver to pick up the returning echoes. The time required for a transmitted pulse to travel from the transducer to a given interface and the echo to return is directly proportional to the distance between the transducer and that interface. If the transmitted pulse is used to trigger an oscilloscope trace on which each returning echo produces a deflection, as shown in Figure 17-5, the distance from the transducer to each interface can be determined directly by the position of its corresponding deflection on the trace. If the transducer and interface both remain stationary, each succeeding oscilloscope trace will be deflected in the same place and will appear to stand still. If, on the other hand, the interface moves with respect to the transducer, the deflection will move along the trace correspondingly. In some systems the returning echoes control the brightness of the trace instead of its deflection. In these cases, the trace appears only when an echo is received.

Ultrasound propagates very poorly through air. For this reason, the transducer must be coupled to the surface of the body by means of a

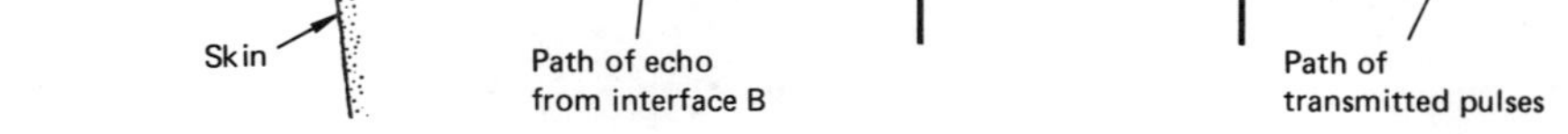

(a)

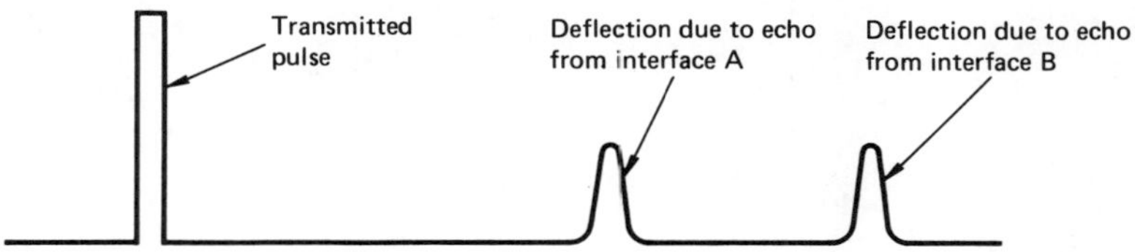

(b)

Fig. 17–5 Principle of pulsed ultrasound technique.

special aqueous gel. Care must be taken that sufficient gel is placed between the probe and the skin to provide efficient transmission of the ultrasound energy.

Two important clinical instruments, the *echoencephalograph* and the *echocardiograph,* utilize pulsed ultrasound. In addition, similar equipment is used for imaging of other organs and for fetal imaging. These instruments are all described in sections below. A different ultrasonic technique is used in blood flow measurement (see Chapter 12) and one type of fetal monitoring (see Section 17.4.2).

17.3.1 Echoencephalography

The *echoencephalograph* utilizes pulsed ultrasound in locating the midline of the brain by simultaneously measuring the distance to the midline from probes at both sides of the head. Midline echoes from the two transducer probes are simultaneously displayed on an oscilloscope, one producing upward deflection of the oscilloscope beam and the other producing a downward deflection, as shown in Figure 17-6. In the normal brain these two deflections line up, indicating equal distance from the midline to each

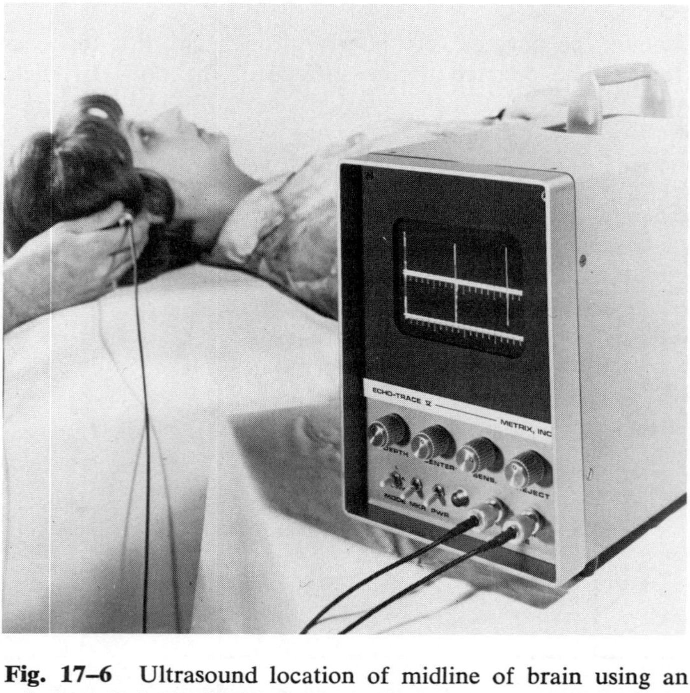

Fig. 17–6 Ultrasound location of midline of brain using an echoencephalograph. *(Courtesy of Metrix, Inc., Denver, Colorado.)*

side of the head. Nonalignment indicates the possibility of a tumor or some other disorder that might cause the midline of the brain to shift from its normal position. In some cases, only a single probe is used, first on one side of the head and then on the other.

An echoencephalograph consists of a source of high-frequency energy to drive the ultrasound transducers, the probe(s) containing the transducer(s), circuitry to amplify the received echoes, and the oscilloscope for display.

17.3.2 Echocardiography

When pulsed ultrasound energy is directed through the precordium into the heart, echoes are received from the wall, valves, and various other structures of the heart. A tracing showing the movement of these structures with respect to time is called an *echocardiogram,* and the techniques of obtaining measurements from the heart using ultrasound constitute the field of *echocardiography.*

A commercially available echocardiograph is shown in Figure 17-7.

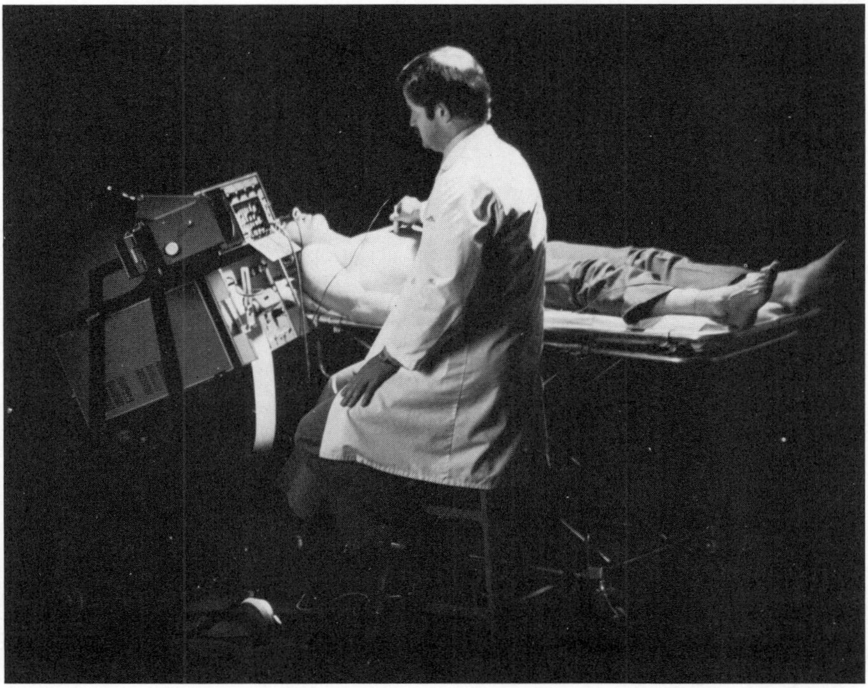

Fig. 17–7 An echocardiograph in use. *(Courtesy of Smith Kline Instruments Inc., subsidiary of Smith Kline Corporation, Philadelphia, Pennsylvania.)*

Basically, it is very similar to that used for echoencephalography, except for the readout. Instead of the received echoes causing a deflection of the electron beam, they cause the beam to be brightened in proportion to the strength of each echo. The beam sweeps across the CRT with each transmitted pulse. However, successive sweeps do not retrace each other. Each sweep produces a line just next to the one preceding it, so that the bright spots representing echoes from a given cardiac structure form a tracing from bottom to top on the screen that shifts from side to side with the movements of that structure. A Polaroid® camera can be used to obtain a permanent record of the measurement. By rotating the Polaroid® picture by 90°, the tracing representing each cardiac structure can be oriented so that time is measured from left to right, as is conventionally done with physiological recordings.

Certain types of strip-chart recorders that produce tracings by moving a beam of light on photographic paper can be used to produce a chart recording directly. For this purpose, however, the brightness of the beam must be controlled by the received echoes and the beam must be made to sweep across the chart from top to bottom with each transmitted ultrasonic pulse.

A typical echocardiogram is shown in Figure 17-8. Traces corresponding to major cardiac structures are labeled.

A successful echocardiogram requires a high degree of skill on the part of the person performing the measurement. The probe must be positioned so that the ultrasound energy is directed toward the region of the heart from which information is desired. Care must be taken to avoid having any bony structure in the path because the ultrasound cannot transverse bone. Also, the ultrasound must be applied to the precordium in order to avoid a path through any air-containing structures.

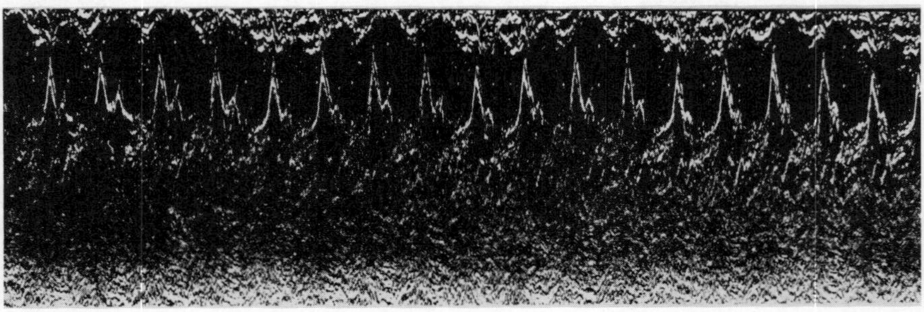

Fig. 17–8 Typical echocardiogram. *(Courtesy of Smith Kline Instruments Inc., subsidiary of Smith Kline Corporation, Philadelphia, Pennsylvania.)*

17.3.3 Other Applications of Pulsed Ultrasound

With the same type of instrumentation used for echocardiography, ultrasonic images of other organs and structures of the body can be produced by scanning an ultrasonic transducer across the surface of the body over the area of interest. At the same time, a pictorial representation of the echoes received appears on an oscilloscope screen similar to that used in echocardiography. The only difference is that an echocardiogram (Figure 17-8) shows variation in the position of certain structures as they change with time, whereas the ultrasonic imaging representation shows a map of the echoes received from a cross section of a region of the body. Ultrasonic scans of the liver, kidney, abdomen, breasts, and various other parts of the body are sometimes able to detect and locate cysts, tumors, and similar internal abnormalities.

Ultrasonic imaging is also useful in determining the size and location of a fetal head from about the 30th week of pregnancy. The measurements can be obtained from a scan of the mother's abdominal region, using the same technique as described above for organ imaging. A simple measurement of the diameter of the fetal skull can be obtained by aiming a hand-held transducer over the fetal head so that the ultrasound passes through both sides of the skull at right angles to produce strong, identifiable echoes.

17.4 Fetal Monitoring

Fetal monitoring is a relatively new and extremely valuable addition to the field of patient monitoring. The period of labor and delivery is extremely critical. Fetal distress, which often occurs during this period, remained unobserved and undiagnosed in the past. However, with modern fetal monitoring techniques, this condition can be detected. The most important indicator of fetal distress is the *fetal heart rate,* commonly abbreviated FHR. In general, electronic monitoring of fetal heart rate is performed using a beat-by-beat technique, in which the FHR is computed and displayed after each heartbeat. This is known as a *nonaveraging method* of computing the heart rate. In contrast, critical care monitors (see Chapter 11) usually indicate the *average* heart rate. Also, in auscultatory methods of determining FHR, the heart rate is averaged over a period of time—typically one minute. The major advantage of the beat-by-beat method over an averaging method is that an indication of instantaneous variation in FHR is possible. Such an instantaneous indication may reveal a distress condition, even though average FHR may appear to be normal. There are two basic methods of FHR monitoring: the *internal* or *invasive* method and the *external* or *noninvasive* method.

Another important parameter in fetal monitoring is *uterine contraction,* abbreviated UC. The time relationships between UC and FHR provide essential information relative to fetal distress.

17.4.1 Basic Principles of Fetal Monitoring

The rate of the normal fetal heart ranges from 120 to 160 beats per minute. Rates above 160 are considered as *fetal tachycardia* and rates below 120 as *fetal bradycardia.* Variations from the normal FHR, depending on their duration and their time relationship with respect to UC, can be important indicators of fetal distress conditions. Figure 17-9 indicates three significant relationships between FHR deviation and UC. Figure 17-9(a) shows a decrease in FHR at the same time as UC is increasing. This condition is known as *early deceleration.* Figure 17-9(b) illustrates *late deceleration,* in which FHR decreases some time after UC has increased. Figure 17-9(c) shows variable deceleration, in which a decrease in FHR seems to be independent of UC.

A fetal monitor is generally a two-channel system by which FHR and UC can be monitored and recorded simultaneously on the same chart with the same time base, to maintain their time relationship. Figure 17-10 shows a block diagram of a fetal monitoring system.

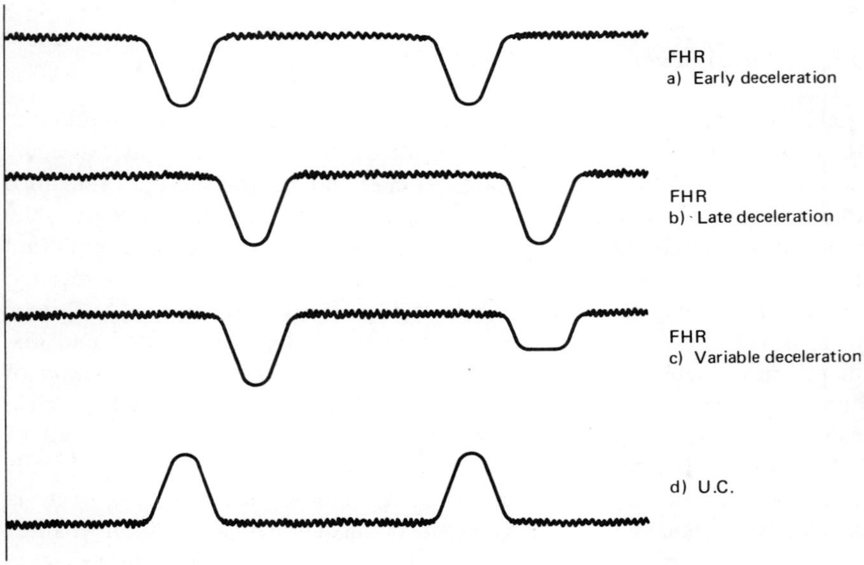

Fig. 17–9 Time relationships between FHR and UC.

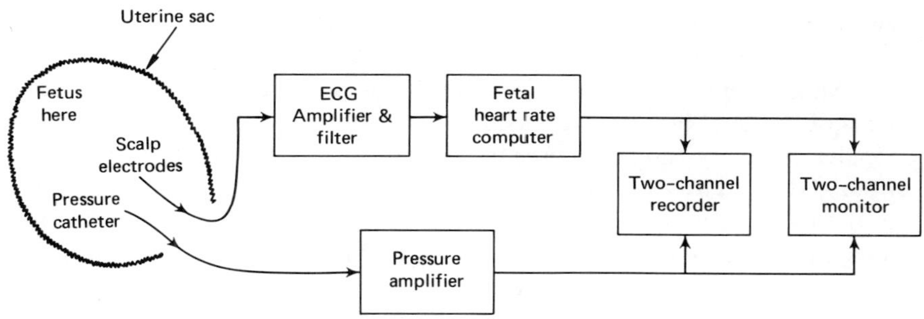

Fig. 17–10 Basic fetal monitoring system–block diagram.

17.4.2 Noninvasive (External) Monitoring

Noninvasive methods of fetal monitoring are those in which it is unnecessary to introduce any catheters into the body of the mother or to attach electrodes or any other apparatus to the fetus. Such methods permit earlier monitoring than the invasive methods described in Section 17.4.3 below, but they are much more susceptible to artifacts and require a greater degree of skill if useful information is to be obtained.

In one type of noninvasive monitoring, a sensitive microphone is strapped to the abdomen of the mother in order to pick up fetal heart sounds. The abdominal surface is first explored with the aid of a stethoscope to determine the location of the fetal heart. Then a microphone is strapped to the location from which the fetal heart can best be heard. The sounds picked up by the microphone are amplified and filtered to remove noise and undesired sounds as much as possible. Special circuitry, called a *heart rate computer,* is used to determine the fetal heart rate, which is displayed on the monitor and recorded on a strip-chart recorder.

Since the microphone and amplifier cannot distinguish the fetal heart sounds from other sounds, the signal entering the fetal heart rate computer may contain, in addition to the desired signal, maternal and other undesirable sounds. Consequently, this system may be unreliable at times. A solution is to use an ultrasonic technique of fetal monitoring. Unlike the pulsed ultrasound systems described in Section 17.3, ultrasonic fetal monitoring utilizes the Doppler effect, described in Chapter 12. In this technique a transducer is strapped to the mother's abdomen to direct the ultrasonic energy toward the fetus. Because the Doppler system responds only to moving structures, such as the fetal heart, echoes from the fetal heart can be distinguished from other echoes and processed to determine the fetal heart rate. By using this ultrasonic method, much of the interference inherent in the microphone system can be eliminated. However, the use of ultrasonic technique requires considerable skill.

Another ultrasonic instrument that can be used to sense the movements of the fetal heart from outside the mother's body is a transcutaneous Doppler device of the type described in Chapter 12 for location of sources of blood flow. This instrument acts as an ultrasonic stethoscope by converting the movements reflected in ultrasonic echoes into audible sounds on a loudspeaker. Although the device does not calculate heart rate, variations in rate can be heard as they occur.

In measuring uterine activity, a different type of external transducer, a *tocodynamometer,* is used. This transducer, which responds to the pressure variations associated with uterine contraction, is also strapped to the abdomen of the mother. Its output, which corresponds to the uterine contractions, is amplified, displayed, and recorded along with the FHR.

17.4.3 Invasive (Internal) Monitoring

Invasive fetal monitoring systems utilize a different approach to obtain the same results as the noninvasive methods. As the name implies, invasive methods require invasion of the mother's body to obtain pressure measurements from the uterus and ECG from the fetus. The fetal ECG is frequently abbreviated *FECG*.

In order to obtain the FECG, a special clip-type electrode is used. (See Chapter 6.) The direct method of monitoring is possible only during the period of labor and delivery, after the membranes have ruptured and the cervix has been dilated. The special clip-type electrode is attached to the fetal scalp (or to the fetal buttocks in the event of a breech). The faint FECG is picked up by the electrodes and amplified. The signal is filtered to remove interference. The amplified FECG is then applied to the fetal heart rate computer for derivation of FHR. Intrauterine contraction is picked up via a fluid-filled catheter inserted into the uterus. The uterine pressure is transmitted via the catheter to a pressure transducer (similar to the transducer used for blood pressure monitoring; see Chapter 9). The signals obtained from the pressure transducer are amplified and displayed on a multichannel monitor and recorded on a two-channel strip-chart recorder. The direct (invasive) method generally produces greater electrical signals than the noninvasive techniques. Interference from artifacts is minimized and good readings can usually be obtained.

When more than one fetal heart rate must be monitored at the same time, as in the case of twins, both the invasive and noninvasive methods can be used simultaneously. In this situation, one FHR is obtained by the direct ECG method, the other by a noninvasive method. Uterine contraction can be measured by either method.

17.5 Temperature Measurements

Devices for measuring body temperatures are among the oldest of diagnostic instruments. As indicated in Chapter 5, the systemic temperature and the skin surface temperature are both of clinical importance.

17.5.1 Measurement of Systemic Body Temperature

The systemic body temperature is one of the vital physiological signs. Although a high degree of accuracy is not important for clinical purposes, methods of measuring the temperature must be reliable and easy to perform. In situations where continuous monitoring of a patient's temperature is necessary, the measuring device must not cause discomfort.

In cases where continuous recording of temperature is not required, the *mercury thermometer* is still the standard method of measurement. Since these devices are inexpensive, easy to use, and accurate, they will undoubtedly remain in common use for many years to come. Even so, electronic thermometers, such as the one shown in Figure 17-11, are available as replacement for mercury thermometers. These instruments, which have disposable tips, require much less time for a reading and are much easier to read than the conventional thermometer. Where continuous recording of the temperature is necessary, or where greater accuracy is needed than can be obtained with the mercury thermometer or its electronic counterpart, more sophisticated measuring instruments must be used.

Most electronic thermometers and instrumentation for continuous temperature monitoring of patients utilize *thermistors.* A thermistor is a temperature-sensing device with the characteristic that its electrical resistance varies with temperature. Electronic circuitry converts the resistance value into a meter reading, digital readout, or pen recording of the temperature.

Another temperature-sensing device sometimes used in medical instruments is the *thermocouple,* which produces an output voltage proportional to the temperature at the junction of two dissimilar metals. The small voltage generated at the thermocouple is amplified to operate a readout device or pen recorder.

17.5.2 Skin Surface Temperature Measurements

Although the systemic temperature remains very constant throughout the body, skin surface temperatures can vary several degrees from one point to another. The range is usually from 85 to 95°F. Exposure to

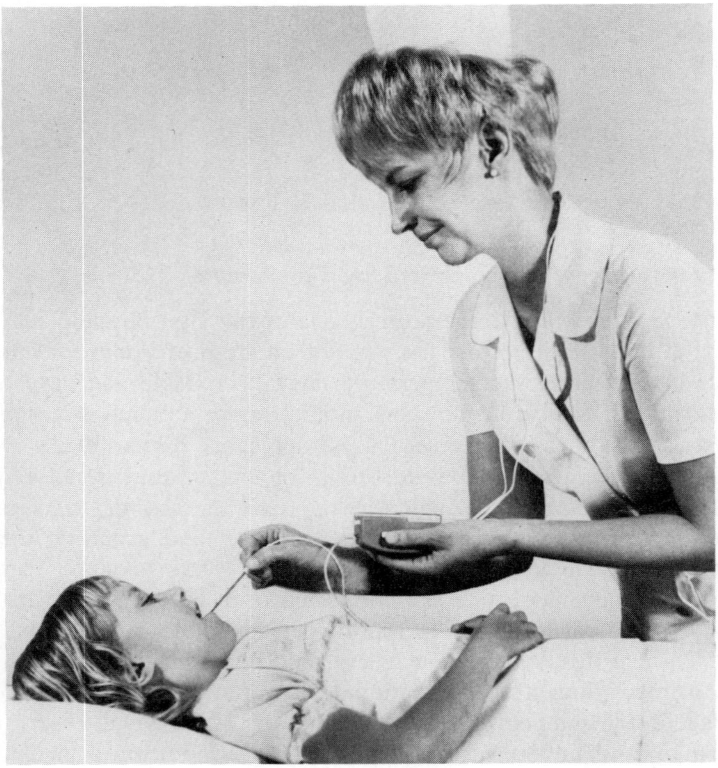

Fig. 17–11 Oral temperature measurement using electronic thermometer. *(Courtesy of Diagnostic, Inc., Indianapolis, Indiana.)*

ambient temperatures, the covering of fat over capillary areas, and local blood circulation patterns are just a few of the factors that influence the distribution of temperatures over the surface of the body. Often skin temperature measurements can be used to detect or locate defects in the circulatory system by showing differences in the pattern from one side of the body to the other.

Skin temperature measurements from specific locations on the body are frequently made by using small, flat thermistor probes taped to the skin. The simultaneous readings from a number of these probes provide a means of measuring changes in the circulatory pattern over a time interval or with a given stimulus.

The human skin has been found to be an almost perfect emitter of infrared radiation. That is, it is able to emit infrared energy in proportion to the surface temperature at any location of the body. If a person is allowed to remain in a room at about 70°F without clothing over the area to be measured, a device sensitive to infrared radiation can accurately read the surface temperature. Such a device, called an *infrared thermometer,* is shown in Figure 17-12. Infrared thermometers in the physiological temperature range are available commercially and can be used to locate breast cancer and other unseen sources of heat. They can also be used to detect areas of poor circulation and other sources of coolness and to measure skin temperature changes that reflect the effects of circulatory changes in the body.

An extension of this method of skin temperature measurement is the *Thermograph,®* shown in Figure 17-13a. This device is an infrared thermometer incorporated into a scanner so that the entire surface of a body, or some portion of the body, is scanned in much the same way that a television camera scans an image, but much slower. While the scanner scans the body, the infrared energy is measured and used to vary the intensity of a light beam that produces a map of the infrared energy on photographic paper. This presentation is called a *thermogram.* Figure 17-13b shows a photograph of two men and a corresponding thermogram. The thermogram shows that each of the two men has an artificial leg. The advantage of this method is that relatively warm and cool areas are immediately evident. By calibrating against known temperature sources, the picture can be read quantitatively.

A similar device, called *Thermovision,®* has a scanner that operates

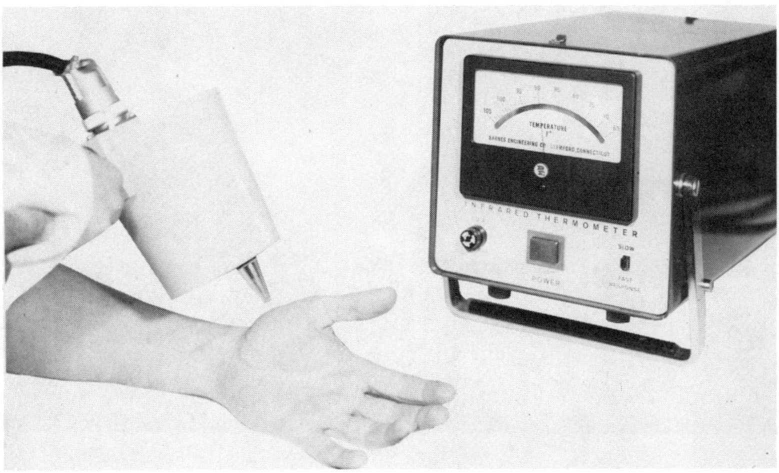

Fig. 17–12 Infrared thermometer. *(Courtesy of Barnes Engineering Co., Stamford, Connecticut.)*

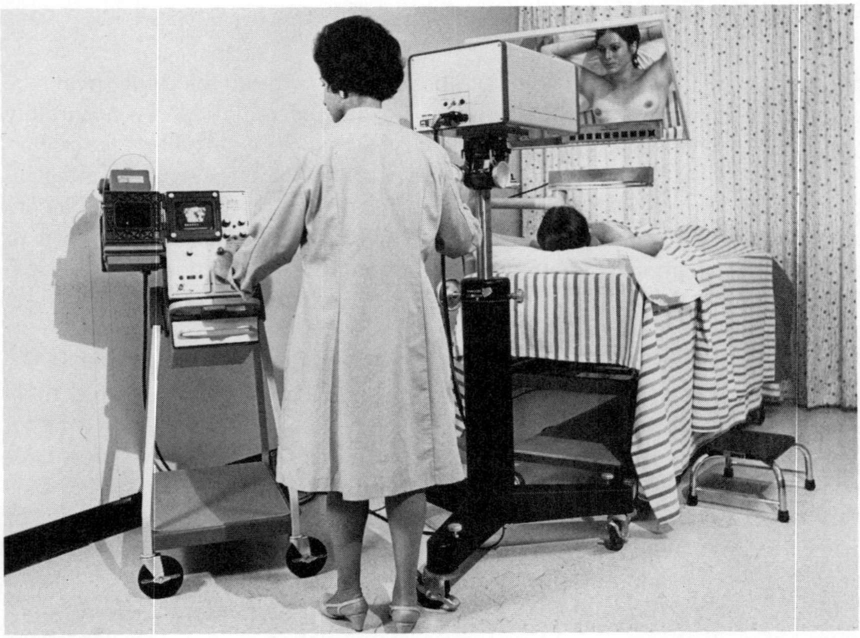

(a)

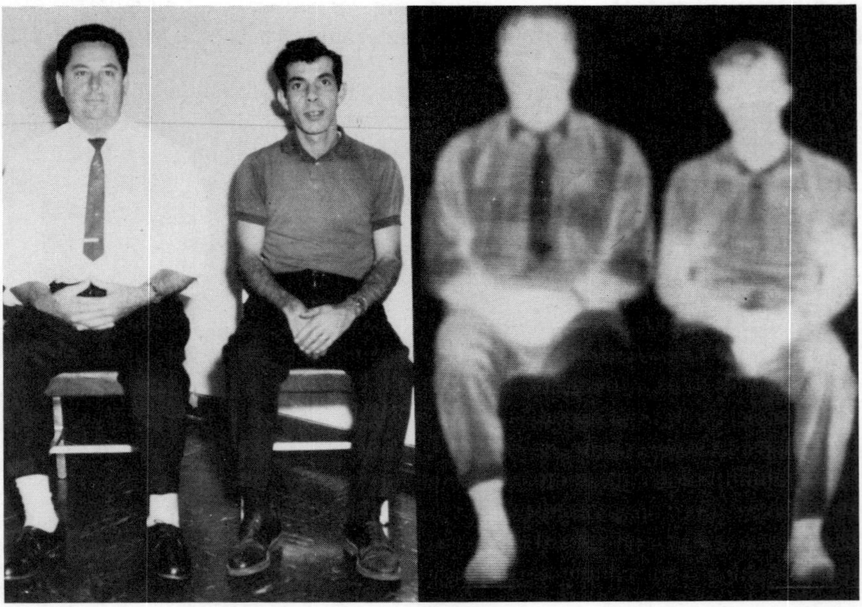

(b)

Fig. 17–13 Thermography: (a) High resolution thermograph; (b) thermogram. (See explanation in text.) *(Courtesy of Barnes Engineering Company, Stamford, Connecticut.)*

at a rate sufficiently high to permit the image to be shown on an oscilloscope. The resulting picture has about 100 vertical lines per frame, and the horizontal resolution is about the same, which seems to be adequate for good representation. The intensity of the measured infrared radiation is reproduced by controlling the brightness of the oscilloscope's electron beam. One advantage of this system is that the picture can be electronically adjusted to bring out specific features. Also, the image can be changed so that warm spots appear dark instead of light, as they do in a thermogram. All these enhancement measures can be performed while the subject is being scanned. A Thermovision® system is shown in Figure 17-14.

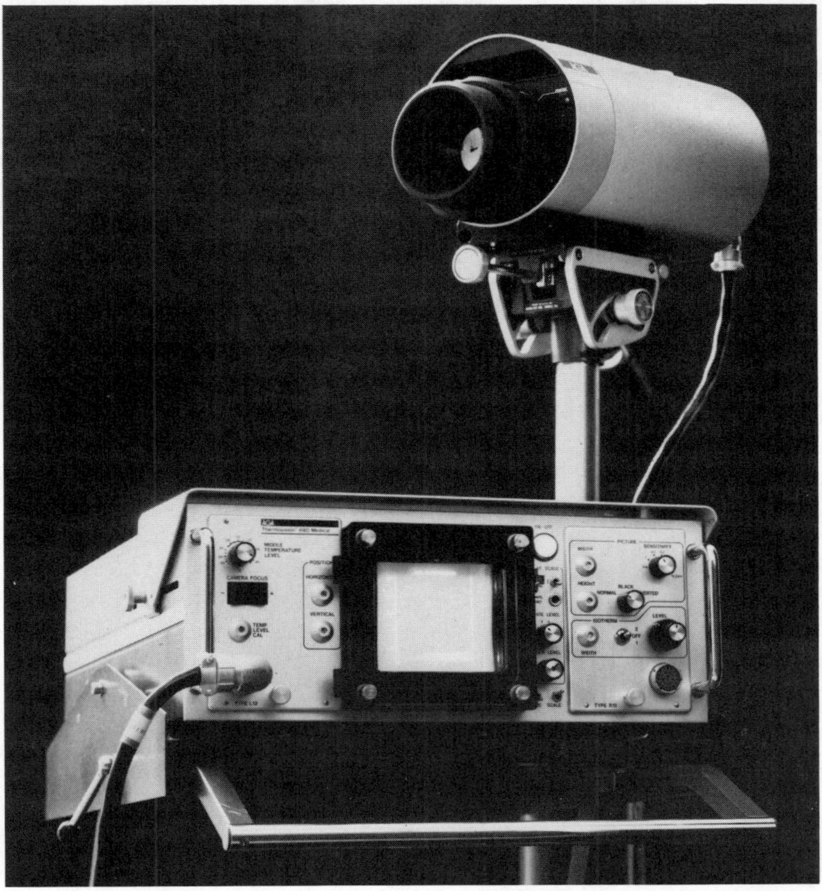

Fig. 17–14 Thermovision system: (a) Thermovision 680 Medical, camera and display unit; (b) Thermovision 680 Medical with accessories. *(Courtesy of AGA Infrared Systems AB, Sweden.)*

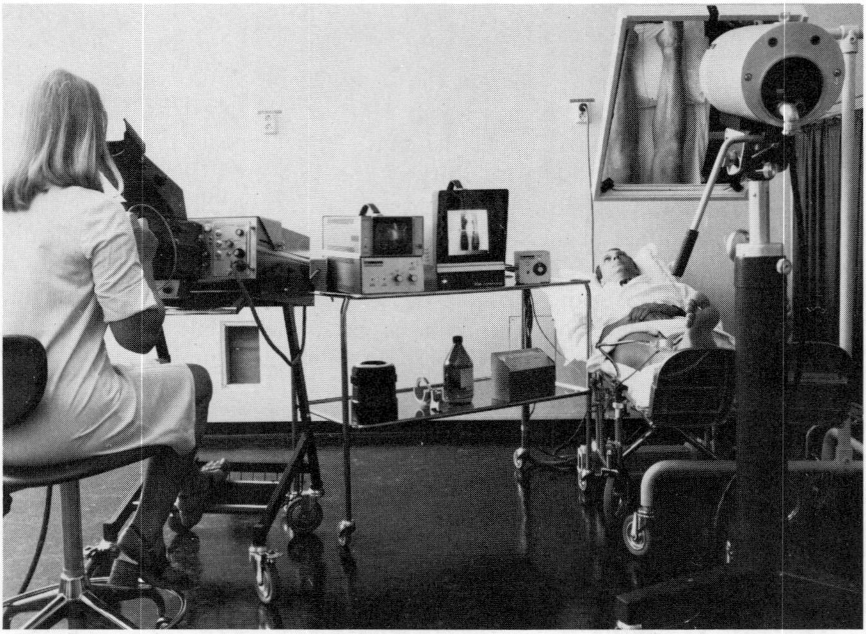

Fig. 17–14 (b) (Continued.)

18

Electrical Safety of Medical Equipment

Each year in the United States about 100,000 people are killed in accidents. About half the fatal accidents occur in motor vehicles, about 20% involve falls, and only about 1% of the fatalities are caused by electric current. The majority of accidental electrocutions occur in industry or on farms. The statistics, which consider medical facilities to be industries, do not specifically show how many of such accidents occur in hospitals, but the number is probably not large. Most electrical accidents, however, are not fatal, but incidents in which staff members or patients receive nonfatal electrical shocks are much more common than the fatality statistics shown.

Recent years have brought a proliferation of electrical and electronic equipment in the hospital. If such equipment is in good working order and used properly, it is relatively safe. Occasionally, however, situations develop in hospitals where equipment is faulty or is used in a way that could precipitate an accident. Usually the personnel using the equipment are not aware of the potential hazard, which in most cases can be avoided with little effort. Thus it is important that all hospital staff be aware of situations that can lead to electrical accidents and become familiar with the simple safety precautions necessary to prevent them.

18.1 Physiological Effects of Electrical Currents

In order for electricity to have any effect on the body, the latter must become part of an electric circuit. At least two connections must exist between the body and an external source of voltage so as to effect a current flow. The magnitude of the current depends on the voltage between the connections and on the electrical resistance of the body. Most body tissue contains a high percentage of water; therefore it is a fairly good electrical conductor. The concepts of resistance and conductors have already been discussed in Chapter 3.

Basically, electric current can affect body tissues in two different ways.* First, the electrical energy dissipated in the tissue resistance can cause a temperature increase. If a high enough temperature is reached, tissue damage (burns) can occur. With household current, electrical burns are usually limited to localized damage at or near the contact points, where the density of the current is the greatest. In industrial accidents with high voltage, as well as in lightning accidents, the dissipated electrical energy can be sufficient to cause burns involving larger parts of the body. In *electrosurgery* the concentrated current from a radio-frequency generator is purposely used to cut tissue or coagulate small blood vessels.

Secondly, the transmission of impulses through sensory and motor nerves involves electrochemical action potentials. An extraneous electric current of sufficient magnitude can cause local voltages that can trigger action potentials and stimulate nerves. When sensory nerves are stimulated in this way, the electric current causes a "tingling" or "prickling" sensation, which at sufficient intensity becomes unpleasant and even painful. The stimulation of motor nerves or muscles causes the contraction of muscle fibers in the muscles or muscle groups affected. A high enough intensity of the stimulation can cause tetanus of the muscle, in which all possible fibers are contracted, and the maximal possible muscle force is exerted, with resulting fatigue and possible injury.

The extent of the stimulation of a certain nerve or muscle depends on the potential difference across its cells and the local density of the current flowing through the tissue. An electric current flowing through the body can be hazardous or fatal if it causes local current densities in vital

* A third type of injury can sometimes be observed under skin electrodes through which a small dc current has been flowing for an extended time interval. These injuries are due to electrolytic decomposition of perspiration into corrosive substances and are, therefore, actually chemical burns.

organs that are sufficient to interfere with the functioning of the organs. The degree to which any given organ is affected depends on the magnitude of the current and the location of the electrical contact points on the body with respect to the organ.

The organ most susceptible to electric current is the heart. If the current is large enough, it can result in complete myocardial contraction, which stops the pumping action of the heart and interrupts the blood circulation. If the circulation is not resumed within a few minutes, first brain damage and then death result, because of the lack of oxygen supplied to the brain's tissues. However, if the current is removed within a short time, the heartbeat resumes spontaneously.

A current of lower intensity that excites only a portion of the heart's muscle fibers can be more dangerous than a current sufficient to cause contraction of the entire heart. This partial excitation can change the electrical propagation patterns in the myocardium, desynchronizing the activity of the heart and causing random, ineffectual muscle activity. This condition is called *fibrillation.* When fibrillation occurs in the ventricles, the heart ceases to pump blood. *Ventricular fibrillation* is normally not reversible, and once induced, regular heart rhythm does not resume even when the current is removed. In order to restore the pumping action of the heart, the heart muscle must be stimulated by a sufficiently strong current pulse from an external *defibrillator.* The complete contraction of all heart muscle fibers resynchronizes the myocardium, after which, hopefully, the heart resumes its normal contractions. Ventricular fibrillation is the most frequent cause of death in fatal electrical accidents.

Respiratory paralysis can also occur if the muscles of the thorax are tetanized by an electric current flowing through the chest or through the respiratory control center of the brain. Such a current is likely to affect the heart also, because of its location.

The magnitude of electric current required to produce a certain physiological effect in a person is influenced by many factors. Figure 18-1 shows the approximate current range and the resulting effects for 1-second exposures to various levels of 60-Hz alternating current applied externally to the body. For those physiological effects that involve the heart or respiration, it is assumed that the current is introduced into the body by electrical contact with the extremities in such a way that the current path includes the chest region (arm-to-arm or arm-to-diagonal leg).

For most people the perception threshold of the skin for light finger contact is approximately 500 μA, although much lower current intensities can be detected with the tongue. With a firm grasp of the hand, the threshold is about 1 mA. A current with an intensity not exceeding 5 mA is generally not considered harmful, although the sensation at this level can be rather unpleasant and painful. When at least one of the contacts with

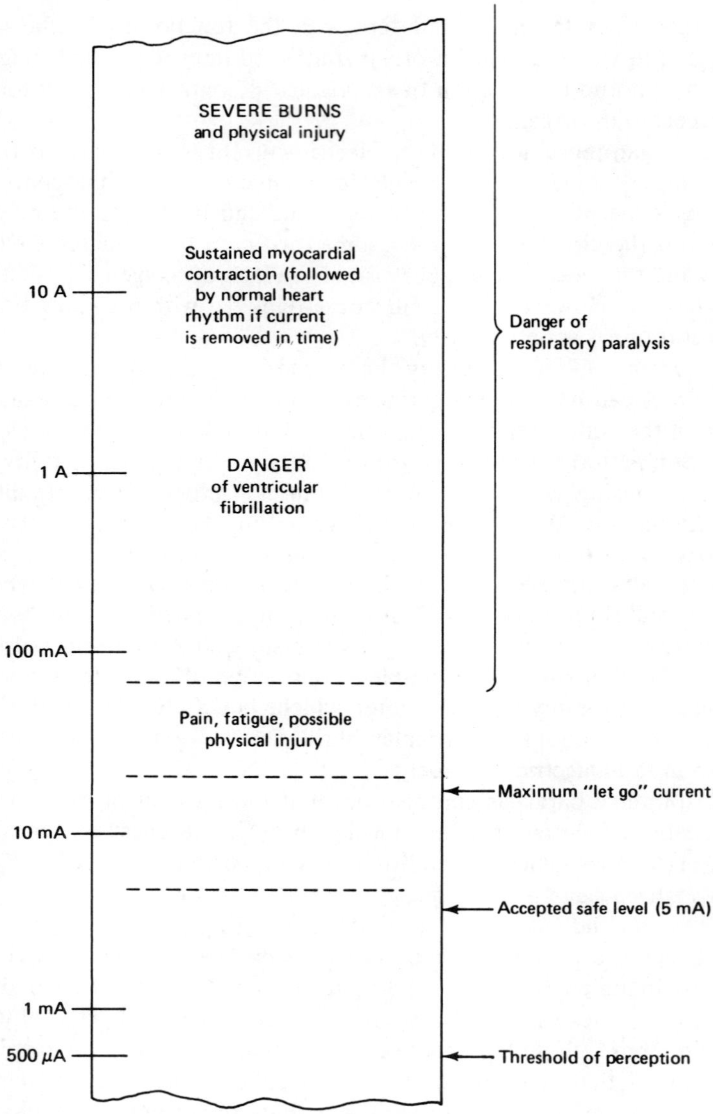

Fig. 18–1 Physiological effects of electrical current (60-Hz line voltage).

the source of electricity is made by grasping an electrical conductor with the hand, currents in excess of about 10 or 20 mA can tetanize the arm muscles and make it impossible to "let go" of the conductor. The minimum current level at which this condition takes place is therefore called the *let-go current*. Ventricular fibrillation can occur at currents above about 100 mA, while currents in excess of about 1 or 2 A cause sustained contraction of the heart, often accompanied by respiratory paralysis.

Data on these effects are rare for obvious reasons and are generally limited to accidents in which the magnitude of the current could be reconstructed, or to experimentation with animals. From the data available it appears that the current required to cause ventricular fibrillation increases with the body weight and that a higher current is required if the current is applied for a very short duration. From experiments in the current range of the perception threshold and let-go current, it is known that the effects of the current are almost independent of frequency up to about 1000 Hz. Above that limit, the current must be increased proportionally with the frequency in order to have the same effect. Thus high-frequency currents are used in electrosurgery to minimize the stimulation of nerves and muscles.

In the foregoing considerations, the electrical intensity is always described in terms of electrical current. The voltage required to cause the current flow depends solely on the electrical resistance that the body offers to the current. This resistance is affected by numerous factors and can vary from a few ohms to several megohms. The largest part of the body resistance is normally represented by the resistance of the skin. Dry, intact skin has a high resistance that is caused mainly by the horny, outermost layer of the skin, the epithelium, which provides a natural protection against electrical danger. When this layer is permeated by a conductive fluid, however, the skin resistance decreases substantially. If the skin is cut or if conductive objects like hypodermic needles are introduced through the skin, the skin resistance is effectively bypassed. Electrode paste used in the measurement of bioelectric potentials also has the effect of reducing the skin resistivity by electrolyte action and mechanical abrasion. Many medical procedures require the introduction of conductive objects into the body, either through natural openings or through incisions in the skin. In many instances, therefore, the hospital patient is deprived of the natural protection against electrical dangers that the skin normally provides. Because of the resulting low resistance, dangerously high currents can be caused by voltages of a magnitude that normally would be rendered safe by the high skin resistance.

To make matters worse, in certain modern medical procedures electrically conductive catheters are introduced not only into the body but also directly into the heart. Such catheters are used for diagnostic purposes (*cardiac catheterization*) to withdraw blood samples from various parts of the heart, to inject radiopaque dye for angiographic procedures, or to measure the blood pressure or cardiac output. In these cases, the catheter provides an electrical connection to the heart through the fluid column that is contained within the insulating catheter. When an externally-worn artificial pacemaker is used in the treatment of heart block, a pacing catheter is inserted into the heart to provide a low-resistance connection. With either type of catheter, the electrically conductive catheter can form one of the two contacts that connect the body to an external electric circuit, as shown in Figure 18-2. When this is the case, all the current flowing through the catheter passes directly through the heart. The current density in the cardiac muscle can, therefore, be several orders of magnitude higher than when the same current is applied to a contact more remote from the heart. As a result, a patient with any type of cardiac catheter is much more sensitive to electric current than he would otherwise be. Such a patient is said to be *electrically susceptible*. The effect of an electric current applied directly to the heart is called *microshock*. In this context, the effect of current when no direct connection to the heart exists is referred to as *macroshock*.

Information on the current necessary to cause ventricular fibrillation when applied directly to the heart is limited. In dog experiments fibrillation could be achieved with as little as 20 μA. In a few measurements on humans whose hearts had to be stopped during open-heart surgery, currents of at least 108 μA were required. To provide a margin of safety, contemporary standards and specifications for medical equipment set much lower limits. For equipment to be used with electrically susceptible patients, the current that accidentally can flow into the patient's heart (*risk current*)

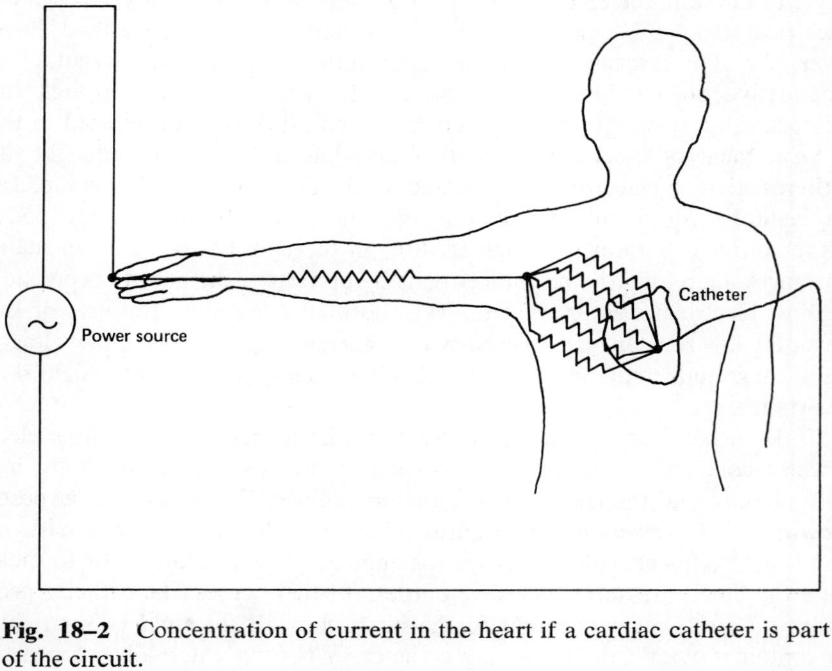

Fig. 18–2 Concentration of current in the heart if a cardiac catheter is part of the circuit.

should not exceed 10 μA. The risk current that can flow in any other patient connection, such as an ECG lead, should be limited to 50 μA. This limit applies to all patients whether electrically susceptible or not. The maximum current that can be obtained by touching the case of an instrument is not to exceed 100 μA if the instrument is likely to contact a patient, and 500 μA if it is not. Under older standards, currents as high as 5 mA were allowed.

18.2 Shock Hazards from Electrical Equipment

In order to be exposed to an electrical shock, the body must be in contact with two electrical conductors that together supply a voltage large enough to deliver a hazardous current. Under normal circumstances nobody would expose himself voluntarily to such a situation. But defective equipment and uninformed users can precipitate hazardous situations rather easily. In order to understand how electrical accidents can happen, it is necessary to understand the principles of the distribution system that brings power to the electrical equipment as it was introduced in Chapter 3.

Electrical power is generated at *power plants* from thermal energy, by burning oil, coal, or gas, from hydroelectric energy or from the nuclear power of an atomic reactor. Through *high-voltage lines* the electricity is then distributed across the country. This high voltage, which is used to reduce the losses on the long lines, is much too dangerous to be brought into households or hospitals. In so-called *substations* (also called *transformer stations*) it is therefore stepped down to safer voltages by means of *transformers*. This stepping down usually occurs in several steps; and a large hospital may have a main transformer station and several local transformer locations, one for each building or floor. One of these transformers is shown in simplified form in Figure 18-3. The high voltage from the main substation enters the transformer, in which it is reduced to 115 V. The output of this transformer actually has two circuits of 115 V each. The two circuits are connected together so that both 115 V and 230 V for larger appliances like portable X-ray machines are available. The normal 115-V wall receptacles are connected to the transformer by two wires that run in a thin steel tube, called a *conduit*. One wire (normally black) connects the contacts in the shorter rectangular slot of the receptacle to one of the 115-V terminals of the transformer. This so-called *hot* wire runs through a circuit breaker located either at the transformer location or on a separate breaker panel.

From the contacts in the longer of the rectangular slots, a white wire runs to the joint terminal for the two 115-V circuits of the transformer. This terminal is connected to the metal enclosure of the transformer as well as to a nearby water pipe or to a metal stake driven into the ground.

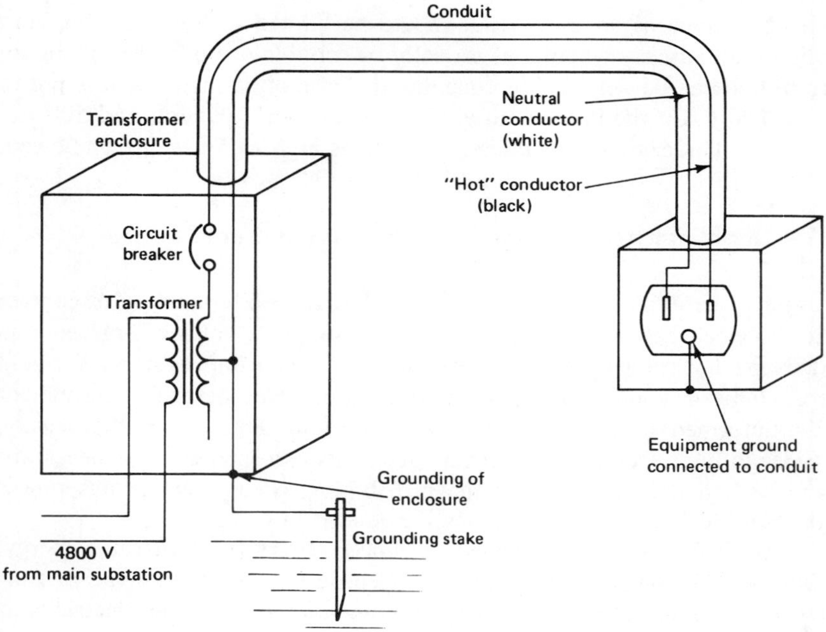

Fig. 18–3 Electric power distribution system (simplified).

Consequently, the white wire, which is called the *neutral* wire, is said to be *grounded* at the transformer. Because the neutral wire is grounded, the line voltage of 115 V exists not only between the hot wire and the neutral wire but also between the hot wire **and any other metallic object that is also connected to ground.** It is this characteristic that is responsible for most electrical accidents. The steel tubing that surrounds the two electrical wires protects them mechanically and serves as a third electrical conductor that connects the grounded metal enclosure of the transformer to the metal boxes in which the receptacles are mounted. The third or U-shaped contact of the receptacle is connected to the receptacle box and is thus grounded through the conduit.

In electrical equipment the heater, transformer, motor, or whatever encompasses its electrical function is connected between the black and the white wires. The electric current therefore comes from the transformer through the hot wire to the equipment and returns through the neutral wire. Both wires, along their way and in the equipment, are carefully insulated with plastic, rubber, or ceramic materials to keep them from coming in contact with each other or with any metal parts that are accessible to the user. Occasionally, however, the insulation becomes defective and one of the two wires comes in contact with the metal case of some piece of equipment or some other exposed metal part. If the wire that makes contact happens to be the hot wire, the dangerous situation shown in Figure 18-4 results. Because the neutral wire is connected to ground, the metal case, which has become "hot" due to the short, can send a dangerous current through the body of any person who touches the case while being in contact with a grounded object at the same time.

Whether this current causes only an unpleasant shock or is large enough to cause an accident due to violent muscle contractions, or even death due to ventricular fibrillation, is determined by the skin resistance at the two points of contact with the body of the victim. If the contact area is large, as it is when one grasps a metallic object, and if the skin is wet from perspiration, water, or any body fluid, the current can be large enough to be dangerous or even fatal. Most electrical accidents in which persons using or operating electrical equipment are killed or injured are the kind that involve simultaneous contact with a faulty piece of equipment and a grounded object. Accidents in which the contacts to the body of the victim are from the hot and the neutral wires of the distribution system are much less frequent. When such accidents occur, they typically involve electricians or servicemen working on power lines or equipment.

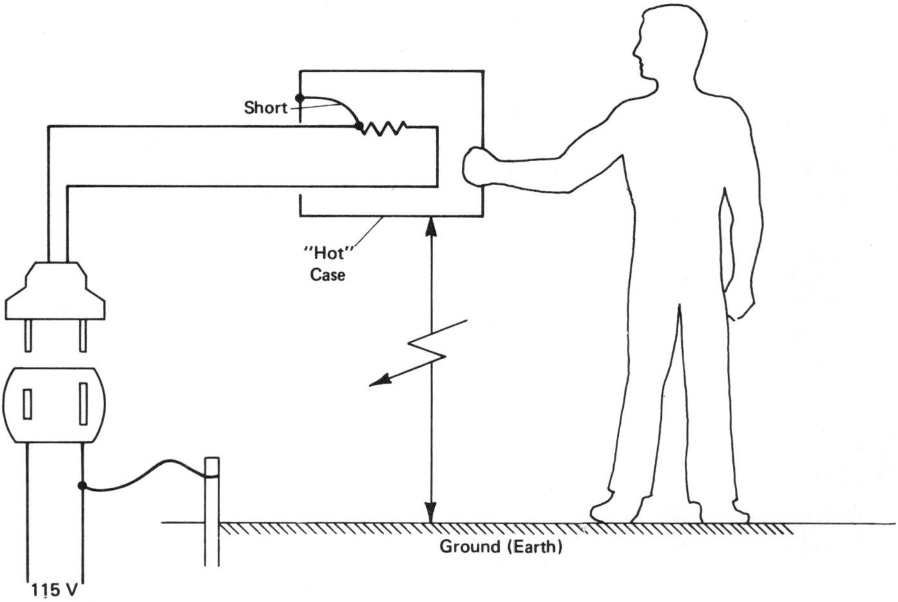

Fig. 18–4 Hazard of ungrounded equipment: short applies line voltage to case.

18.3 Methods of Accident Prevention

In order to reduce the likelihood of electrical accidents, a number of protective methods have evolved. Some are used universally, some are required only in areas that are considered especially hazardous, and still others have been developed especially for use in hospitals.

18.3.1 Grounding

The method of protection used most frequently is the *grounding* of equipment. Its principle is shown in Figure 18-5. In this method the metal case of the equipment is connected to ground by a separate wire. In cord-connected electrical equipment this ground connection is established by the third, round, or U-shaped contact in the plug. If a short occurs in a device whose case has been grounded in this way, the electrical current flows through the short to the case and returns to the substation through the ground wire. Ideally, this short circuit current will be large enough to cause the circuit breaker to trip immediately. This action removes the power from the faulty piece of equipment and thus limits the hazard.

Protection by grounding, however, has several shortcomings. Obviously it is effective only as long as a good ground connection exists. Experi-

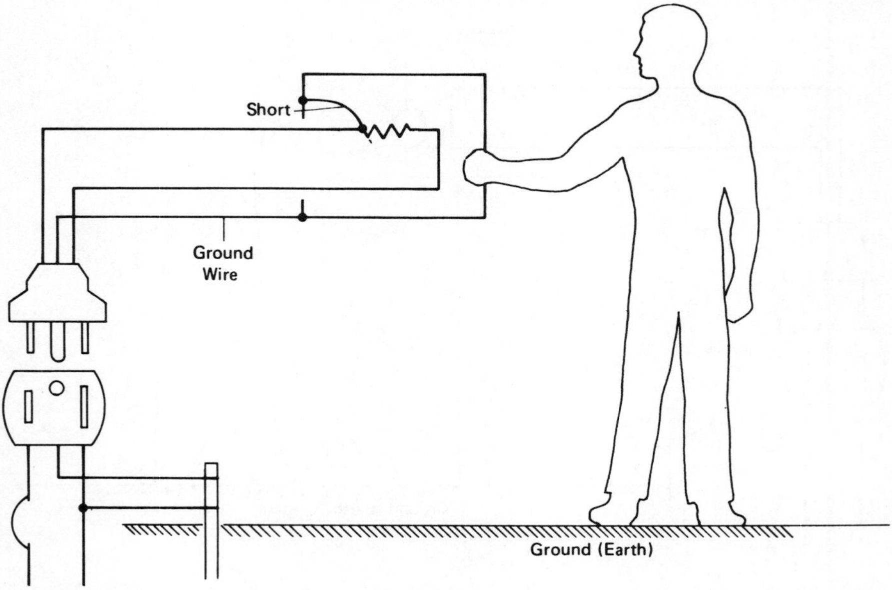

Fig. 18–5 Case of equipment grounded by ground wire and ground pin of line plug.

ence has shown, however, that many electrical receptacles, plugs, and line cords fail, to some degree, under the hard use experienced in a hospital, and an alarmingly high percentage of hospital equipment is not reliably grounded. Also, in order to cause immediate tripping of the circuit breaker, the resistance of the grounding system must be very low. If the resistance is higher, as is sometimes the case when the steel conduits are used instead of ground wires, it may take seconds or even minutes after a short until the circuit breaker trips. During this time the defective equipment is still hazardous. If a fault occurs in such a grounded piece of equipment, safety is achieved by removing power from the whole branch circuit to which the faulty device is connected. In hospitals this removal of electrical power can itself be dangerous if life-sustaining equipment depends on power provided by the same circuit.

18.3.2 Protection by Low Voltage

The higher the voltage, the higher the current that will flow through a person in an electrical accident. By operating equipment from a voltage much lower than the powerline voltage, the potential electrical hazards can be reduced substantially. One way of achieving this situation is to operate equipment from batteries. Aside from the use of a lower voltage, there is the additional advantage that the equipment does not have to be grounded. Although battery operation is generally limited to small devices like razors or toothbrushes, equipment as large as portable X-ray machines sometimes uses this method of protection. Another way of obtaining a lower operating voltage is by means of a small transformer, which, as shown in Figure 18-6, can be located directly in the plug of the equipment. This

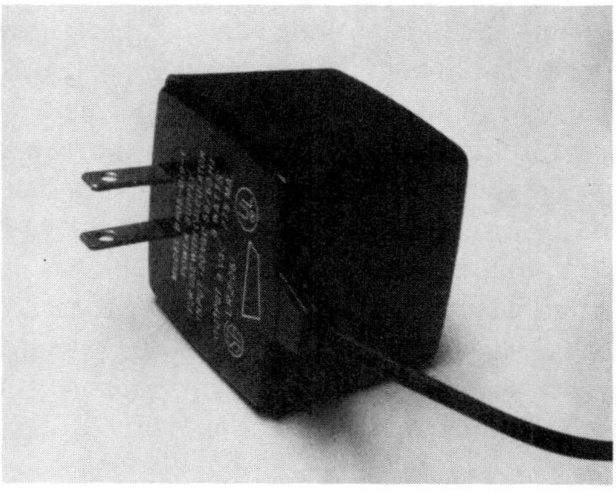

Fig. 18–6 Line plug with built-in low-voltage transformer. *(Courtesy of Veterans Administration Biomedical Engineering and Computing Center, Sepulveda, California.)*

method is often used in medical equipment that contains only a small lamp, like ophthalmoscopes and endoscopes. To provide an additional safety factor, the transformer is normally also utilized to isolate the low-voltage part of the circuit from ground.

18.3.3 Double Insulation

In double-insulated equipment the case is made of a nonconductive material, usually a suitable plastic. If accessible metal parts are used, they are attached to the conductive main body of the equipment by a separate (protective) layer of insulation in addition to the (functional) insulation that separates this body from the electrical parts. Double-insulated equipment need not be grounded, and therefore it is equipped with a plug that does not have a ground pin. Equipment of this type must be labeled "Double Insulated." Double insulation is now widely used as a method of protection in hand-held power tools and electric-powered garden equipment like lawn mowers. Often electric razors can also be considered double insulated even if they are not especially labeled as such. Double insulation, however, is only of limited value for equipment found in a hospital environment. Unless the equipment is also designed to be waterproof, the double insulation can easily be rendered ineffective if a conductive fluid like saline or urine is spilled over the equipment or if the equipment is submerged in such a fluid.

18.3.4 Isolation of Patient-Connected Parts

In many types of medical equipment electrodes or transducers are connected to the body of the patient. Examples are ECG equipment, pressure recorders that connect to indwelling catheters, and electrosurgical machines. In order to simplify the electronic circuits, it was once standard practice to connect one of the electrodes and the metal case of the transducer to ground. In doing so, however, one of the two electrical connections necessary for an electrical accident was automatically provided. Such equipment, therefore, brought with it an inherent safety hazard. To avoid this potential danger, modern equipment of this type has discarded the practice of grounding patient leads and transducers. Modern circuit techniques have made possible the design of amplifiers that are completely isolated from ground. Modern pressure transducers are designed essentially like the double-insulated equipment described earlier without exposed metal parts.

18.3.5 Ground-Fault Circuit Interrupter

Another protection method is the ground-fault circuit interrupter. Its principle is based on the fact that all the current that normally flows into equipment through the hot wire returns through the neutral wire. If, however, a person touches some defective piece of equipment and current returns to ground through his body, the current in the neutral wire will be somewhat smaller than that in the hot wire. The ground-fault circuit interrupter monitors the difference between these two currents, and if it senses a certain difference (usually 5 mA), it interrupts the power like a circuit breaker. This kind of protection is now required for outdoor receptacles and bathrooms in private homes and motels but is also occasionally found in hydrotherapy rooms and renal dialysis units in hospitals.

18.3.6 Isolated Power Distribution Systems

Electrical accidents that occur because the body of the victim is in contact with ground are possible only because the neutral wire is grounded. If both wires of the distribution system were isolated from ground, accidents of this type could be prevented. Although such distribution systems are possible, the method can be used only in very small systems where the distance between the transformer and receptacles is short. Consequently, isolated power systems are seldom used. Exceptions are operating rooms and sometimes intensive care units where isolated power systems are used to provide additional protection. Isolated power systems will be described in more detail in Section 18.6.1.

18.4 Safety Precautions

The method of accident prevention used in a given situation or in a certain type of medical equipment is determined at times by standards and regulations that are set by agencies and institutions on the federal or state level. Sometimes it is up to the manufacturer of the equipment to choose one of several methods of protection, to ensure the continuing effectiveness of the safety measures. Preventive maintenance, on the other hand, is the duty of the technical and engineering staff of the hospital or of companies contracted for this purpose. Hospital personnel who actually use the equipment, however, can render almost any of the safety preventive methods ineffective if they abuse the equipment. Conversely, with sufficient care, the staff can not only maintain a high degree of safety but can also help uncover potentially hazardous defects before they endanger patient or staff. The correct way of using equipment safely can be summed up in a number of Do's and Don'ts.

DON'TS:

DON'T remove plugs from receptacles by pulling on the line cord. Pulling the line cord can cause the ground wire to break or become loose, thus rendering the grounding protection ineffective.

DON'T use "cheater plugs" (adapters) in the hospital. In older hospital buildings where two-wire receptacles without a hole for the ground pin are still encountered, they should be replaced with new receptacles. The use of adapters, in most cases, makes the grounding protection ineffective.

DON'T use extension cords except in an emergency. Properly designed electrical distribution systems for hospitals and other medical facilities should provide a sufficient number of receptacles at the appropriate locations to make the use of extension cords unnecessary. The use of extension cords often jeopardizes the grounding protection and, in addition, presents a tripping hazard. If an extension cord is absolutely necessary, only heavy-duty three-wire cords with connectors providing ground connections should be used. Two-wire extension cords with molded connectors sold for household use are unsuitable for rough usage and thus should never be employed in a medical facility.

DON'T run carts over electrical cables or connectors and don't step on cables or connectors.

DON'T use any electrical equipment without being thoroughly familiar with its operation and the hazards that it might create.

DO's:

DO familiarize yourself with all electrical equipment on the ward, in the operating room, or the medical office by studying the instruction manuals and letting an experienced person explain the proper use of the equipment.

DO observe always the correct operating procedures.

DO report immediately equipment that shows any irregularity, such as shocking the operator, intermittent operation, or loose controls.

DO observe any special instructions or regulations established for certain procedures by the hospital administration.

DO observe any special instructions or labels attached to the instrument.

18.5 Special Safety Precautions in Surgery

Because of the hazards associated with surgery, special safety precautions are necessary for operating rooms, emergency rooms, delivery rooms, and certain related areas of the hospital. Three hazards, in particular, make such precautions necessary to protect patient and staff:

1. Most surgical procedures require incisions in the skin of the patient. In other procedures, objects like endoscopes or probes

are inserted into the body of the patient through natural openings. In either case, the protection otherwise provided by the high resistance of dry, intact skin is effectively bypassed. During surgery a patient is therefore exceptionally vulnerable to electrical hazards.

2. Many surgical procedures require general anesthesia, which is introduced by agents in the form of gases or volatile liquids. Some anesthetics are flammable and, when mixed with air in a certain ratio, can form highly explosive mixtures. Anesthetic explosions have killed and maimed patients and hospital staff on several occasions. Extreme care must be exercised to avoid the introduction of any possible source of igniting sparks when such anesthetics are in use.
3. Electrosurgical machines (commonly called "Bovies" after one particular make) are used in many surgical procedures. This type of device may be the most hazardous of all hospital instruments. Not only has it been the cause of many anesthetic explosions, it can also cause a particular type of burn injury to the patient. Special safety precautions necessary to prevent this type of burn are treated in Chapter 16.

Safety precautions for surgery are specified in a *"Standard for the Use of Inhalation Anesthetics"* (NFPA Standard No. 56A), which has been prepared by the National Fire Protection Association. This standard is followed by virtually all hospitals in the United States. Despite its title and despite the name of the preparing organization, it deals not only with the explosion hazard created by the use of flammable anesthetics but also with electrical shock hazards. The safety measures described below are selected from those required by Standard 56A at the time of writing. The standard is revised at certain intervals, and so the reader is advised to consult the current version of Standard 56A if in doubt about any safety problem.

Many of the safety measures described in NFPA Standard 56A are intended to prevent electrostatic discharges that could ignite explosive mixtures or they concern devices for handling gases. Since neither subject is related to electrical and electronic equipment, they are not covered in this book. The rules of Standard 56A apply to what are referred to as *"Anesthetizing Locations."* These include all areas in which any type of inhalation anesthetics may be used. Because more and more nonflammable anesthetic agents are used today, the standard also differentiates between *Nonflammable Anesthetizing Locations*, where the hazards are mainly of an electrical nature, and *Flammable Anesthetizing Locations,* where the explosion hazard requires additional safeguards.

18.5.1 Isolated Power System

Standard 56A for anesthetizing locations requires that all receptacles for cord-connected electrical equipment as well as the ceiling-suspended operating lamps be powered from an isolated distribution system. As mentioned in Section 18.3.6, such systems are more effective if they are small. The power for the isolated distribution system, therefore, is not supplied from the transformer substation directly but is obtained from a separate isolation transformer for each operating room. This transformer, together with the associated circuit breaker and the line isolation monitor described below, is mounted in a separate enclosure, either in the operating room or adjacent to it. The panel of such an installation is shown in Figure 18-7.

If a short between the case and one of the two wires occurs in a piece of equipment powered from an isolated system, the result will be quite different from that of the grounded system described earlier. Even if the case of the equipment is not grounded properly, someone touching the equipment and a grounded object simultaneously will not receive a shock, for neither of the power conductors is connected to a ground. Nevertheless, a small current can flow through the body of such a person because of the capacity between the conductors of the system and ground. This current, however, will be of a magnitude of at most 1 or 2 mA, which may be perceived without being harmful. If the equipment in which the short occurs is properly grounded, this *leakage current* will return through the ground connection. In this case, however, the short in the faulty equipment effectively grounds one of the conductors of the isolated distribution system. As a result, the isolated system is changed back to a grounded distribution system and all the protection provided by the isolated system is obviated. In order to provide a warning in the event that this situation occurs, isolated power systems employ *line isolation monitors* (LIM). This device alternately checks the two wires of the distribution system for isolation from ground. The degree of isolation, expressed as the so-called *risk current* or *fault hazard current,* is indicated on an electric meter.

In addition to the meter, two warning lamps are provided. When the system is adequately isolated, a green lamp (sometimes labeled "SAFE") will be on. If the isolation begins to deteriorate or if a short occurs between one of the wires and ground anywhere in the system, a red lamp (sometimes labeled "HAZARD") will light up. At the same time, an acoustical alarm will begin to sound. This hazard alarm merely indicates that the system has lost its protective properties. It still requires a second fault before an actual hazard can arise. If the alarm occurs while an operation is in progress, it is therefore possible to complete the procedure before attempt-

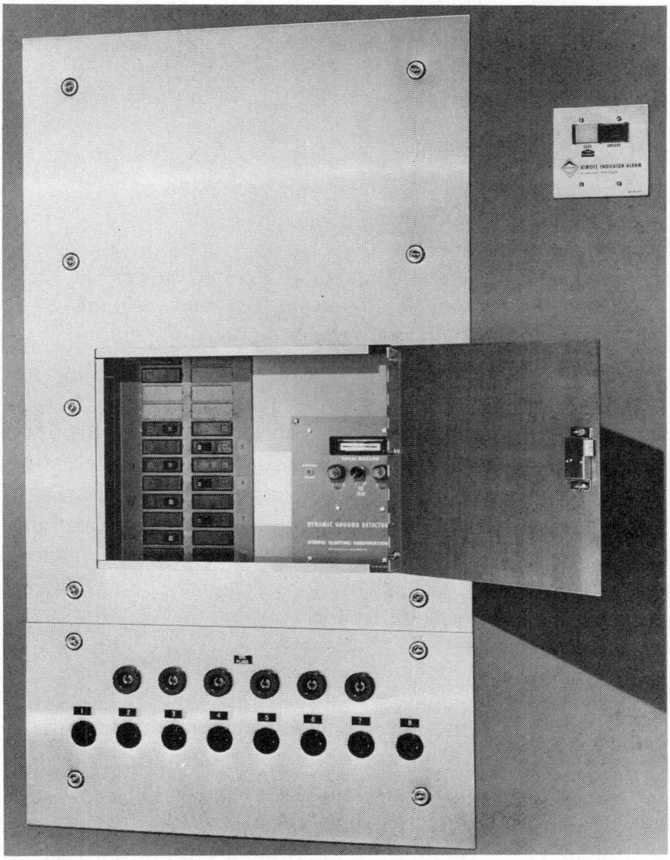

Fig. 18–7 Panel of isolated power distribution system. *(Courtesy of Sorgel Electric Corporation, subsidiary of Square D Company, Oshkosh, Wisconsin.)*

ing to find the cause of the alarm. For this situation, the line isolation monitor has a button with which the acoustical alarm can be silenced. Even if the acoustical alarm is turned off, the red warning lamp remains on, indicating the continued presence of an alarm condition. The line isolation monitor also has a button that allows it to be tested for proper functioning. Pressing this button simultates a short. Both the red lamp and acoustical alarm should come on within a few seconds.

Receptacles powered from an isolated system are not the common three-prong type but are a special locking type, shown in Figure 18-8(a). Where 230 V are required, such as for portable X-ray machines, a similar

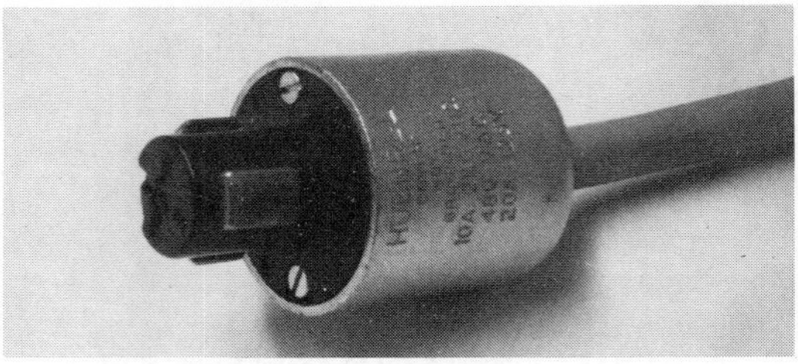

Fig. 18–8 Locking plug for isolated power distribution system. *(Courtesy of Veterans Administration Biomedical Engineering and Computing Center, Sepulveda, California.)*

type is employed. Both types of plugs are connected to the receptacle by lining up the keylike part of the plug with the receptacle, pressing the plug into the receptacle (which requires considerable force), and turning the plug clockwise about one quarter turn. The plug is disconnected by turning it counterclockwise, whereupon it is ejected from the receptacle by spring force.

18.5.2 Grounding System

In addition to the isolated distribution system, NFPA Standard 56A requires a special high-quality grounding system for all anesthetizing locations. This system not only protects the patients and staff by shunting all leakage currents to ground but is also necessary for the proper functioning of the line isolation monitor described in Section 18.6.1. The special grounding system is called an *equipotential grounding* system because it keeps all metallic objects in the area that could possibly come in contact with staff or patient at the same electrical potential. For this purpose, not only the enclosures of electrical equipment but also all other metal objects —operating tables, anesthesia machines, and instrument tables—that might come in contact with electrical equipment must be interconnected by the grounding system. Portable items of this kind may require the use of separate ground wires that are connected to a common grounding point near the head of the operating table. Special bayonet-type plugs are used on this ground wire. It should be noted that all ground wires and associated connectors are of a green color.

The NFPA Standard also requires that an ohmmeter or similar device be provided in each operating room in order to ascertain electric continuity of the equipotential ground, especially to portable devices. Similar equipotential grounding systems are also required for the protection of electrically susceptible patients, as described in Section 18.6. Figure 18-10 shows such a system as it is used in an intensive care unit.

18.5.3 Other Safety Measures

Because of the particular hazards of surgical procedures, Standard 56A requires that any electrical device or part of such a device that may be taken into the operating field by design or accident must be constructed so that spillage of or immersion in a fluid will not result in a shock hazard.

18.5.4 Use of Flammable Anesthetics

The safety measures described thus far are required for all anesthetizing locations; however, additional precautions are necessary in locations where flammable anesthetics may be used. The purpose of these additional measures is to avoid any possibility of sparks, arcs, or high temperatures where an explosive gas mixture may be present. Because the vapors of anesthetics are heavier than air and tend to accumulate at the floor level, all electrical wiring, switches, plugs, and receptacles installed less than 5 ft above the floor must be of a special explosion-proof design. All portable equipment must be designed especially for the hazardous environment and must be labeled so explicitly. The staff must take special care to prevent any equipment not so labeled from being in such a location. Other sections of Standard 56A cover measures that are intended to prevent sparks from electrostatic discharges. Such measures range from conductive flooring to specifications for the textiles used in outer garments to be worn by the staff in flammable anesthetics locations. Because a description is beyond the scope of this book, however, the reader is referred to Standard 56A of the National Fire Protection Association or to the rules and regulations in effect at his place of employment.

18.6 Special Measures for the Protection of Electrically Susceptible Patients

If the current is applied to the body through the skin, a current of at least 100 mA is necessary to cause ventricular fibrillation. Accidents of this type normally occur only if defective equipment or gross negligence is involved. If one of the electrical conductors is applied directly to the heart, however, the patient becomes *electrically susceptible,* and much smaller electrical currents can be hazardous. Currents of a magnitude likely to be dangerous to such patients can be received from perfectly intact equipment due to *capacitive leakage.*

This type of leakage exists whenever energized metal structures—transformers, motors, heaters, and even normal wiring—are surrounded by metal enclosures and the equipment is powered by alternating current. The magnitude of the leakage current depends on the type and physical size of the equipment and can vary from less than 20 μA for small equipment-like examination lamps up to several hundred microamperes for such equipment as portable X-ray machines or certain types of respirators. Because these currents are below the 500-μA level, they cannot be perceived. They are large enough, however, to endanger electrically susceptible patients if they should flow through the electrical connection to the heart. Thus patients of this kind are more endangered, and special measures must be taken in the design of power distribution systems and equipment used with electrically susceptible patients. Since these measures can sometimes fail, special precautions should be taken by the hospital personnel who work around such patients.

18.6.1 Pacing Catheters

Electrical conductors that lead directly to the heart and thus render the patient electrically susceptible can occur in several different medical procedures. When a pervenuous pacing catheter is inserted for temporary pacing with an external electrical pacemaker, the electrical connection to the heart is created intentionally. The resistance of the pacing catheter is very low, and even small voltages that might accidentally come in contact with the external connection of the catheter could endanger the patient. For this reason, the external connection of such pacing catheters should be treated with extreme care. Early external pacemakers were line operated, and the medical literature reports several incidents in which faulty or ungrounded pacemakers caused fibrillation.

Most modern external pacemakers are battery operated to prevent accidents of this kind, although a properly designed line-operated pacemaker should be equally safe. The dangers associated with external pacemakers have only been fully appreciated since the early 1970s. Pacemakers built before that time made no effort to prevent accidental contact with the pacing leads, and they have terminals with easily accessible metal parts, as shown in Figure 18-9. Where pacemakers of this kind are still in use, great care should be taken to avoid accidental contact with any metal parts of the pacemaker and the pacing catheter. If necessary, insulating covers should be used. If the terminals of the pacing leads must be handled, either during insertion of the catheter or when the pacemaker has to be changed or adjusted, they should be touched only while wearing dry, intact, surgical-type rubber gloves.

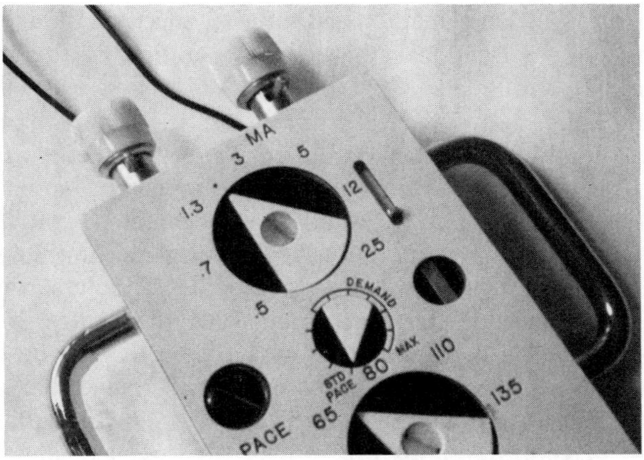

Fig. 18–9 Older pacemaker with terminals that expose metal parts. Great care should be exercised to avoid touching the conductive parts. *(Courtesy of Veterans Administration Biomedical Engineering and Computing Center, Sepulveda, California.)*

Pacing catheters are normally inserted under fluoroscopic control, either in the cardiac catheterization laboratory or using a portable fluoroscope ("C-arm") at the bedside. As an emergency procedure, however, they can be inserted without a fluoroscope by watching the ECG signal on a monitor or recorder that is connected to the terminals of the catheter. For this purpose, however, only modern ECG monitors or ECG recorders with isolated patient leads (see Section 18.3.4) should be used. Older devices, in which the RL lead is grounded, could inject hazardous currents into the catheter and thus endanger the patient.

18.6.2 Fluid-Filled Catheters

Fluid-filled catheters are inserted into the heart to establish a hydraulic connection for the injection of dyes in angiography and cardiac output determinations or for the measurement of intracardiac pressures. Because the catheter for this procedure is made of electrically insulating materials while the fluid in the catheter is electrically conductive, an electrical connection is also established. Although the electrical resistance of the fluid-filled catheter is much higher than that of the metallic pacing catheter, fluid-filled catheters can nevertheless endanger the patients on which they are used. Therefore modern power injectors for angiographic procedures have their syringes designed in such a way that the radiopaque dye does not come in contact with the metal parts of the injector. In addition, some injectors have safety interlocks that allow operation of the injector only when it is properly grounded.

Similarly, modern pressure transducers are designed with plastic bodies to prevent the fluid in the catheter from coming in contact with metal parts that could possibly inject a current into the catheter. An elecrical connection to the heart can also be established accidentally without the staff being aware of it. In a study published in the medical literature, 300 patients in whom 16-gauge, 24-in. disposable catheters were inserted through an arm vein for the measurement of the central venous pressure were examined radiologically. It was found that in not fewer than 13% of the patients the end of the catheter had inadvertently been positioned in the right atrium or right ventricle. Patients with catheters for the measurement of central venous pressure or for fluid exchange procedures should, therefore, also be considered as electrically susceptible.

18.6.3 Protective Measures

Patients for which a connection to the heart has been established in one of the ways described above must be given special protection from electrical hazards. All the safety precautions recommended for general care and described in Section 18.5 should be followed with great care. Current standards require that new installations for the care of electrically susceptible patients (intensive care and coronary care units) be equipped with equipotential grounding systems of the type used in operating rooms described in Section 18.5.2. The purpose of such a system, shown in Figure 18-10, is to ensure that no hazardous voltages can exist in the vicinity of the patient. Some hospitals even use isolated power distribution systems of the type described in Section 18.5.1 in intensive and coronary care units, although this practice has been subject to controversy. No matter which additional safety measures are employed for electrically susceptible patients, the most important protection is obtained through the alertness of the hospital staff and the attention given to the external end of any catheter which is likely to provide an electrical connection to the heart of the patient.

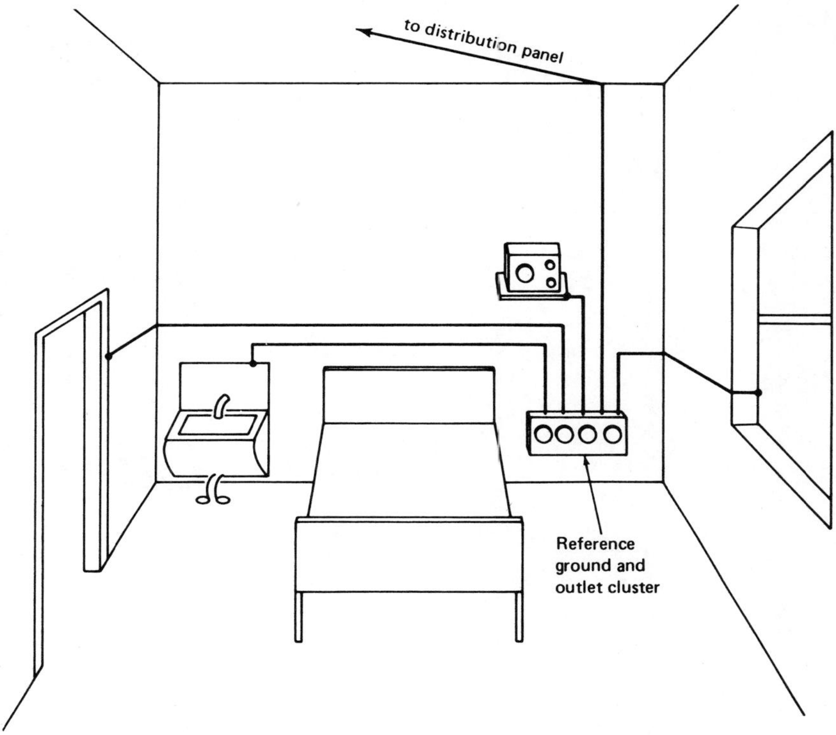

Fig. 18–10 Principle of an equipotential grounding system in one cubicle of a modern intensive care unit.

19

Computers in Health Care

The development of the digital computer and the application of computer techniques to medicine and allied fields have ushered in a new era of progress in patient care. In fact, it may be shown someday that no other single event will have had the impact on the practice of medicine that the computer has created. Coupled with recent developments in medical instrumentation, the advent of the computer has placed a powerful new tool in the hands of the physician and medical practitioner, one by which they can greatly enhance their capabilities.

Anyone involved in patient care is apt to encounter a computer, or at least some aspect of automatic information processing, at some point along the way. Consequently, a basic knowledge of computer terminology and some of the more widely used applications of computers in clinical medicine is important in the training of the modern practitioner. The purpose of this chapter is to provide this background and an appreciation of the capabilities of the digital computer without overwhelming the reader with technical details. Personnel who actually program or operate computerized medical equipment will, of course, require specialized training in the specific instrumentation system with which they will become involved.

19.1 Basic Computer Terminology

Although it may appear that some degree of intelligence or magic is involved, it must be realized that a computer is nothing more than an elaborate machine capable of rapidly carrying out a set of instructions that has previously been worked out by a human mind. This set of instructions is called a *computer program,* and the person who writes the instructions is called a *programmer*. In writing a computer program, certain strict rules of format and punctuation must be followed so that the computer can interpret the instructions. A set of these rules constitutes a *programming language*. Programming languages have names like *FORTRAN* (derived from *FOR*mula *TRAN*slation), *BASIC*, and *COBOL* (derived from *CO*mmon *B*usiness *O*riented *L*anguage). All these languages are widely used in the writing of programs for various computer applications associated with patient care.

All the programs used by a computer in carrying out its functions are called *software*. By contrast, the *hardware* of a computer system consists of all the physical equipment involved. The computer itself is often called the *central processing unit (CPU)*. However, the computer hardware also includes any number of *peripheral devices,* such as typewriters, printers, and TV-type displays.

Regardless of its size or complexity, a computer generally consists of four basic parts: an *arithmetic unit* in which mathematical computations and decision-making processes take place; a *memory* in which information and programs are stored; one or more *input* or *output (I/O) devices* through which the computer is able to communicate with its users; and a *control unit,* which interprets the instructions of the program, one by one, and coordinates all the other parts of the system.

The primary memory in most computers consists of a vast array of tiny doughnut-shaped magnetic devices, called *cores,* that are magnetized by electric current applied to wires running through their centers. In an increasing number of cases, however microscopic electronic *integrated circuits* are used instead of the cores. In either type of memory, information can be stored or retrieved, often in less than a millionth of a second. Additional memory is frequently provided by magnetic disks or special tapes that have greater storage capacity than the primary memory but that are slower in their operation.

Because numbers and letters of the alphabet are stored and manipulated in electronic circuits and magnetic cores, they must be handled in a form that is compatible with such devices. Thus each number or letter in the computer is represented by a *binary code,* a group of digits, each of which can be either a "one" or a "zero." Each binary digit is called a *bit.* The group of bits used to represent a letter or number is called a *character,* and the group of bits that the computer stores and handles as a unit is called the *computer word.* A character may be six or eight bits, while typical computer word length ranges from 12 to 32 bits. Some computers operate with variable word lengths. In such cases, the information is organized into eight-bit segments, called *bytes.* Each word is therefore some number of bytes.

In the primary memory of the computer, a core or electronic circuit is required for each bit of storage. In a 16-bit computer with a core memory, for example, 16 cores are required for each word. The *memory size* of a computer is given as the number of words that can be stored in the primary memory. For instance, a small computer may be designated as having an 8K core memory. This means that the computer has a core storage capacity of about 8000 words. Large computer systems, by contrast, may have nearly a million words of core storage. Such systems also have additional tape and disk storage with a capacity of many millions of words.

The size and complexity of a computer system are determined by the assortment of peripheral devices and the capability of its arithmetic unit as well as its storage capacity. A large, versatile system will usually have a variety of input and output devices and can serve a large number of users. If it is able to serve several users simultaneously, the computer is said to be a *time-sharing* system. Because of the speed at which it can operate, a time-sharing system is capable of servicing each of its users as though he were the only one using the computer at the time. Each user has an input-output device called a *remote terminal,* which is connected to the computer by means of a direct hookup or via a telephone line (see Chapter 13). The terminal may consist of a simple keyboard and typewriter, such as the *Teletype®* machine shown in Figure 19-1, or it may be much more elaborate. Many computer terminals have *cathode-ray-tube (CRT)* displays of the type shown in Figure 19-2. The CRT display also has a keyboard from which information and instructions can be entered into the computer.

A hospital utilizing a time-sharing system may have its own computer, or it may subscribe to a commercial time-sharing service. Where a hospital has its own equipment, terminals at various locations throughout the hospital are usually connected directly to the computer by means of wires or cables. Hospitals that are spread among several buildings may utilize telephone lines to interconnect some of the more distant terminals

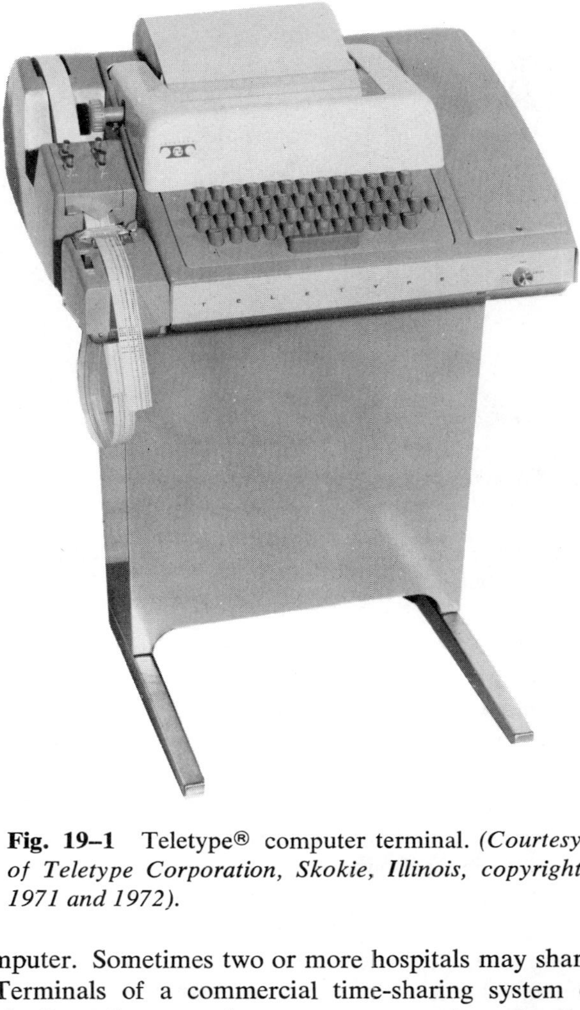

Fig. 19–1 Teletype® computer terminal. *(Courtesy of Teletype Corporation, Skokie, Illinois, copyright 1971 and 1972).*

with the computer. Sometimes two or more hospitals may share a common computer. Terminals of a commercial time-sharing system can be connected by telephone lines to a large computer, perhaps hundreds of miles from the hospital.

In some hospitals, instead of a time-sharing system, a small computer is used for each individual application. For example, one such computer may be used to process test results from the clinical laboratory and another may be incorporated in the patient-monitoring system in the intensive and coronary care units. Computers of this type are said to be *dedicated* to a specific task and are programmed just for that task. In most cases they are connected directly to the instrumentation system they serve. Sometimes, the computer is built into the instrumentation.

Small computers of this type are generally designated as *minicomputers,*

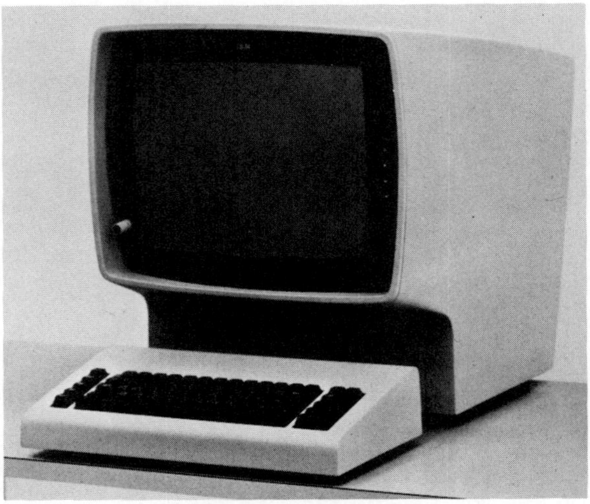

Fig. 19–2 Cathode-ray-tube computer terminal. *(Courtesy of IBM Corporation.)*

although that term can also be used for smaller computers used in time-sharing applications.

When a computer accepts information as it is being generated by instrumentation in the hospital, it is said to be *on line*. If the information is recorded and later taken to the computer, the system is *off line*. If the computer is able to perform its calculations and process the information as rapidly as it is received, it is said to operate in *real time*. With an on-line computer operating in real time, results of a clinical procedure can be provided while the patient is still connected to the instrumentation. In this situation, any required repetitions of the procedure can be performed without having to recall the patient.

As stated in Chapter 13, the output signals from most medical instruments are in *analog* form, in which the variable being measured is represented by a voltage that varies with time. However, because a digital computer handles and stores information in *digital* form (numbers or letters of the alphabet), the analog signals must be converted into digital form, or *digitized*. Where this process is necessary, an *analog-to-digital* converter is required to measure or *sample* the signal voltage at a sufficiently high rate to keep up with all possible variations and provide a digital value for each sample. By means of a special switching device, called a *time-multiplexer,* the output signals from several instruments can be digitized simultaneously by a single analog-to-digital converter.

19.2 Capabilities of a Digital Computer

Applications of the digital computer in clinical medicine and related fields are so numerous that even listing all of them is beyond the scope of this book. Most of these applications, however, utilize a few basic capabilities of the computer that provide an insight to ways in which computers can be used in conjunction with biomedical instrumentation. These basic capabilities are listed below.

1. *Data acquisition.* The reading of instruments and transcribing of information can be done automatically under control of the computer. The results are a substantial saving in time and effort and a reduction in the number of errors in the data. When data are expected at irregular intervals, the computer can continuously scan all input sources and accept information whenever it is produced. If the data originate in analog form, the computer can control the sampling and digitizing process as well as the identifying and formatting of the data. In some cases, the computer can be programmed to reject unacceptable readings and provide an indication of possible trouble in the associated instrumentation. Sometimes the computer provides automatic calibration of each input source.
2. *Storage and retrieval.* The ability of the digital computer to store and retrieve large quantities of data is well known. The biomedical field provides ample opportunities to use this capability. In a modern hospital large amounts of data are accumulated from many sources. These sources include admission and discharge information, physicians' reports, laboratory test results, and several other kinds of information associated with each patient. In addition, the hospital also generates a considerable amount of non-patient-oriented data, such as pharmacy records, inventories of all types, and accounting records. Without a computer, the storage of this vast amount of information is both space and time consuming. Manual retrieval of the data is tedious and, for some types of information, almost impossible. The digital computer, however, can serve as an automated filing system in which information can be automatically entered as it is generated. These files can be stored as long as necessary and updated whenever appropriate. Any or all of the information can be retrieved on command whenever desired.

3. *Assimilation and organization of information.* In addition to simply storing and retrieving data, the digital computer can be programmed to organize the stored information in various ways. For example, data related to a given patient can originate at various times and from many different sources within the hospital. To generate a patient data file, the computer must assimilate all information from each patient as it arrives and file it with data already in the computer for that patient. The computer can then organize the data and prepare a complete report, including all tests for the day. Furthermore, if desired, any given test result can be reported along with similar data from previous days to permit the physician to observe day-to-day changes. The data can also be manipulated in other ways for special purposes as appropriate. While these types of data manipulation are relatively simple with a computer, they can be extremely cumbersome if performed manually, particularly where large amounts of data are involved.
4. *Data reduction and transformation.* The sequence of numbers resulting from digitizing an analog physiological signal such as the ECG or EEG would be quite useless if retrieved from the computer in their original form. To obtain meaningful information from such data, some type of data reduction or transformation is necessary to represent the data as a set of specific parameters. For example, the values and durations of the various features of the ECG waveform must be derived from the raw ECG signal and average values must be obtained over several heart cycles. These types of data reduction can easily be accomplished by the computer.
5. *Mathematical operations.* Many important physiological variables cannot be measured directly but must be calculated from other variables that are accessible. For example, many of the respiratory parameters described in Chapter 14 can be calculated from the results of a few simple breathing tests and gas concentration measurements. Where a digital computer is connected on-line with the measuring instruments, the calculated results can be obtained while the patient is still connected to the instruments. As a result, the physician is able to conduct further tests if the results so indicate and knows immediately if any measurements were not properly made and require repetition.
6. *Pattern recognition.* In order to reduce certain types of physiological data into useful parameters, it is often necessary that important features of the physiological waveform be identified.

For example, analysis of the ECG waveform requires that the important peaks and intervals of the electrocardiogram be recognized and identified. Digital computer programs are available to search the data representing the ECG signal for certain predetermined characteristics that identify each of the important peaks. Similar methods are used in other pattern recognition problems, but since each type of pattern has unique features that must be identified, programming for pattern recognition is a highly specialized process.

7. *Limit detection.* In applications involving monitoring and screening, it is often necessary to determine when a measured variable is outside certain normal limits. For example, in the analysis of the electrocardiogram, each important parameter of the ECG can be checked to determine whether it falls within a preestablished "normal" range. By comparison of the measured parameter with the upper and lower normal limits, the computer can indicate which parameters are outside the normal range and the amount by which they deviate from normal. Using this technique, patients can be screened to select those with ECG irregularities that should receive further attention. In most cases, the "normal" range is defined in advance, but sometimes the computer is programmed to establish normal ranges for each patient based on the averages of repeated measures taken under specified conditions.
8. *Statistical analysis of data.* In the diagnosis of disease it is often necessary to select one most likely cause out of a set of possible causes associated with a given set of observed symptoms, measurements, and test results. Similarly, medical research investigators must decide at times whether an observed change or condition in a person or animal is due to some treatment imposed by the researcher or whether the result could be attributed to some other cause or just to chance alone. Both situations require the use of inferential statistical procedures, some of which are quite complex. Fortunately, most statistical methods lend themselves well to computer techniques, especially when large numbers of variables must be analyzed together or where data from a large number of patients are used. Even simple descriptive statistics, such as means, standard deviations, and frequency distributions, can be computerized, thus resulting in significant savings of time and effort.
9. *Data presentation.* An important characteristic of any instrumentation and data processing system is its ability to present the

results of measurements and analyses to its users. Through appropriate output devices, a digital computer can provide information in a number of useful forms. Table printouts, graphs, and charts can be produced automatically, with features clearly labeled using both alphabetic and numeric symbols. If the necessary computer peripherals are available, plots and cathode-ray-tube displays can also be generated. In addition to controlling the output devices, the computer can be programmed to organize the data for presentation in the most meaningful form possible, thus providing the user with a clear and accurate report of his results.

10. *Control functions.* Digital computers can be equipped to provide analog or digital output signals that can be used to control other devices. In this case, the computer can be programmed to influence or control the physiological, chemical, or other measurement process from which its input data are being generated. In essence, the computer can be used to provide feedback to the source of its data. For example, while reading and analyzing the results of a chemical process, the computer can be made to control the rate, quantity, or concentration of reagents added to the process, or it could control the heating element of a temperature bath. By controlling these and other possible inputs, the process can be regulated to achieve desired results. In addition, the computer can be programmed to recognize certain characteristics of the measured results that would indicate possible sources of error. Sometimes other parameters are monitored in addition to the actual results in order to increase the sensitivity of the computer to conditions that may result in erroneous measurements. The computer can be made to automatically compensate for some sources of error, such as a gradual drift in the baseline, by either altering the process itself or by mathematically adjusting the results before printing them out. When more serious types of error occur, the computer can alert the operator to the condition, or if necessary, can automatically stop the process.

The extent to which each of these capabilities can actually be utilized in a given situation depends on the available *hardware* (equipment and circuitry in the computer and associated devices) and *software* (computer programs) in the system. Obviously some of these capabilities require greater resources than others.

19.3 Computer Applications in Clinical Medicine

For many years the principal function of the computer in the hospital was connected with billing, accounting, and other business applications. Only recently has it found a role in direct patient care. Following are descriptions of some of the more common clinical applications.

19.3.1 Computerized Patient Monitoring

Instrumentation for the monitoring of patients in special care units was described in Chapter 11. When the patient-monitoring system includes a digital computer, its ability to detect physiological situations that require attention and to provide useful information to the physician can be greatly increased.

Commercially available computerized patient-monitoring systems are just beginning to appear in hospitals around the United States. In some cases, the computer does little more than store and retrieve the monitored information and display trends in certain variables. More elaborate systems perform some analysis of the data for detection of arrhythmias and determination of certain parameters, such as systolic, diastolic, and mean blood pressure values.

Each of the monitored variables is sampled and digitized at an appropriate rate under computer control. These variables usually include the ECG waveform (or, in some cases, only heart rate), arterial and possibly venous blood pressure from indwelling catheters, temperature and sometimes respiration rate. Patient information (identification, weight, height, age, etc.), blood gas values, and other manually obtained information are entered into the computer by keyboard.

In addition to the continuous display of ECG and blood pressure waveforms and the indication of alarm conditions, a computerized patient-monitoring system serves as a valuable source of information to the physician or nurse. Whenever desired, past or present information, either measured or derived, can be printed out or displayed on a cathode-ray-tube screen. In some systems, curves showing day-to-day or hour-to-hour changes in certain parameters can be displayed.

Some large hospitals have more elaborate computerized patient-monitoring systems that are able to calculate such parameters as stroke volume, cardiac output, and peripheral vascular resistance. Such systems are also able to perform much more elaborate analyses of data in order to detect situations in which the attention of the nurse or physician is required. Trends in certain parameters as well as current values are sometimes considered in such analyses. Some of these capabilities will undoubtedly be included in new systems that will become commercially available in the future.

Two basic types of computerized patient-monitoring systems are available. The type shown in Figure 19-3 incorporates a general-purpose minicomputer that is programmed specifically for the patient-monitoring task. Analog-to-digital conversion and appropriate devices are included to obtain data from the various monitor channels. A CRT display is provided for presentation of data and curves. In some systems, the CRT display is also used for display of ongoing ECG or pressure waveforms.

The other type of system does not include a general-purpose computer but instead incorporates computer circuitry to control the display of waveforms and to store and retrieve information. A patient-monitoring system of this type is shown in Figure 19-4. The manufacturer describes the system as a "noncomputer computer patient-monitoring system."

The system shown in Figure 19-4 has a nonfade display in which the waveforms move across the screen with uniform brightness. An alphanumeric display of the value and alarm limits for each parameter and patient identification for each tracing on the screen are provided with

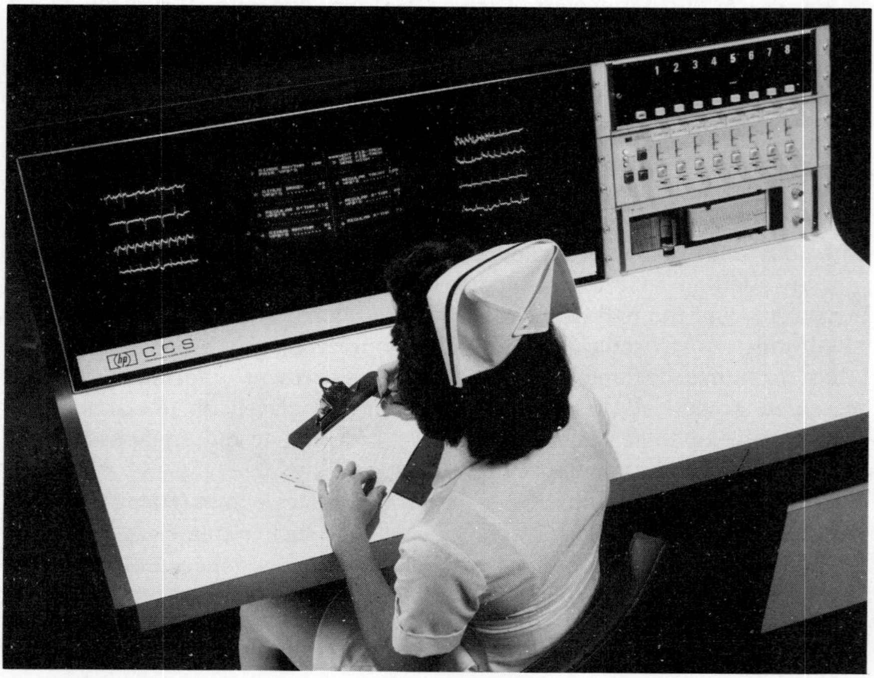

Fig. 19–3 Nurses' station of computerized patient-monitoring system. *(Courtesy of Hewlett-Packard Company.)*

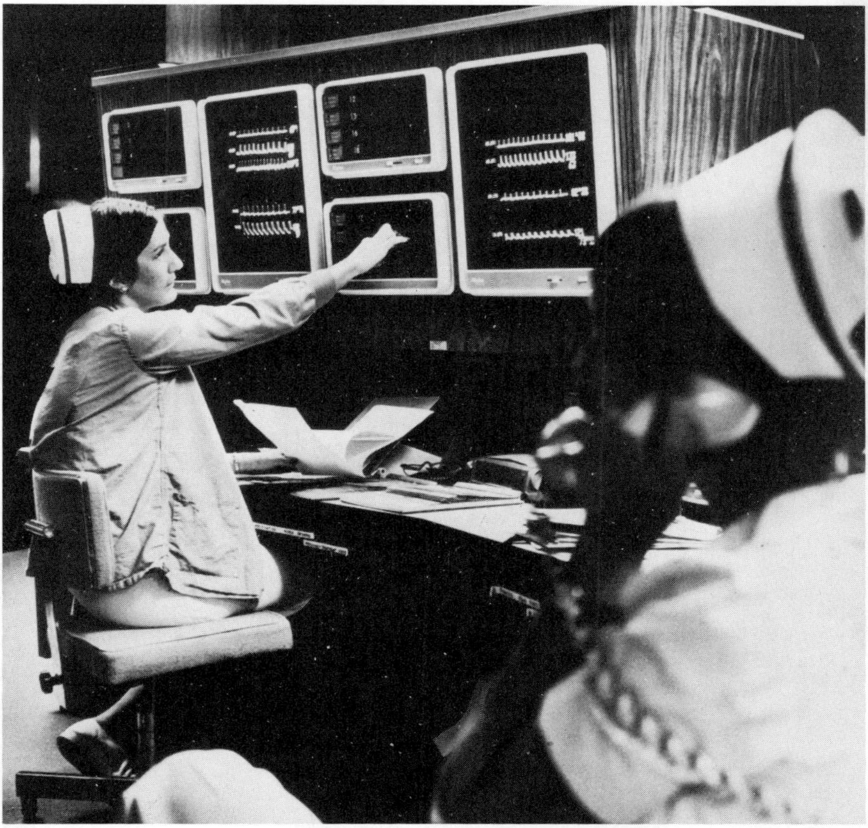

Fig. 19–4 Patient monitoring system utilizing computer-type circuitry to provide nonfade display: (a) Nurses' station. *(Courtesy of Spacelabs, Inc., Chatsworth, California.)*

the waveforms. Scales and identification information are also given for each trend plot.

19.3.2 Computer Analysis of the Electrocardiogram

The greatest progress to date in the use of computers for the clinical analysis of physiological data has occurred in the field of cardiology. There are several reasons. First, ECG potentials are relatively easy to measure. Secondly, the ECG is an extremely useful indicator for both screening and diagnosis. In addition, certain abnormalities of the ECG are quite well defined and can be readily identified.

Measurement of the electrocardiogram for computer analysis is essentially the same as in manual ECG interpretation except that some

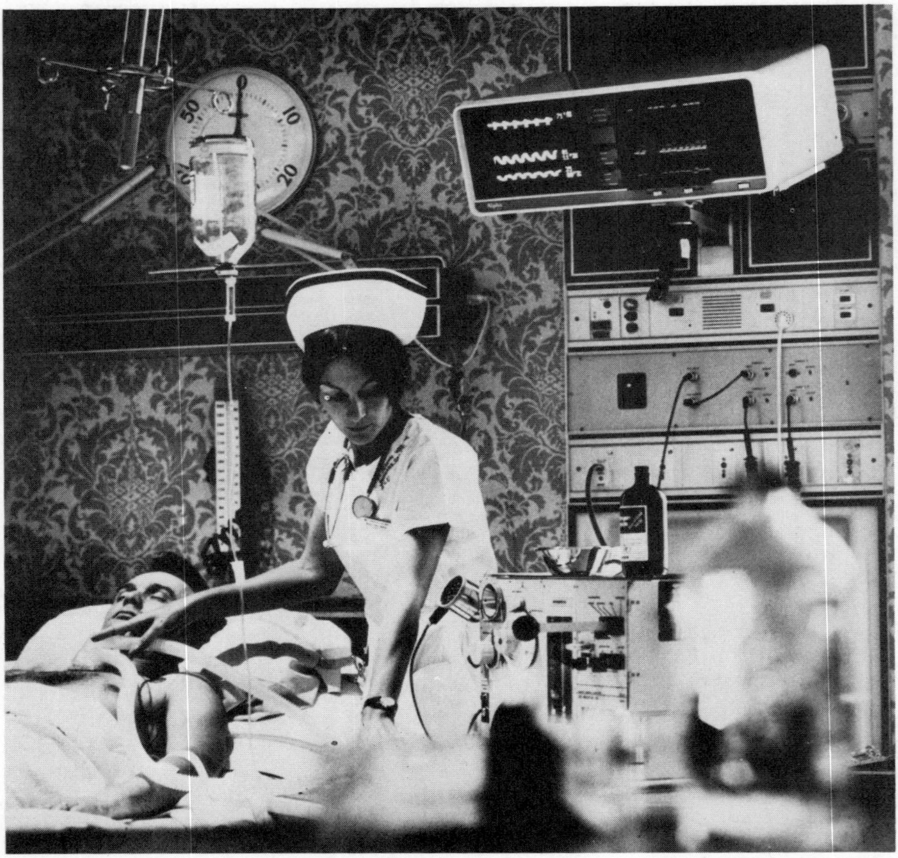

Fig. 19–4 (Continued.) (b) Bedside unit.

presently used computer systems utilize special equipment for acquisition of the ECG waveform. This equipment, which simultaneously obtains ECG signals from three leads and transmits the information by telephone line to the computer for analysis, is described in Chapter 7. Telephone-line transmission of ECG signals is covered in Chapter 13.

Entry of the ECG into a digital computer requires that the analog ECG signals be converted into digital form at a sampling rate of between 100 and 1000 readings per second. Electronic filtering (see Chapter 4) is often used ahead of the converter to eliminate noise and interference.

The computer is then required to recognize each of the important features of the ECG waveform and measure its amplitude and duration. The clinically significant intervals between features are also measured. For screening of the ECGs, each of these parameters is checked to see if it falls within normal limits, and a report is prepared by the computer, listing the values of all amplitudes and durations and pointing out any abnormalities. Heart rate is also determined and printed out with a special indication if it is outside the normal range.

19.3.3 Other Applications

Computers are also used in a number of other applications in hospitals and clinics. Some of these are described below.

Processing of Test Results from Clinical Laboratories. In this type of system, the physician or nurse on the ward enters test requests via a remote computer terminal or on special computer-readable order forms and receives test results on a computer-printed form or a CRT display. In such a system, the computer prepares blood-drawing lists and loading lists for automated chemistry equipment. Test results from automated equipment are automatically read by the computer and assimilated with patient data and the results of manually performed tests. All results are checked and verified by the computer before the report is presented on the CRT and printed out. Such systems have provisions by which emergency requests can be entered at any time and by which a physician can request the results of a specific test as soon as that test has been completed.

Axial Radiographic Tomography for Three-Dimensional Visualization of the Brain. In this system, radiography and computer techniques have been combined to produce a much more detailed view of the internal structures of the brain than is possible by ordinary X rays. Views are made of several horizontal slices through the brain by scanning each slice from 180 different vantage points, 1 degree of rotation apart. Information from the 180 scans is combined using the appropriate mathematical rules so as to produce the final image. See Chapter 15 for information regarding instrumentation for radiography.

Computerized Pulmonary Function Laboratory. Signals from a pneumotachograph, various gas analyzers, and other instrumentation in the pulmonary laboratory are fed into the computer on-line. The patient is asked to perform a set of breathing tests as described in Chapter 14. Airflow data, gas analyzer readings, and pertinent curves are immediately displayed to permit the physician or technician to judge whether the patient's performance is satisfactory. If not, the test can be stopped and rerun while the patient is still in the laboratory. In one commercially available system, the computer performs all necessary calculations and provides a report that includes patient data (identification, height, weight, age, etc.) and a number of calculated test results. These parameters include forced vital capacity, FEV_1, FEV_3, ratios of these FEVs to the forced vital capacity, maximum midexpiratory flow rate, inspiratory capacity, residual volume, FRC, total lung capacity, maximum voluntary ventilation, anatomic dead space, minute volume, diffusing capacity, and nitrogen washout data. All results are compared with normal values stored on tape for future reference. Definitions of all these measurements are given in Chapter 14.

In addition to the preceding clinical applications, computers are used in a number of other ways in health care. These applications include radiotherapy, planning, billing, outpatient appointment scheduling, acquisition and processing of data for multiphasic screening clinics, pharmacy control, and the cardiac catheterization laboratory. As time goes on and as new hardware and software systems become available, this list of applications will continue to grow.

20

Care and Use of Electronic Equipment

Modern electronic equipment in general has the reputation of being very reliable and the electronic equipment found in the hospital is no exception. However, on occasion, all electronic equipment can suddenly behave strangely or refuse to work completely. When such a malfunction occurs in a TV set or transistor radio, it results only in a minor inconvenience. Breakdown of electronic equipment used in the hospital can have serious consequences and can sometimes even endanger the lives of patients. Knowledgeable action on the part of the hospital staff who use the equipment, however, can reduce the likelihood of equipment failure and can aid in quickly returning the equipment to working order in the event of a breakdown.

This chapter provides the hospital staff with a set of practical instructions for the care and use of electronic equipment. Preventive measures are treated first, followed by instructions on what to do if an equipment malfunction is suspected. Attempts to service or repair malfunctioning equipment should normally be left to hospital technicians or engineers, or to service personnel brought in from the outside. In the rare event that repair service is not available on short notice when important equipment malfunctions, efforts to restore equipment to operation may be justifiable that otherwise should not be attempted. Instructions for such emergency repair attempts are given in the last part of the chapter.

20.1 Proper Use of Equipment

Equipment breakdown can be caused or accelerated by abuse or certain environmental conditions. Simple precautions can sometimes prevent either situation from occurring.

20.1.1 Mechanical Damage

Everyone knows that electronic instruments should not be dropped and no one would drop equipment on purpose. Nevertheless, accidental dropping is often the cause of damage. Equipment placed on narrow shelves, for instance, has frequently been sent crashing down by somebody stumbling over attached leads. Shelves of this kind, should therefore have a ridge or some type of interlock to prevent equipment from being pulled off easily.

Equipment is also in danger of being dropped accidentally when it is used on caster-equipped carts, such as crash carts for emergencies. Carts of this type should be as wide and low as possible to keep them from turning over, and their wheels should be as large as practical to prevent them from being caught on thresholds. Even when carts are built in this way, it is still a good policy to use two persons in moving them, one pulling and one pushing, so that the cart can be lifted over obstacles like thresholds or gaps in elevator doors.

Before such carts are moved, however, it should be ascertained that all line cords are unplugged. When an equipment cart is moved while a line cord is still connected to a receptacle, the forceful removal of the plug from the receptacle will usually damage both the cord and receptacle and may also pull equipment from the chart.

Should any electrical equipment be accidentally dropped despite these precautions, it is imperative that each device be examined by a technician or serviceman for possible damage before it is used with a patient. Not only can the mechanical shock of the fall cause damage that may interfere with the operation of the equipment, it could also dislodge internal parts. The result could cause dangerous voltages to appear on the case of the equipment or on parts that are connected to the patient.

Experience shows that equipment malfunctions are frequently caused by defective line cords, patient cables, and pressure transducers. Damage to these parts is often the result of carelessness or abuse. Care should be exercised when unplugging line cords or patient cables to grasp the plug rather than pull the cable. Stepping on cables or plugs or allowing carts to run over them should also be avoided. Pressure transducers should be handled carefully, since they can be damaged by banging or dropping them on table tops or the floor.

20.1.2 *Fluid Spillage*

Most electronic equipment is provided with vent holes or jalousies to permit circulation of air and prevent overheating. When such vents are located on the top of an equipment case, there is the danger that any kind of liquid spilled on the equipment can drip onto the sensitive electronic circuits inside and cause damage. Even if the manufacturer of the instrument was considerate enough to locate such vents on the side and back of the case, it is still considered good practice to avoid placing bowls, IV bottles, and other fluid-filled containers on electronic equipment. In the crowded environs of a hospital ward, however, this practice is sometimes not easily observed, and it has occasionally been proposed that medical instruments be built with slanted "roofs" to discourage using them as depositories for other utensils (Figure 20-1).

20.1.3 *Overheating of Equipment*

Although vents in an equipment case can provide undesirable entry ports for spilled fluids, they are necessary to prevent overheating as noted. For this reason, the vents should never be blocked by drapes or other obstructions. For the same reason, electronic equipment should never be placed directly on radiators or other heaters. A fan or blower is used on some equipment to provide adequate air circulation. Where this is the case

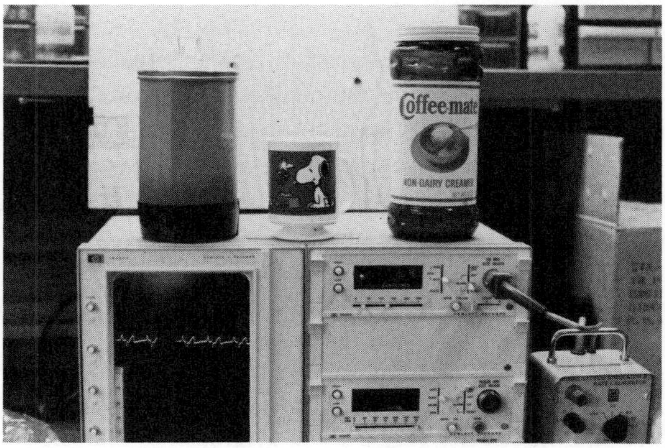

Fig. 20–1 Even though space is usually scarce in a hospital, fluid-filled containers should never be placed on top of electronic equipment.

an air filter similar to the filters in window air conditioners prevents lint and dust from entering the equipment. Such filters must be washed at certain time intervals, about every 6 to 12 months, a task normally performed by the technician who services the equipment. If the air filter is not cleaned, it can clog and cause overheating of the equipment.

20.1.4 Cleaning and Sterilization of Electronic Equipment

Electronic equipment can suffer damage if unsuitable materials or methods are used for cleaning and sterilizing. Electronic equipment and associated parts, such as cables and transducers, should normally never be autoclaved; cold gas sterilization is used instead. The only exceptions may be certain patient cables, transducer domes, and temperature probes, provided that the manufacturer specifically approves the use of sterilizing fluids or autoclaving.

If detergents or antibacterial solutions are used to clean the outside of electronic equipment, care should be taken to prevent any excess fluid from entering the case through vents and other openings. Certain solutions may, however, stain or discolor the equipment cabinets. Denaturated alcohol should not be used for cleaning electronic equipment because it often contains acetone, which can damage plastic parts and paint.

20.2 Equipment Malfunctions

Even if all such precautions are followed carefully, a piece of equipment can still suddenly fail to operate properly. When this situation occurs, the person using the equipment must take appropriate steps to restore it to operation.

The normal procedure in the event of a suspected equipment malfunction is to call a serviceman. Quite frequently, however, an apparent equipment malfunction is not caused by faulty equipment but is the result of an operator error or a power interruption. Before a service call is placed, it is therefore suggested that these two possibilities be ruled out by the methods described in the following sections.

There are, however, two conditions in which one should not attempt any of the described measures to restore the equipment to service:

1. If a piece of equipment emits smoke or the acrid, chemical smell of overheated insulation material.
2. If the equipment delivers electrical shocks to staff or patients.

Static shocks, however, which occur during dry weather and especially after walking on nylon rugs, should be differentiated from shocks caused by faulty equipment. To determine whether a shock is due to a static discharge or to faulty equipment, one should touch the place from which the shock was received a second time. A static discharge will deliver a shock only the first time that the equipment is touched, whereas faulty equipment will deliver a shock every time it is touched.

If either of the indicated conditions is observed, the equipment should be immediately disconnected from the patient and unplugged. The equipment should be labeled "Defective—Do not Use" until it has been checked by a serviceman or technician.

20.2.1 Operator Errors

A study conducted in 1972 on the causes of trouble calls in cardiac monitoring systems had some interesting results. This study was limited to one particular group of equipment, but other types of equipment can be expected to give similar results. In no fewer than 58% of the 197 problems encountered in 190 trouble calls, the apparent malfunction was not caused by equipment failure but was due to human errors. In 11.4% of the cases, the equipment was actually functioning properly and the operator merely thought it was malfunctioning. Other common operator errors were improper adjustments of controls or errors in the connection or placement of electrodes. In view of these results, it seems to be important first to rule out the human element in the case of a suspected equipment malfunction. If the operator has rather limited experience with a particular piece of equipment, it is a good idea to have a more experienced operator check the instrument to verify that it has been adjusted and connected properly. In equipment connected to a patient with electrodes, the electrodes should be inspected and checked to be sure that they adhere properly and are supplied with electrode jelly. Patient cables often cause problems by bad contact either where they are connected to the electrodes or where they are plugged into the equipment. By observing the display while touching the cable or electrodes, instabilities caused by bad connections can often be detected. When a pressure transducer is used, the dome and catheter should be inspected for air bubbles, and the flushing mechanism should be examined for proper operation to ensure that the catheter has not become plugged. All equipment should be examined for proper adjustment of all controls. No general recommendations can be given for that procedure other than to refer to the instruction manuals for the equipment.

20.2.2 Power Interruption

In the previous section it was assumed that the equipment showed some "sign of life"—that is, that pilot lights were on or that displays showed some kind of pattern. Sometimes, however, the equipment appears to be completely dead and devoid of power. If such is the case, it should be determined whether the equipment is turned on, whether its line cord is plugged into a receptacle, and whether the other end of the line cord has separated from the equipment (if it is of the removable type). If these inspections do not reveal the cause of the problem, the receptacle into which the equipment is plugged should be checked to be sure it has power. This test can easily be done by plugging some other electrical device, such as a lamp, into the same receptacle to see if it works. If it does not, the *circuit breaker* for the receptacle may have tripped, thus cutting off the power. Circuit breakers occasionally trip for no apparent reason. In most cases, however, their tripping is caused by faulty equipment. For this reason, some hospitals have a policy that circuit breakers may be reset only by a technician or electrician. As a result, the access door for the circuit breakers may be kept locked. Where this policy does not exist and when an electrician is not on duty, the person operating the malfunctioning equipment should try to reset the circuit breaker. Circuit breakers for a given hospital area are usually mounted together in a wall panel, as shown in Figure 20-2. The panel might be covered by an access door. It is important to know where the breaker panel for a given ward or laboratory is located, for these panels are sometimes hidden in broom closets or utility rooms. The circuit breakers should be clearly marked as to which room or part of a room they belong and as to whether they are for the lights or receptacles, which normally have separate circuit breakers.

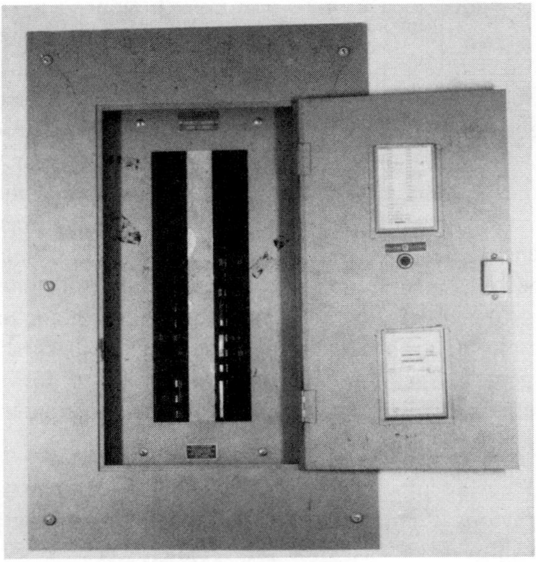

Fig. 20–2 Circuit breaker panel.

In practice, however, these markings are often not very clear. It should be noted that circuit breakers for 220-V circuits often used for receptacles for portable X-ray machines have two connected handles or a handle that is of double width. Every panel also has a main circuit breaker that controls the power to all the other circuit breakers on the panel. This main breaker is normally the topmost (or bottom-most) breaker of the panel, has two connected handles, and may be of a different color than the other circuit breakers. The handles of circuit breakers can be in one of three positions: ON, OFF, and a TRIP position located about halfway between the other two positions, as shown in Figure 20-3.

A tripped circuit breaker is reset by moving the handle first to the OFF position and then to the ON position. If the circuit breaker for the dead receptacle cannot be identified from the markings, one should look for a breaker with a handle that is in the TRIP position. In some makes of circuit breakers, however, this position is not easily visible because it is close to the ON position.

Two procedures should be avoided when trying to find and reset a tripped circuit breaker.

1. Never try to find the tripped circuit breaker by arbitrarily moving the handles of other circuit breakers to OFF and then to ON. Doing so would momentarily remove power from other pieces of equipment or turn off lights and create hazards.

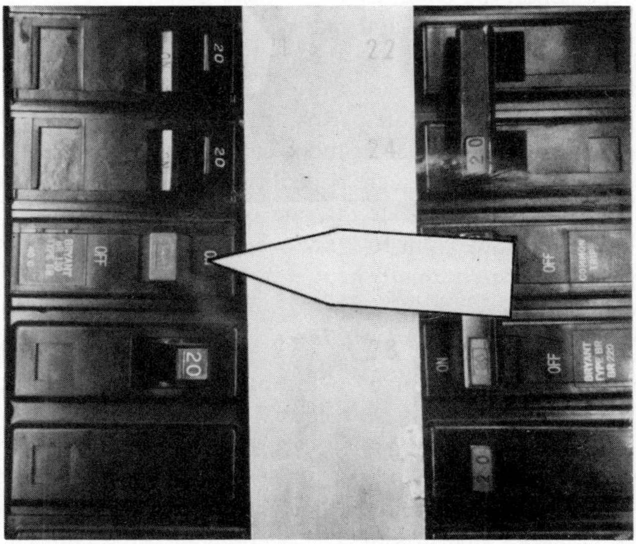

Fig. 20–3 Close-up of a circuit breaker panel. The circuit breaker indicated is in the tripped center position.

2. If a circuit breaker is reset and immediately trips again (indicated by a "clack" sound), do not try to reset it a second time. Tripping of a circuit breaker while trying to reset it indicates that the malfunction that tripped it in the first place still persists.

20.3 Service Calls for Repair of Faulty Equipment

If a piece of equipment is obviously faulty, as indicated by smoke or the delivery of shocks, or if operator error and power interruption have been ruled out as being the cause of the malfunction, it is time to place a service call. Hospital policy and the type of equipment involved will determine whom to call. Large hospitals usually have equipment repairmen, technicians, and even engineers on their staffs to service all or most of the equipment. Other hospitals may have contracts with maintenance companies that service equipment of different manufacturers. If no arrangements of this kind exist, the manufacturer of the equipment or his local representative can usually be called to service the equipment. In any event, it is important that the staff members using the equipment know whom to call for service.

The extent of the problem created by a piece of equipment being out of service depends on the circumstance. If the defective instrument is only one of several identical items and if the others are not being used at the time, a simple exchange can solve the problem. Occasionally similar, but not identical, equipment can be substituted. In some situations, it may be possible to replace the function performed by the equipment temporally with additional staff attendance without sacrificing the quality of patient care. Life-saving equipment, such as defibrillators and pacemakers, should be available at least in duplicate. If one of these instruments fails, it is important for the hospital staff to know where alternate instruments of the same or similar types are normally kept.

20.3.1 Reporting of Equipment Malfunctions

The work of the repairman or technician responding to the service call can often be simplified if he receives a detailed report on the cause of the call. The statement "it does not work" is not sufficient; it can mean all kinds of things from absolutely dead equipment to equipment that works but is just marginal in one particular aspect of its function. Unusual events or observations that preceded or accompanied the equipment failure should be reported, for they can help in diagnosing the cause of the malfunction. Observations that should be reported include difficulties in calibrating the equipment and unusual artifacts noticed on the display. Events that might have caused or contributed to the equipment malfunction are incidents in which the equipment was dropped or bumped or a situation in which the equipment was connected to a patient during defibrilliation.

It should also be noted that some equipment will malfunction or show marginal performance when the line voltage drops to an unusually low level, as in the case of a so-called brownout. If the line voltage has returned to its normal value when the equipment is checked out, it will function properly again and will frustrate the serviceman trying to diagnose the reported malfunction.

A marginal performance can also be caused by abnormally high or abnormally low ambient temperature, although most equipment is designed to operate over a range of at least 60 to 90°F (16 to 33°C). Such unusual operating conditions should, however, be reported to the serviceman because they might have contributed to the malfunction.

20.4 Emergency Procedures if Repair Service Is Not Readily Available

Many hospitals in the United States and Canada are located in rural or isolated areas where service calls for malfunctioning equipment can be very expensive and where it may take days until a serviceman can respond even to an urgent call. In such a situation, the hospital staff should try the following measures to restore the equipment to service, which under different circumstances should be left to a serviceman.

20.4.1 Changing Fuses in Medical Equipment

In addition to the circuit breaker that protects the receptacle into which equipment is plugged, most electrical equipment contains one or more fuses of its own. In equipment with more than one fuse, some of the fuses may blow without the equipment appearing completely "dead." Fuses are normally located somewhere on the rear panel of the equipment, often near the point at which the line cord enters or connects to the equipment case.

Before personnel attempt to check the fuses, the equipment should be unplugged from the receptacle. The fuses themselves are small glass tubes, less than one inch long, with a shiny metal cap at each end. Fuses are contained in one of two different types of fuse holders. The screw (or bayonet) type, shown in Figure 20-4a, is opened by turning the round knob to the left. Sometimes a slot for inserting a coin or screwdriver is provided in case the knob is too tight for removal with the fingers. The fuse comes

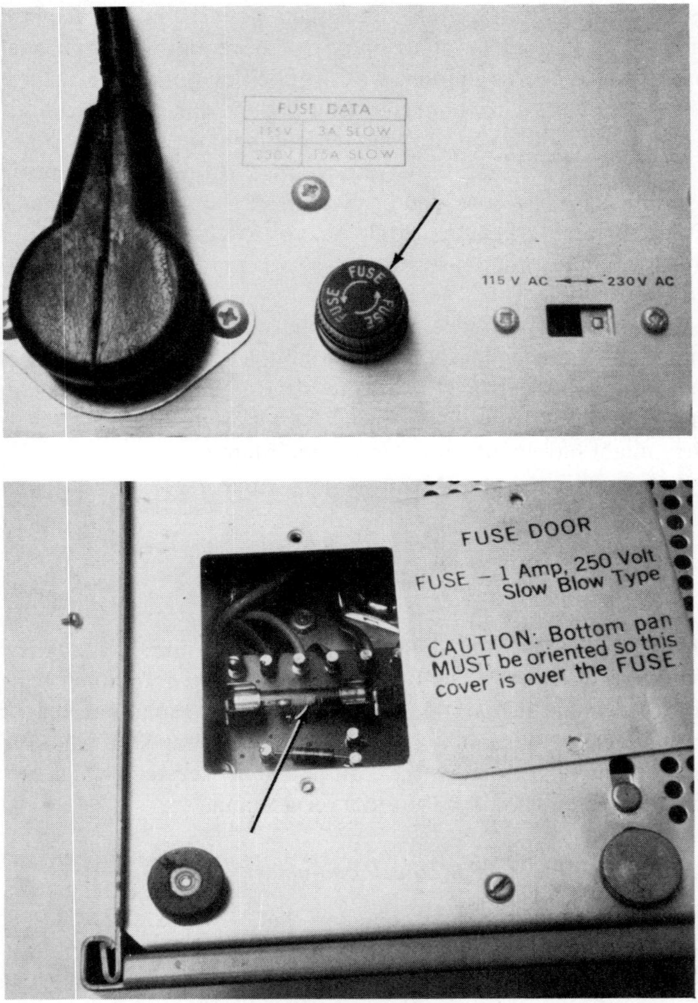

Fig. 20–4 Two different types of fuse holders: (a) bayonet type; (b) clip-type (fuse indicated by arrow) normally hidden behind a removable "door."

out with the knob and can be removed from the knob by pulling it out straight. The clip-type fuse holder, shown in Figure 20-4b, is often hidden behind a protective cover plate made of metal or plastic (sometimes transparent). A screwdriver might be required to remove the cover. The fuse can then be removed from the two clips that hold it by its metal caps. If the clips are very tight, this process may not be easy. Removal can be simplified by slipping a piece of tape (e.g., 1-in. surgical adhesive tape, folded lengthwise with the sticky side together to prevent it from sticking) behind the fuse to pull it out. It can also be pried out with a narrow tongue depressor or a similar tool, but care should be taken not to break the glass of the fuse. Some fuse holders have a plastic lever to simplify removal of the fuse. If the equipment has more than one fuse, only one fuse should be removed at a time to prevent mixups.

Fuses come in two different basic types, as shown in Figure 20-5. In the so-called fast fuse a thin wire is stretched between the metal caps inside the glass tube. These wires are sometimes thinner than a human hair and may not be easily visible. When the fuse blows, the wire melts or disintegrates and sometimes—but not always—leaves a shiny or whitish deposit on the inside of the glass tube. In the other type of fuse, the so-called slow-blow type, a tiny coil spring is stretched from one of the caps and connected to a wire from the other cap with a glob of solder. When the fuse blows, the solder melts and the coil spring snaps back, leaving a gap in the center. With this type of fuse, it is fairly easy to see when the fuse has blown.

In larger equipment, especially in types that contain motors or heaters, fuses of a different type are sometimes found. Here the glass tube is filled with fine sand or the tube is made of ceramic. It is not possible to determine by visual inspection whether this type of fuse has blown.

Because each fuse is rated to blow at a certain current level, a fuse should be replaced only with a fuse of the same rating. Also, a fast fuse should be replaced only with a fast fuse and a slow-blow fuse only with a slow-blow fuse. Generally the current rating of a fuse is stated next to the fuse holder or on the cover over the clip-type holders, but sometimes it is only listed in the instruction manual. The current rating is also listed on the metal caps of the fuses and on the little boxes in which they are packed

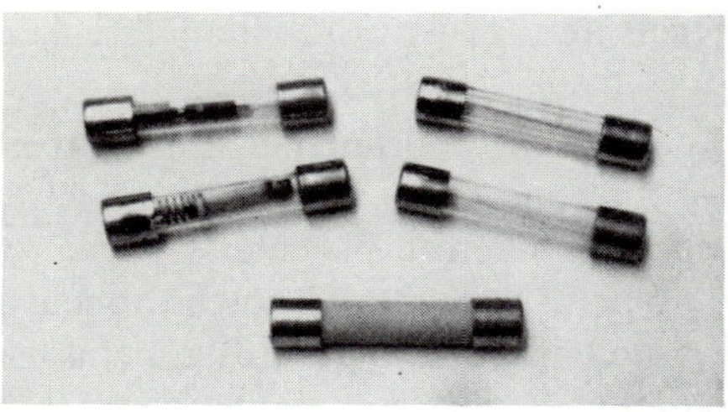

Fig. 20–5 Various types of fuses: left, two slow-blow fuses; right, two fast fuses with glass bodies. The thin fuse wire is not visible in this photo. Front, a fuse with ceramic body which cannot be inspected visually.

—often, however, in a rather confusing way. It is therefore suggested that spare fuses be kept in separate boxes or envelopes that are clearly marked. Some manufacturers ship their equipment with a set of spare fuses, and some even go so far as to provide a holder for the spare fuses next to the equipment fuse holder.

Replacing the fuses may restore the equipment to working order. Sometimes the blown fuse, however, is merely the symptom of some other malfunction of the equipment, and when replaced, it will immediately blow again.

20.4.2 Identifying Shorted Equipment

Section 20.2.2 noted that if a circuit breaker trips again when it is reset, it should not be reset a second time. The tripping indicates that the malfunction that caused it to trip still persists. This malfunction is usually a short, which can be located in the electrical distribution system. More frequently, however, the short circuit is not in the distribution system itself but in one of the pieces of equipment connected to the system. If the faulty instrument can be identified, it can be disconnected and all other instruments connected to the same power circuit can be restored to operation. The following steps will help in identifying the shorted piece of equipment.

1. Turn off and unplug all equipment from the "dead" circuit.
2. Disconnect any patient connections (leads, transducers) from the equipment.
3. Reset the circuit breaker. (If it should trip again, the fault is not in the equipment but in the wiring.)
4. Plug in and turn on the equipment, one piece at a time, and observe which item causes the circuit breaker to trip.

In certain kinds of equipment malfunction, line voltage can momentarily appear on the case of the equipment or on the plug (if the plug has a metal case). Such plugs should therefore be held with a dry towel while being plugged in. The equipment case should not be touched while it is turned on. If the ON-OFF switch is of the type with a metal handle, a nonmetallic object, like a wooden tongue depressor, should be used to operate it.

Sometimes the circuit breaker trips some time after it has been reset, in some cases as long as half an hour. This situation can indicate that the circuit is overloaded, which is probable if such equipment as heaters, air conditioners, or hyperthermia-hypothermia equipment is in use. In this case, some of the equipment should be turned off and, if necessary, plugged into other receptacles powered from a different circuit breaker. The use of extension cords should be avoided, however, for any patient-connected equipment.

20.4.3 Last Effort

If the procedures described fail to restore the equipment to operation, one last step can be tried. Occasionally equipment malfunctions are caused by loose internal connections. These connections can sometimes be restored, at least temporarily, by a mechanical shock. To apply such a shock, the equipment case should be dealt a sharp blow with the fist or the flat hand, either at the top or on the side. Although the chances of success for this procedure are quite small, the blow is unlikely to damage the equipment and is therefore worthwhile trying as a last effort. Should it be successful, however, it should be kept in mind that this type of "repair" is apt to be only temporary and does not rule out a service call.

Bibliography

General

The following works may be considered as general references throughout the book. Other references are cited for particular chapters.

BEST, C. M. and N. B. TAYLOR, *Physiological Basis of Medical Practice,* 9th Ed. Brobeck, John K., *Editor,* Baltimore, Md.: The Williams & Wilkins Co., 1973.

BROWN, J. H. U., J. E. JACOBS, and L. STARK, *Biomedical Engineering.* Philadelphia: F. A. Davis Company, 1971.

CROMWELL, L., F. J. WEIBELL, E. A. PFEIFFER, and L. B. USSELMAN, *Biomedical Instrumentation and Measurements.* Englewood Cliffs, N.J.: Prentice-Hall, Inc., 1973.

EVANS, W. F., *Anatomy and Physiology, the Basic Principles.* Englewood Cliffs, N.J.: Prentice-Hall, Inc., 1971.

GEDDES, L. A., and L. E. BAKER, *Principles of Applied Biomedical Instrumentation,* 2nd Ed. New York: John Wiley & Sons, Inc., 1975.

GUYTON, A. C., *Textbook of Medical Physiology*. Philadelphia: W. B. Saunders Company, 1971.

RAY, C. D. (Ed.), *Medical Engineering*. Chicago: Year Book Medical Publishers, Inc., 1974.

SCHMIDT-NIELSEN, K., *Animal Physiology*. Englewood Cliffs, N.J.: Prentice-Hall, Inc., 1974.

STRONG, P., *Biophysical Measurements*. Beaverton, Oreg.: Tektronix, Inc., 1970.

WEISS, M. D., *Biomedical Instrumentation*. Philadelphia: Chilton Book Company, 1973.

YANOF, H. M., *Biomedical Electronics*, 2nd edition. Philadelphia: F. A. Davis Company, 1972.

Chapter 3

Electricity in Patient Care Facilities. Boston: National Fire Protection Association, 470 Atlantic Ave., 1973.

MARCUS, A., and MARCUS, W., *Basic Electricity*. Englewood Cliffs, N.J.: Prentice-Hall, Inc., 1974.

ROBINSON, VESTER, *Basic Principles of Electricity*. Reston, Va.: Reston Publishing Company, 1973.

Chapter 4

HERRICK, C. N., and DEEM, W. R., *Introduction to Electronics*. Pacific Palisades, Ca.: Goodyear Publishing Company, 1973.

KAHN, M., *The Versatile Op. Amp*. New York: Holt, Rinehart & Winston, Inc., 1970.

Chapter 5

ADOLPH, E. F., "The Heart's Pacemaker," *Scientific American*, Vol. 216 (March 1967), pp. 32–37.

BEST, C. M., and N. B. TAYLOR, *The Living Body, a Text in Human Physiology*. New York: Holt, Rinehart & Winston, Inc., 1971.

BRAZIER, M., "The Analysis of Brain Waves," *Scientific American*, Vol. 206, No. 6 (June 1962), pp. 142–143.

BRAZIER, MARY A. B., *The Electrical Activity of the Nervous System*. Baltimore, Md.: The Williams & Wilkins Co., 1968.

DUBIN, DALE, *Rapid Interpretation of EKGs.* Tampa, Fl.: Cover Publishing Company, 1970.

MOUNTCASTLE, V. B. (*Editor*), *Medical Physiology,* 12th edition, Vols. I and II. St. Louis, Mo.: The C. V. Mosby Co., 1968.

SCHER, A., "The Electrocardiogram," *Scientific American,* Vol. 205, No. 5 (November 1961), pp. 132–141.

WIGGERS, C. J., "The Heart," *Scientific American,* Vol. 196, No. 4 (May 1957), pp. 75–82.

WINSON, TRAVIS, *The Electrocardiogram in Myocardial Infarction.* Summit, N.J.: Ciba Pharmaceutical Company, 1968.

ZWEIFACH, B. W., "The Microcirculation of the Blood," *Scientific American,* Vol. 200, No. 1 (January 1959), pp. 54–60.

Chapter 6

GEDDES, L. A., *Electrodes and the Measurement of Bioelectric Events.* New York: John Wiley & Sons, Inc., 1972.

Chapter 7

Technicians Guide to Electrocardiography. Waltham, Mass.: Hewlett-Packard Company.

BURCH, G. E., and T. WINSOR, *A Primer of Electrocardiography,* 4th edition. Philadelphia: Lea & Febiger, 1960.

Chapter 8

BURCH, G. E., and N. P. DE PASQUALE, *Primer of Clinical Measurement of Blood Pressure.* St. Louis, Mo.: The C. V. Mosby Co., 1962.

GEDDES, L. A., *The Direct and Indirect Measurement of Blood Pressure.* Chicago: Year Book Medical Publishers, Inc., 1970.

Recommendations for Human Blood Pressure Determination by Sphygmomanometers. New York: American Heart Association, 1967.

Sphygmomanometers—Principles and Precepts. Copiague, N.Y.: W. A. Baum Company, 1965.

Chapter 9

ASPINALL, MARY JO, *Nursing the Open-Heart Surgery Patient.* New York: McGraw-Hill Book Company. A Blakiston publication, 1973, pp. 105–111.

BELL, J. A., "Malpositioning of Central Venous Catheters," *Lancet,* Vol. 1 (January 13, 1973), p. 105.

CHUN, G. M. H., and M. H. ELLESTAD, "Perforation of the Pulmonary Artery by a Swan-Ganz Catheter," *New England Journal of Medicine,* Vol. 284 (May 6, 1971), p. 1041.

GERNERT, CAROLYN F., and STEPHANIE SCHWARTS, "Pulmonary Artery Catheterization," *American Journal of Nursing,* Vol. 73, No. 7 (July 1973), p. 1182.

HENZEL, J. H., and M. S. DE WEESE, "Morbid and Mortal Complications Associated with Prolonged Central Venous Pressure Cannulation," *American Journal of Surgery,* Vol. 121 (1971), p. 600.

HUDAK, CAROLYN, M., et al., *Critical Care Nursing.* Philadelphia: J. B. Lippincott Co., pp. 128–129.

JOBIN, GARY, "Pitfalls, of Pressure Monitoring." Presented at the Los Angeles County Heart Association's 11th Annual Spring Symposium, March 27, 1974.

KONIGSBERG, E., "A Pressure Transducer for Chronic Intravascular Implantation," *Fourth National Biomedical Sciences Instrumentation Symposium,* Anaheim, Ca.: May 1966.

LAPIN, E. S., and J. A. MURRAY, "Hemoptysis with Flow-Directed Cardiac Catheterization," *Journal of the American Medical Association,* Vol. 220, No. 9 (May 29, 1972).

LONG, MADELEINE, et al., "Complications of Central Venous Pressure Monitoring: Cardiac Arrhythmias and Conduction Disturbances," *Heart and Lung,* Vol. 2, No. 3 (May–June 1973), p. 416.

NIELSEN, MARY, A., "Intra-arterial Monitoring of Blood Pressure," *American Journal of Nursing,* Vol. 74, No. 1 (January 1974), p. 48.

PIEGAS, LEOPOLDO, et al., "Use of the Swan-Ganz Catheter in the Diagnosis of Ventricular Septal Defect after Myocardial Infarction. A Report." *Heart and Lung,* Vol. 2, No. 4 (July–August 1973), p. 539.

RUTHERFORD, BARRY D., et al., "The Value of Monitoring Pulmonary Artery Pressure for Early Detection of Left Ventricular Failure Following Myocardial Infarction," *Circulation,* Vol. 43 (May 1971), p. 655.

SCOTT, MEREDITH L., et al., "Clinical Application of a Flow-Directed Balloon-Tipped Cardiac Catheter," *The American Surgeon* (December 1972), p. 690.

SHINE, KENNETH J., "Measurement of Pulmonary Artery and Pulmonary Capillary Wedge Pressure." Presented at the Los Angeles County Heart Association's 11th Annual Spring Symposium, March 27, 1974.

SWAN, H. J. C., and W. GANZ, et al., "Catheterization of the Heart in Man with Use of a Flow-Directed Ballon-Tipped Catheter," *New England Journal of Medicine,* Vol. 283 (August 27, 1970), p. 447.

WELL, MAX HARRY, and HERBERT SHUBIN, *Diagnosis and Treatment of Shock.* Baltimore, Md.: The Williams & Wilkins Co., 1967, pp. 61–66.

Chapter 10

An Overview of Pacing. Minneapolis: Medtronic, Inc., 1973.

ANDREOLI, K. G., et al., *Comprehensive Cardiac Care.* St. Louis, Mo.: The C. V. Mosby Co., 1971.

Cardiac Pacemaking. Somerville, N.J.: Hoechst Pharmaceuticals, Inc., 1974.

GIBBONS, JOLIN H., et al., *Surgery of the Chest.* Philadelphia: W. B. Saunders Company, 1969.

LOWN, B., "Intensive Heart Care," Scientific American, Vol. 219, No. 1. (July 1968), pp. 19–27.

Chapter 11

BUKSTEIN, E. J., *Biomedical Electronics,* 1st edition. New York: Howard W. Sams Company, 1973.

"Coronary Arteriography," *Directions in Cardiovascular Medicine,* Vol. 1. Somerville, N.J.: Hoechst Pharmaceuticals, Inc., 1970.

"The Coronary Care Unit," *Directions in Cardiovascular Medicine,* Vol. 3. Somerville, N.J.: Hoechst Pharmaceuticals, Inc., 1970.

A Guide to Fetal Monitoring. Waltham, Mass.: Hewlett-Packard Company, 1973.

KARSELIS, T., *Descriptive Medical Electronics & Instrumentation.* Thurofare, N.J.: Charles B. Slack, Inc., 1973.

KLEIN, B., *Introduction to Medical Electronics.* Blue Summit Ridge, Pa.: Tab Books, 1973.

Planning a Patient Monitoring System. Waltham, Mass.: Hewlett-Packard Company, Medical Electronics Division, 1973.

Note: Many instrument manufacturers have published description booklets on patient-monitoring systems.

Chapter 12

CAPPELEN, C. (Ed.), "New Findings in Blood Flowmetry," *Universitetsforlaget,* Oslo, Norway, 1968.

The Measurement of Cardiac Output by the Dye Dilution Method. Monograph available from Lexington Instruments Corporation, 241 Crescent Street, Waltham, Mass., 1963.

ZIERLER, K. L., "Circulation Times and the Theory of Indicator Dilution Methods for Determining Blood Flow and Volume." In *Handbook of Physiology,* Sec. 2, Vol. 1, J. Field (Ed.), American Physiological Society, 1959, pp. 585–615.

Chapter 13

CACERES, C. A. (Ed.), *Biomedical Telemetry.* New York: Academic Press, 1965.

CROMWELL, LESLIE, "Use of Telemetry in Cardiovascular Research," *Proceedings of the 1968 National Conference IEEE,* Houston, Texas, April 1968.

HANISH, H. M., *Biolink Telemetry Systems Application Notes.* Biocom., Inc., Culver City, Ca., 1968.

MACKAY, R. S., *Bio-Medical Telemetry.* New York: John Wiley & Sons, Inc., 1968.

Chapter 14

BASS, B. H., *Pulmonary Function in Clinical Medicine.* Springfield, Ill.: Charles C Thomas, Publisher, 1964.

BELINKOFF, S., *Introduction to Inhalation Therapy.* Boston: Little, Brown and Company, 1969.

BUIST, A. S., "Clinical Significance of Pulmonary Function Tests: Early Detection of Airways Obstruction by the Closing Volume Technique," *Chest,* Vol. 64, No. 4 (1973), pp. 495–499.

CHERNIAK, R. M., and L. CHERNIAK, *Respiration in Health and Disease.* Philadelphia and London, England: W. B. Saunders Company, 1963.

COMROE, JULIUS H., et al., *The Lung: Clinical Physiology and Pulmonary Function Tests.* Chicago: Year Book Medical Publishers, Inc., 1963.

EGAN, D. F., *Fundamentals of Inhalation Therapy.* St. Louis, Mo.: C. V. Mosby Co., 1969.

FILLEY, GILES F., *Pulmonary Insufficiency and Respiratory Failure*. Philadelphia: Lea & Febiger, 1968.

SCHOLANDER, P. F., "Analyzer for Accurate Estimation of Respiratory Gases in One-half Cubic Centimeter Samples," *Journal of Biological Chemistry*, Vol. 167 (1947).

Chapter 15

"Cardiac Catheterization," *Directions in Cardiovascular Medicine*, Vol. III. Somerville, N.J.: Hoechst Pharmaceuticals, Inc., 1973.

JAUNDRELL-THOMPSON, F., and W. J. ASHWORTH, *X-Ray Physics and Equipment*. Philadelphia: F. A. Davis Company, 1970.

JOHNS, W. E., *The Physics of Radiology*. Springfield, Ill.: Charles C Thomas, 1961.

Chapter 16

The reader is referred to the Travenol Company, Morton Grove, Illinois, for references on the heart-lung machine and oxygenators. "Solid State Electrosurgery," service manual, Valleylab, Boulder, Colorado, 1972 is a reference for electrosurgery.

Chapter 17

BARNES, R. B., "Thermography of the Human Body," *Science*, Vol. 140, No. 3569 (May 24, 1963), pp. 870–877.

BRAZIER, MARY, A. B., *The Electrical Activity of the Nervous System*, 3rd edition. Baltimore: The Williams & Wilkins Co., 1968.

FEIGENBAUM, H., *Echocardiography*. Philadelphia: Lea & Febiger, 1972.

SEGAL, B. L., "Echocardiography, Clinical Application in Mitral Stenosis," *JAMA*, Vol. 1951 (January 17, 1966), pp. 161–166.

VENABLES, P. H., and MARTIN, I. (Eds.), *A Manual of Psycho-Physiological Methods*. New York: John Wiley & Sons, Inc., 1967.

Chapter 18

BRUNER, J. M. R., "Hazards of Electrical Apparatus," *Anesthesiology*, Vol. 28 (1968), pp. 396–424.

LANGSDON, C. S., "The Aberrant Central Venous Catheter and Its Complications," *Radiology, Vol.* 100 (1971), pp. 55–59.

Manual for the Safe Use of Electricity in Hospitals, 76B-T. Boston: National Fire Protection Association (NFPA), 470 Atlantic Avenue, 1973.

National Electrical Code 1975. Boston: National Fire Protection Association, 60 Batterymarch Street, 1974.

Patient Safety, Application Note AN 718. Waltham, Mass.: Hewlett-Packard Company, Medical Electronic Division, 1970.

Standard for the Use of Inhalation Anesthetics, 56A. Boston: National Fire Protection Association, 470 Atlantic Avenue, 1973.

Chapter 19

"The Computer, Wilhelm Röntgen, and the EMI Scanner," *Computers and Medicine,* AMA, Vol. 11, No. 5 (1973).

MARTIN, J. N. (Ed.), "Special Section on Medical Data Processing," *Medical Electronics and Equipment News,* Vol. 13, No. 12 (1973), pp. 11–32.

STACY, R. W., and B. D. WAXMAN (Eds.), *Computers in Biomedical Research,* Vols. I, II, III, and IV. New York: Academic Press, 1965–1974.

WARE, W. H., *Digital Computer Technology and Design,* 2 volumes. New York: John Wiley & Sons, Inc., 1963.

Chapter 20

HASLAM, K. R., and BRUNER, J. M., "The Epidemiology of Failures in Cardiac Monitoring Systems," *Medical Instrumentation,* Vol. 5 (1973), pp. 293–296.

APPENDIX A

Glossary of Electrical and Instrument Terms

Throughout this book many technical terms have been used, terms that are perhaps unfamiliar to the reader. To help achieve a better understanding, the following glossary is presented in alphabetical order for easy reference. There are many sources for these definitions, including the authors' own interpretation. However, two major sources should be recognized. The first is the *Glossary of Instrument Terms* published by Gould Instrument Systems Division, Cleveland, Ohio; and the second is a textbook, *Basic Electric Circuits,* by Leslie Cromwell (W. C. Brown Co.).

Accuracy: The capability of an instrument to follow the true value of a given phenomenon.

Admittance: The reciprocal of impedance. Symbol: Y. Unit = mho.

Ambient temperature: The prevailing temperature in the immediate vicinity or the temperature of the medium surrounding an object.

Ampere: The practical unit of current. Abbreviation: A.

Amplitude: The magnitude of variation in changing quanity from its zero value. The word must be modified with an adjective, such as "maximum," that designates the specific amplitude in question.

Analog: An adjective that has come to mean continuous, cursive, or having an infinite number of connected points. The instrumentation industry uses the words "analog" and "digital" where the more precise language would be "continuous" and "discrete." Short for "analogous."

Attenuation: Reduction or division of signal amplitude—retaining the characteristic waveform; implies deliberately throwing away or discarding a part of the signal energy for the sake of reduced amplitude.

Balanced bridge: A bridge circuit, which has an output voltage of zero.

Balanced input: A symmetrical input circuit having equal impedance from both input terminals to ground.

Bandwidth: The range of frequencies over which a given device is designed to operate within specified limits.

Bonded strain gauge: Strain-sensitive elements arranged to facilitate bonding to a surface in order to measure applied strain on that surface.

CGS system of units: A system of physical units in which the centimeter, gram, and second are the fundamental units.

Calibration: The process of comparing a set of magnitudes of a continuously varying magnitude with another set previously established as a standard.

Capacitance: The property of a body, by virtue of which a potential difference exists between it and surrounding bodies, when a quantity of electricity is imparted to it. It is measured by the quantity of electricity required to raise its potential by one unit. Symbol: C. Unit = farad.

Charge: The total quantity of electricity on a conductor. An excess or deficiency of electrons on a body.

Conductance: The reciprocal of resistance. Symbol G. Unit = mho.

Coulomb: A unit of quantity of electricity. It is equivalent to one ampere flowing for one second.

Current: The flow of electricity round a circuit. It is measured by the quantity of electricity that flows past a cross section per second. Symbol: I. Unit = Ampere.

Current density: The current flowing in a conductor per unit area of cross section. It is usually expressed in amperes per square inch or per square centimeter.

dc amplifier: One that has a frequency response band that goes down to dc. This definition includes direct-coupled amplifiers but is not restricted to them.

Demodulator: A device that extracts the modulation information from a modulated carrier. In most cases, it rectifies the incoming modulated carrier frequency and separates the desired modulation signal from the carrier.

Differential input: An input circuit that rejects voltages that are the same at both input terminals and amplifies the voltage difference between the two input terminals. May be either balanced or floating and may also be guarded.

Differential transducer: A device that is capable of following simultaneously the voltages across or from two separate signal sources and providing a final output proportional to the difference between the two signals.

Digital output: An output quantity consisting of a set of discrete magnitudes coded to represent digits in a system of notations. Most common example of digital output is an electric typewriter.

Discriminator: A device in which the properties of a signal, such as frequency or phase, are converted into amplitude variations.

Distortion: An unwanted change in waveform. Principal forms of distortion are inherent nonlinearity of the device, nonuniform response at different frequencies, and lack of constant proportionality between phase shift and frequency.

Distributed capacity: Capacitance evenly distributed over the entire length of a signal cable. Includes capacitance between signal conductors and from each conductor to ground.

Drift: A gradual and unintentional deviation of a given property—in the case of a recording pen, usually the deviation from zero rest position.

Electrode: 1. A conductor, by means of which a current passes into or out of a fluid or an organic material, such as human skin; often one terminal of a lead.

2. The emiter, collector, or base of a semiconductor.

3. The cathode, grid, or anode of a vacuum tube or gas discharge lamp.

4. A metallic conductor, such as in an electrolytic cell, which conduction by electrons is changed to conduction by ions or other charged particles.

5. A device that combines definitions (1) and (4)—for example, a calomel half-cell.

It is conceivable that under definition (4) an electrode could be a kind of transducer.

Electromotive force: The force that tends to make a current flow. Symbol: E.

Electron: The fundamental unit of negative electricity.

Electrostatic coupling: Coupled by means of capacitance so that charges on one circuit influence another circuit owing to the capacitance between the two.

Floating: The condition of a device or circuit that is not grounded and not tied to any established potential.

Frequency: The number of cycles per second. Symbol: f. Unit = Hz.

Frequency-modulated signal: A signal where the intelligence is contained in the deviation from a center frequency. In a recording instrument, this deviation is proportional to the applied stimulus.

Frequency response: The portion of the frequency spectrum that can be covered by a device within specified limits of amplitude error.

Full scale: The total interval over which an instrument is intended to operate. Also, the output from a transducer when the maximum rated stimulus is applied to the input.

Gain stability: The extent to which the sensitivity of an instrument remains constant with time. The property reported in specifications should be instability, which is the maximum change in sensitivity from initial value over a stated period of time under stated conditions.

Ground: 1. A point in a circuit used as a common reference or datum point in measuring voltages.

2. The conducting chassis or framework on which an electrical circuit is physically mounted and to which one point in a circuit is often connected.

3. The earth or a low-resistance conductor connected to the earth at some point and having no potential difference from another conductor connected to the earth at the same point.

Please remember that the first definition does not necessarily have anything to do with the other two.

Ground loop: The generation of undesirable signals within a ground conductor caused by circulation currents within the conductor that originate from a second source of potential, frequently as a result of connecting two separate grounds to a signal circuit.

Guarded input: An input that has a third terminal that is maintained at a potential near the input-terminal potential for a single-ended input or near the mean input potential for differential input. It is used to shield the entire input circuit.

Guard shield or "guard": An internal floating shield that surrounds the entire input section of an amplifier. Effective shielding is achieved only when the absolute potential of the guard is stabilized with respect to the incoming signal.

Harmonic: An oscillation of a periodically varying quantity, having a frequency that is an integral multiple of the fundamental frequency. A harmonic having three times the fundamental frequency is called the third harmonic and so on.

Hybrid: 1. An electronic circuit having both vacuum tubes and transistors.

2. A mixture of thin-film and discrete integrated circuits.

3. A computer that has both analog and digital capability.

Impedance: An indication of the total opposition that a circuit or device offers to the flow of alternating current at a particular frequency.

Inductance: The property of a circuit by virtue of which electromagnetic induction occurs. It may be self- or mutual inductance or a combination of both.

Inductive pickup: Signals generated in a circuit or conductor owing to mutual inductance between it and a distributing source.

Insulated: A condition when the substance between one conductor, circuit, or device and another cannot conduct current at operating voltage and beyond (to the limit of breakdown voltage).

Internal calibration: Calibration by an internal voltage source (provided with the instrument) rather than an external standard.

Lead: 1. An electrical conductor or wire used to connect a test point to an electronic device or instrument; a wire terminated by an electrode.

2. A particular connection scheme for the input leads in an electrocardiogram; for example, voltage between right arm and left arm constitutes "lead I." Number of leads taken during an electrocardiogram may vary between 8 and 12, normally designated I, II, III, aVR, aVL, aVF, and V_1—V_6 (first three are the most significant).

3. The particular oscillogram resulting from one of the connections above.

Linearity: The "straight-lineness" of the transfer curve between an input and an output; that condition prevailing when output is directly proportional to input.

Lowpass filter: A filter that transmits alternating current below a given cutoff frequency and substantially attenuates all other currents.

Magnetic field: Any space or region in which magnetizing forces are of significant magnitude with respect to conditions under consideration. A magnetic field is produced by any current flow or a permanent magnet, including the earth itself.

Marking: Impressing or causing to appear on some surface a visible trace, line, dot, or symbol. Handwriting is one form of cursive marking.

Mho: A practical unit of conductance. It is the conductance of a body having the resistance of one ohm.

Microfarad. 10^{-6} farad. Symbol: μF.

Natural frequency: The frequency at which a system with a single degree of freedom will oscillate on momentary displacement from rest position by a transient force in the absence of damping.

Noise: Any unwanted electrical disturbance or spurious signal that modifies the transmission, measurement, or recording of desired data.

Null-balance: A condition of balance in a device or system that results in zero output or zero current input.

Ohm: The practical unit of resistance. Abbreviation: Ω

Ohm's law: The ratio of the steady direct potential difference between any two points in a circuit to the resulting steady direct current is constant, provided that the physical conditions remain unaltered.

Operating temperature: The temperature or range of temperatures over which an instrument is expected to operate within specified limits of error.

Pen centering: An electrical or mechanical adjustment by which an oscillograph pen is positioned to channel center.

Pen positioning: An electrical or mechanical adjustment by which an oscillograph pen is positioned to any desired amplitude grid mark on the chart to represent zero signal.

Period: The time for a complete oscillation or for a single cycle of events. The reciprocal of frequency.

Phase: In a periodic function or wave, the fraction of the period that has elapsed, measured from some fixed origin. If the time for one period is represented at 360° along a time axis, the phase position is called the phase angle.

Potential difference: An electrical condition existing between two points and tending to cause a movement of electricity from one point to the other. It is measured by the work done in moving a unit charge of electricity from one point to the other. Symbol: V. Unit = volt.

Power: The rate of doing work. Symbol: $\boldsymbol{P}$. Units: watt, kilowatt, or horsepower.

Range: A statement of the upper and lower limits between which an instrument's input may be received and for which the instrument is calibrated.

Rated range: The nominal operating range within which a device can be operated and still maintain the performance characteristics specified by its manufacturer.

Reliability: A statistical term having to do with the probability that an instrument's repeatability and accuracy will continue to fall within specified limits. The attribute that makes an instrument work day after day, the way it is supposed to work.

Resistance: That property of a substance by virtue of which it resists the flow of electricity through it. Symbol: R. Unit = ohm.

Resistance balance: The amount of resistance that is required to null the output of certain transducers or input systems.

Resistance strain gage: A metallic wire or foil grid or crystal that produces a resistance change directly proportional to its change in length (strain). Its output is often calibrated in terms of other quantities that vary with strain.

Resolution: The smallest change in applied stimulus that will produce a detectable change in the instrument output.

Scale factor: 1. The amount by which a quantity being measured must change in order to produce unit pen deflection.

2. The ratio of real to analog values.

Sensitivity: The property of an instrument that determines scale factor. As commonly used, the word is often short for "maximum sensitivity," or the minimum scale factor with which an instrument is capable of responding.

Signal conditioner: A device placed between the signal source and the pen-drive amplifier to condition the signal. Examples: damping networks, attenuator networks, preamplifiers, excitation and demodulation circuitary, signal converters (for changing one electrical quantity into another—e.g., volts to amperes), instrument transformers, equalizing or matching networks, filters, and so on.

Single-ended (amplifier): An amplifier with one input terminal and one output terminal tied to a common point and therefore operating at a common potential. This point may or may not be connected to ground.

Single-phase: A system in which there is only a single alternating voltage.

Stability: 1. Independence or freedom from changes in one quantity as the result of a change in another.

2. The absence of drift.

Temperature effect: The change in performance owing to changes in temperature. It is specifically the difference between output at room temperature and at some other specified temperature from the same stimulus value when all other conditions are constant. It is generally specified as a percentage of full-scale output per interval of temperature.

Thermistor: A semiconductor whose resistance is extremely temperature sensitive. Like carbon (formerly alone among conductors), thermistors have negative temperature coefficients. Thermistors are used to compensate for temperature variations in other parts of a circuit, and they are also used as transducers.

Time base: 1. A reference time signal recorded at given intervals with the information signal.

2. The axis of chart motion.

3. The abscissa of many plotted curves.

Transducer: A device for translating faithfully the changing magnitude of one kind of quantity into corresponding changes of another kind of quantity. The second quantity often has dimensions different from the first and serves as the source of a useful signal. It is convenient to think of the first kind of quantity as an "input" and the second as an "output." Thus the input quantity to a dynamic microphone is air pressure; the output quantity is voltage.

Transient: Phenomena that take place in a system owing to a sudden change of conditions and that persist for a relatively short time.

Tuned filter: An arrangement of electronic components that either attenuates signals at a particular frequency and passes signals at other frequencies, or vice versa.

Turns ratio: The ratio of the number of turns in one winding of a transformer to the number of turns in another winding.

Vernier: Any device, control or scale used to obtain fine adjustment or more accurate measurement than the main measuring scale.

Voice frequency: The frequency range of ordinary speech, usually considered to be a band from 100 Hz to 3 kHz.

Volt: The practical unit of potential difference. It is the potential difference that produces a current of one ampere when applied steadily to a conductor, the resistance of which is one ohm. Abbreviation: V.

Voltage: Emf or potential difference expressed in volts.

Watt: The practical unit for power and therefore the rate at which energy is converted to work or dissipate as heat. In the case of electricity, power P in watts equals the product of voltage times in-phase current. Abbreviation: W.

Waveform: The graphical representation of a wave, formed by plotting amplitude versus time. Waveshape.

Zero adjustment: Bringing the pointer or pen of an instrument to zero when the input signal is zero.

Zero-line stability: Absence of drift when the instrument is at pen zero.

APPENDIX **B**

A Suggested Approach to Calibration and Balancing of an Amplifier-Transducer System

1. *Warm up the equipment:* Plug in the transducer and amplifier/display system and allow 15 minutes before using to ensure maximum stability. A small amount of drift will occur on the readout during warmup but will usually not be more than a few mm Hg.

2. *Position transducer on infusion manifold:* Make standard fluid reservoir and flush system connections; this can be done during the warmup period.

3. *Balance the transducer:* Open the transducer to atmosphere and set the desired range on the amplifier, depending on the numerical values of the parameter being measured. With the *balance control* compressed, adjust the amplifier readout to zero by using position control. Release the *balance indicator* and then compress it again so that readout returns to zero. Some equipment is automatically balanced when the amplifier readout is adjusted to zero.

4. *Calibrate the transducer:* Ascertain the calibration factor, which should be noted somewhere on the transducer cable. The calibration factor

corrects for slight individual differences between transducers that occur even with transducers of the same type. With one manufacturer, the *calibration indicator* is compressed on the amplifier. The readout then indicates 100 times the calibration factor on a 0 to 200 mm Hg scale, or 20 times the calibration factor on a 0 to 40 mm Hg scale. The readout position is then adjusted to this desired value and the calibration indicator is again compressed to recheck that the readout again indicates that value.

5. *Adjust monitor sweep to desired position.*
6. *Connect transducer to the patient:* Or place a sterile cap over the opening to prevent contamination.

APPENDIX C

Problems and Exercises

Introduction

This book is both a reference and a textbook. In the latter function, problems and exercises are needed to aid the student. In a book of this nature, which is primarily descriptive, quantitative problems are not as necessary as in the usual technical book. A few have been provided, but most of these exercises are designed to test the student's knowledge of the key portions of the text, as well as provide an opportunity to expand on it. The problems are relatively short and do not include long essay-type questions. Such questions are left to the instructor to pose.

Chapter 1

1.1 In your hospital setting, outline all the monitoring and interventive equipment of which you are aware; list the kinds of personnel directly involved with such equipment. Which of these personnel need be concerned with troubleshooting? Which ones are also involved in direct patient intervention on the basis of such monitoring?

1.2 Trace the historical development of nursing's involvement in patient instrumentation.

1.3 Make a list of all the possible uses for biomedical instrumentation in the field of health maintenance (e.g., case finding, genetic counseling, follow-up).

1.4 Make a list of all medical instruments to which you would be exposed in a typical working week and cite the section of this book where you would find information on this equipment.

Chapter 2

2.1 Give three examples of physiological variables that provide useful diagnostic information.

2.2 What is the purpose of a transducer in a medical instrument? Give an example of a transducer commonly used in clinical medicine.

2.3 What is the difference between the range and sensitivity of an instrument?

2.4. A given ECG is displayed on a monitor screen that has sensitivity settings of ½ and 1 mV per centimeter deflection on the screen. At which setting is the ECG pattern largest on the screen? Why?

2.5 Why is proper calibration important in the use of a medical instrument?

2.6 What effect would you expect an inadequate frequency response to have on the waveform recorded by an electrocardiograph?

2.7 Describe movement artifact and tell what should be done to reduce it.

Chapter 3

3.1 What is meant when a particle or an object is said to be electrically charged?

3.2 How may an object become electrically charged?

3.3 Sketch a representation of the electric field surrounding an isolated negative electric charge. A positive charge.

3.4 Sketch a representation of the electric field surrounding two proximate unlike electric charges and the field around two proximate charges that are alike.

3.5 When two unlike electric charges become proximate, how will they behave?

3.6 When two like charges become proximate, how will they behave?

3.7 Describe the two basic kinds of energy and give an example of each.

3.8 What is an ion? A cation? An anion?

3.9 In terms of atomic structure, what is a key difference between good conductors of electricity and poor conductors?

3.10 How may static electricity be hazardous in the operating room? How may this hazard be minimized?

3.11 How many microamps are there in 1 mA?

3.12 What is electric current?

3.13 Define (a) potential difference, (b) equipotential, (c) isopotential, (d) voltage, (e) coulomb, and (f) ampere.

3.14 What are the hemodynamic analogies of electric current, voltage, and resistance?

3.15 Assume that a metal sphere is charged to +7 V with respect to an uncharged sphere and that a third sphere is charged to +9 V with respect to the uncharged sphere. What is the value of the voltage between the two charged spheres?

3.16 In order for an electric current to exist, two basic conditions must be met. What are they?

3.17 What value of current will flow when a difference of potential equal to 5 V is applied to a resistor whose value is 500 Ω.

3.18 A 1000-Ω resistor conducts 5 μA of current. Determine the value of the applied voltage.

3.19 When 3000 V are applied to a conductor, a current of 60 A results. Determine the value of the conductor's resistance.

3.20 What is the difference between (a) direct current, and (b) pulsating dc and ac?

3.21 Sketch some examples of alternating current waveforms.

3.22 Name the three basic functions of the capacitor.

3.23 Explain how the capacitor is able to perform its three basic functions.

3.24 How does an isolation transformer function?

3.25 What is meant by overcurrent protection?

3.26 How may a short circuit occur in electric wiring.

3.27 How may closely spaced energized insulated wires pass alternating current between them?

3.28 What is the difference between electric energy and power? Give one example of each.

3.29 Give the units of electric current, voltage, resistance, power, and energy.

3.30 The 120-V 60-Hz power distribution system is a three-wire system, one wire of which is the equipment grounding wire (or conduit). Name the other two.

3.31 What color insulation is used to identify the equipment ground wire in the power distribution system?

3.32 Name the insulation colors used to identify the wires connected to a typical 120-V 60-Hz wall outlet.

3.33 What is the purpose of the equipment ground wire?

3.34 What is leakage current? How may it occur?

3.35 What is a typical value of leakage current for a battery-operated external pacemaker?

Chapter 4

4.1 Describe the function of the input terminal of an electronic amplifier.

4.2 An undesirable electrical signal is generally referred to as ________.

4.3 In a vacuum tube, the electron current flows through a vacuum. Describe the medium through which current flows in the transistor.

4.4 When comparing vacuum tubes, transistors, and integrated circuits, which is the one device that is most complex and most useful in medical applications?

4.5 Describe, in detail, the advantages of a differential amplifier for use in medical applications.

4.6 If a differential amplifier is used in medical applications, which amplifier will be better—one with high CMRR or one with low CMRR? Explain why.

4.7 Describe the function of the isolation amplifier as well as its main purpose.

4.8 What is the electronic device that can be used to select a certain frequency segment of an electronic signal?

4.9 The cathode-ray tube utilizes an electron beam to write electrical waveforms on the face of the tube. What are the means by which the beam is moved across the face of the tube?

4.10 What is the name by which a solid-state lamp is known?

Chapter 5

5.1 What are the relative charge concentrations (for sodium and potassium ions) inside and outside an excitable cell at rest?

5.2 What are the value and polarity of the voltage *outside* (with respect to the inside) a heart muscle cell at rest?

5.3 Briefly describe the depolarization-repolarization process of an excited nerve cell.

5.4 What is an action potential? What is its typical value?

5.5 What is the *all-or-nothing law?*

5.6 How do pacemaker cells differ from neuronal cells?

5.7 What is meant by a cell's absolute and relative refactory period?

5.8 What is the duration of the absolute refactory period for a heart muscle cell?

5.9 What is the difference between an electrocardiogram and an electrocardiograph?

5.10 Describe one cycle of the heart's electric activity.

5.11 What is the electrical and mechanical significance of the recorded P wave? Q wave? R wave? T wave? QRS complex?

5.12 What is the typical value of the ECG (in millivolts) recorded at the surface of the body? Within the heart?

5.13 Name the ECG segments and intervals.
5.14 What is a synapse? An excitatory synapse? An inhibitory synapse?
5.15 List the values of the common EEG rhythms.
5.16 What is the dicrotic notch?
5.17 A patient's blood pressure is recorded as 190/70. Define these values.
5.18 What are cardiac output, stroke volume, total blood volume, and mean circulation time?
5.19 What is the significance of the heart sounds?
5.20 What is the difference between internal respiration and external respiration.
5.21 What is the value of alveolar pressure during normal inspiration? During normal expiration?
5.22 What is meant by airway resistance?

Chapter 6

6.1 What is a transducer?
6.2 Why is an electrode called a transducer?
6.3 What is a half-cell potential? How is it formed?
6.4 What is meant by electrode offset voltage?
6.5 What may cause baseline drift or wandering in the recorded ECG?
6.6 What are some advantages in using Ag/AgCl electrodes? Electrolytic jelly?
6.7 Name some types of electrodes used to record the ECG and the EEG.
6.8 What is the principal advantage in using the floating electrode? Disposable electrodes?
6.9 What is meant by the term "artifact"?
6.10 What is the difference between unipolar and bipolar electrodes?
6.11 Describe how the spiral-type fetal monitoring electrode is constructed and used.

Chapter 7

7.1 Before taking an ECG recording, the recorder is *standardized*. Describe this procedure and explain its purpose.
7.2 The term "lead" in electrocardiography has actually two different meanings. Describe the two connotations of the word.
7.3 What are the five electrodes used for a normal clinical electrocardiogram?
7.4 A patient monitor has malfunctioned and in order to get an ECG trace in a hurry you are connecting the patient cable of an ECG recorder to the three electrodes placed on the patient in the Modified Chest Lead (Marriott) configuration. Which of the five electrode connectors of the patient cable must be used and in which position should the lead selector switch of the ECG recorder be placed?

7.5 When recording an electrocardiogram, you notice a widening of the baseline of the recording. What measures should you take to obtain a usable recording?

7.6 You are to take the electrocardiogram of a patient who has both legs in plaster casts that extend to above the knee. Where would you place the RL and LL electrodes?

Chapter 8

8.1 What is meant by "systolic" and "diastolic" blood pressure?

8.2 Discuss the common routine method of measuring blood pressure indirectly.

8.3 Do you consider the method discussed in Problem 8.2 to be an accurate method? Explain your answer.

8.4 What is meant by the following words or terms: (a) auscultation, (b) Korotkoff sounds, (c) sphygmomanometer, and (d) hypertension?

8.5 Discuss the precautions necessary (a) in use of the stethoscope, (b) on the size of a blood pressure cuff, and (c) in measurements on children.

Chapter 9

9.1 Explain the differences between direct and indirect blood pressure determinations; include the advantages and disadvantages of each, as well as a discussion of relative accuracy and clinical situations that dictate the use of one over the other.

9.2 Explain the basic operation of the physiological resistance or strain gauge transducer. What precautions should be taken to prolong life and ensure accurate monitoring?

9.3 Draw a schematic representation of a typical direct pressure monitoring system, including infusion manifold, flushing solution and syringes, transducers, and so on.

9.4 Explain the terms calibration and balancing. How are they accomplished on most equipment?

9.5 Discuss the nature of the vascular compartment being monitored, the type of instrumentation involved, and the special approaches to ensure accuracy and safety for the following parameters:

Central venous pressure
Pulmonary artery pressure
Pulmonary capillary wedge pressure
Central arterial pressure

9.6 What are the specific advantages of monitoring pulmonary capillary wedge pressure versus central venous pressure and left atrial pressure?

9.7 Discuss the steps you would take during troubleshooting of a damped arterial tracing. What specific errors in equipment selection and placement will contribute to this and related problems, fostering inaccuracy?

9.8 Describe the physiological or mechanical basis for each of the following arterial tracings and artifacts:

Tubing movement
Whip
Damping
Premature ventricular contractions (PVCs)
Decreased cardiac output
Atrial fibrillation
Changes in intrathoracic pressure on pulmonary artery tracings
Cardiac tamponade

9.9 Draw typical waveforms encountered in the above.

Chapter 10

10.1 What is bradycardia? Tachycardia? First-degree heart block? Third-degree heart block?

10.2 Name the component parts of a pacemaker system.

10.3 Describe some uses for the external pacemaker.

10.4 Name some types of power sources for implantable pacemakers and their typical life expectancies.

10.5 Name the two principal modes of pacing.

10.6 Describe the operation of a fixed-rate pacemaker.

10.7 Describe the operation of a demand pacemaker. A standby pacemaker. An atrial programmed pacemaker.

10.8 What is meant by the terms capture, threshold, sensitivity?

10.9 Describe the common type of pacing electrodes.

10.10 Why should wearers of implanted pacemakers avoid obvious sources of electromagnetic interference?

10.11 What is the physiological result of ventricular fibrillation? Atrial fibrillation?

10.12 What is the difference between ac defibrillation and dc defibrillation? Which method is preferred? Why?

10.13 Sketch and label the lown waveform. The dual-peak waveform. The truncated waveform.

10.14 What is the difference between a defibrillation procedure and a cardioversion procedure?

10.15 In a defibrillation procedure, should the defibrillator be synchronized to the patient's ECG? Why?

10.16 Name the common types of defibrillator paddles.

10.17 In a clinical application, a defibrillator was set to produce an energy output of 160 W-s. When applied to a patient, the output was found to equal 120 W-s. Explain the reason for this difference.

10.18 Why must a saline-soaked gauze pad or conductive jelly be used when defibrillator paddles are applied to the skin of a patient?

10.19 What is meant by the heart's vulnerable period? When does it occur?
10.20 What part may telemetry play in mobile emergency care?

Chapter 11

11.1 Describe the main function and application of electronic instrumentation in the critical care unit.
11.2 Name and briefly describe at least four criteria items that are necessary for a good critical care instrumentation system.
11.3 What is the most common and widely used instrument for critical care monitoring, and what type of information does this instrument provide?
11.4 An ECG monitor has a calibrate button for use in calibrating the monitoring system. What is the magnitude of this calibration signal?
11.5 An ECG monitor can display the ECG patterns of the upper and lower limbs only. The patient is connected to four electrodes. The lead selector switch has three positions. What leads are they?
11.6 Describe the difference between a digital and a conventional heart rate indicator.
11.7 When it becomes necessary to make a detailed analysis of the patient ECG for such details as S-T segment depression, the monitor should be used on which mode of operation? Describe why.
11.8 Describe the purpose of the defibrillator in the critical care unit.
11.9 Describe the typical central station monitoring equipment and name some special requirements for this equipment.
11.10 When monitoring blood pressure, it becomes necessary to convert the physical parameter of pressure into an electrical signal. What is the device used for this conversion?
11.11 External pacemakers fall under two basic categories, the continuous and the demand type. Describe the differences and similarities of these devices.
11.12 Briefly describe the difference between the bouncing ball and the nonfade type of patient monitor.
11.13 The most common method for measuring respiration via the ECG leads and electrodes measures certain characteristics of the chest. What is it?

Chapter 12

12.1 Name three methods used to determine blood flow. Which one of the methods can also be used to measure the blood volume?
12.2 What are the requirements for a substance to be used an indicator in dilution methods? What indicators are used most frequently?
12.3 Describe the principle of a cardiac output determination using the Swan-Ganz® catheter.

12.4 What is the major limitation of ultrasonic and magnetic blood flow meters?

12.5 What is a plethysmograph and how can it be used to measure the blood flow in a leg?

Chapter 13

13.1 What is meant by the term biotelemetry?

13.2 List some advantages and disadvantages of biotelemetry.

13.3 Draw a block diagram of a system to send an electrocardiogram from an ambulance to a hospital by telemetry.

13.4 What do you see as some of the problems of telemeterized systems in the future?

13.5 It is desirable to monitor the temperature of a man very accurately while he is climbing a mountain and then record the data on tape for later computer analysis. You are to remain in a cabin at the foot of the mountain. Explain how you would do this accurately and draw a block diagram of any equipment stages used in your system.

13.6 Explain how four physiological parameters can be monitored and telemetered simultaneously.

13.7 If subdermal needles connected to a telemetry transmitter are implanted into a muscle, explain how a trained physician might recognize different effects from another room by using a sense other than vision to monitor.

13.8 Design a hospital with a telemetry system, explaining why you would telemetrize the functions you have selected.

Chapter 14

14.1 Name and describe four important lung volumes and capacities.

14.2 What is a spirometer? For what types of measurements is it used?

14.3 Describe a body plethysmograph. Name two measurements for which it is used.

14.4 Name a pulmonary volume or capacity measurement that cannot be obtained directly with a spirometer. Why? Name a method by which this measurement can be obtained.

14.5 What is the closing volume? Why is it important? How is it determined?

14.6 How are the partial pressures of oxygen and carbon dioxide measured in blood?

14.7 What is the difference between an inhalator and a respirator? Under what circumstances should each be used?

14.8 Explain the three modes of operation of an assistor-controller (assist mode, control mode, and assist-control mode). When should each be used?

14.9 How does a volume respirator differ from a pressure-cycled ventillator?
14.10 What is IPPB and for what purpose is it used?
14.11 Describe a nebulizer and its function. What is the advantage of an ultrasonic nebulizer?

Chapter 15

15.1 How are X rays generated and what happens when they travel through an object?
15.2 Describe two methods used to visualize the intensity distribution of X rays that have passed through a body section.
15.3 What are the three controls usually found on an X-ray machine and how do they affect the properties of the X rays?
15.4 What are contrast media used for?
15.5 Which effect of X rays is utilized in radiation therapy?
15.6 Describe the safety precautions used to limit the radiation exposure to hospital staff.

Chapter 16

16.1 Describe the difference between the electrosurgical generator and the ECG monitor.
16.2 What can happen if an electrosurgical generator is used on a patient where the electrical current flows from the generator through an ECG monitor and then back to the generator?
16.3 What are the advantages or disadvantages of the isolated-type electrosurgical generator?
16.4 Describe the characteristics that are important for an efficient patient plate.
16.5 One of the instruments in a normal operating room is considered a good generator of electrical noise. What is this instrument? What is affected by this noise?
16.6 How does a fibrillator work?
16.7 Briefly describe how a Doppler flow indicator works.
16.8 Consider that grounded types of ECG monitor and electrosurgical generators are used on a patient. Assume that the patient plate of the ESU is *not* connected to the patient. Describe what will happen.

Chapter 17

17.1 Discuss the advantages and disadvantages of surface electrodes versus subdermal needle electrodes for EEG measurement.
17.2 What is a photic stimulator? For what purpose is it used?

17.3 Give three causes of noise or artifact in an EEG recording.

17.4 Name two important ways in which EMG is normally displayed. How does this differ from the usual EEG readout? Why is the method of displaying EMG different from that of EEG?

17.5 Nerve latencies were measured at two electrodes placed 30 cm apart along a nerve. Latencies measured 20 and 30 ms, respectively. What was the nerve conduction time between the two electrode locations? What was the nerve conduction velocity?

17.6 What is the difference between unipolar and bipolar measurement of EMG potentials? Describe the electrodes used for each type of measurement.

17.7 Explain the principle of echocardiography. Why is this technique so useful as a clinical tool?

17.8 Name two important measurements associated with fetal monitoring and explain why they are important.

17.9 Discuss the differences between invasive and noninvasive methods of fetal monitoring and the relative advantages and disadvantages of each.

17.10 What is a thermistor and how does it function? In what type of clinical instrument is it utilized?

17.11 Discuss the principles involved in thermography. How is this technique used clinically?

17.12 What is the difference between fetal heart rate monitoring and the intensive heart rate monitoring?

17.13 In monitoring fetal heart rate by the direct (invasive) method, special clip-type electrodes are used. What is the device used to pick up the fetal heart rate in the noninvasive method?

17.14 Fetal heart rate is normally compared to a maternal physiological parameter. What is the maternal parameter?

17.15 What is the one big restriction in using the clip-type fetal electrodes?

Chapter 18

18.1 Name two effects of electrical current on the body. What is the most frequent cause of fatal electrical accidents?

18.2 Which condition or conditions are the most frequent cause of electrical accidents?

18.3 Name three methods used to reduce the dangers of electrical accidents.

18.4 Why are transistor radios and flashlights normally considered safe with respect to electrical shock?

18.5 While a surgical procedure is in progress, a buzzer suddenly goes of and a red light labeled "HAZARD" appears on a panel at the wall of the operating room. The circulating nurse goes to the panel and presses a button, whereupon the buzzer stops while the light remains. What happened? What are the implications of the event and what should be done after the procedure is completed?

18.6 What special considerations should be followed when a patient is paced from an external pacemaker by means of a pacing catheter inserted through a vein?

Chapter 19

19.1 Explain the difference between hardware and software in a computer system.

19.2 Define each of the following terms in your own words.
(a) bit
(b) byte
(c) character
(d) computer word
(e) terminal
(f) time sharing
(g) off line
(h) real time

19.3 What functions does the computer perform in a computerized patient-monitoring system?

19.4 Name three applications of computers in clinical patient care, other than patient monitoring, and describe the role of the computer in each.

19.5 Give an example of how computerized pattern recognition is used in clinical diagnostic screening.

Chapter 20

20.1 Describe some of the precautions that should be used to prevent electronic equipment from being dropped accidentally. What should be done if equipment has been dropped?

20.2 What method is normally used to sterilize electrical equipment or its parts?

20.3 A hard rain is pounding against the hospital windows, and you notice that you receive a slight electrical shock when touching a patient monitor. What would you do?

20.4 You have just started work in a hospital that uses a type of patient monitor with which you are unfamiliar. You suspect that one of the units is faulty. What do you do?

20.5 What is a "brownout" and how can it affect the function of medical equipment?

Index

A

D

F

G

H

I

J

K

L

Q

R